THE PINEAL GLAND

THE PINEAL GLAND

A Ciba Foundation Symposium

Edited by
G. E. W. WOLSTENHOLME
and
JULIE KNIGHT

CHURCHILL LIVINGSTONE
Edinburgh and London
1971

First published 1971

Containing 134 illustrations

I.S.B.N. 0 7000 1502 7

Contents

CONTENTS

Membership

L. Martini (Chairman)	Istituto di Farmacologica e di Terapia, Università degli Studi, Via Vanvitelli 32, 20129 Milano, Italy
F. Antón-Tay	Instituto de Investigaciones Biomédicas, Universidad Naçional Autonoma, Apartado Postal 70228, Mexico City 20, D.F., Mexico
A. Arstila	Laboratory of Electron Microscopy, University of Turku, Turku 3, Finland
J. Axelrod	Mental Health Intramural Research Programme, National Institute of Mental Health, 9000 Rockville Pike, Bethesda, Maryland 20014, U.S.A.
J. P. Collin	Laboratoire de Biologie Animale, Université de Clermont-Ferrand, Complexe Scientifique des Cézeaux, B.P. No. 45, 63 Aubière, France
E. Dodt	William G. Kerckhoff-Herzforschungsinstitut der Max-Planck-Gesellschaft, 6350 Bad Nauheim, Germany
Virginia M. Fiske	Department of Biological Sciences, Wellesley College, Wellesley, Massachusetts 02181, U.S.A.
F. Fraschini	Istituto de Farmacologia e di Terapia, Università degli Studi, Via Vanvitelli 32, 20129 Milano, Italy
J. Herbert	Department of Anatomy, University of Cambridge
J. A. Kappers	Nederlands Centraal Instituut voor Hersenonderzoek, Ijdijk 28, Amsterdam-O, The Netherlands
D. E. Kelly	Department of Biological Structure, University of Miami, School of Medicine, P.O. Box 875, Biscayne Annex, Miami, Florida 33152, U.S.A.
C. Kordon	Laboratoire d'Histophysiologie, Collège de France, 4 Avenue Gordon-Bennett, Paris 16e, France
A. B. Lerner	Section of Dermatology, School of Medicine, Yale University, New Haven, Connecticut, U.S.A.
B. Mess	Department of Anatomy, University Medical School, Dischka utca 5, Pécs, Hungary
S. M. Milcu	Institutul de Endocrinologie, Academia de Stiinte Medicale, Bulevardul Aviatorilor 34, Bucharest, Rumania
R. Miline	Medicinski fakultet, Institut za histologiju i embriologiju, Novi Sad, Yugoslavia
A. Moszkowska	Laboratoire d'Histophysiologie, Collège de France, 4 Avenue Gordon-Bennett, Paris 16e, France

Marcella Motta — Istituto di Farmacologia e di Terapia, Università degli Studi, Via Vanvitelli 32, 20129 Milano, Italy

I. Nir — Department of Applied Pharmacology, Hebrew University Medical School, Jerusalem, Israel

A. Oksche — Anatomisches Institut, Justus Liebig-Universität, Friedrichstrasse 24, Giessen 63, Germany

C. Owman — Institute of Anatomy and Histology, Department of Anatomy, University of Lund, Biskopsgatan 7, 223 62 Lund, Sweden

Amanda Pellegrino de Iraldi — Instituto de Anatomia General y Embriologia, Facultad de Medicina, Universidad de Buenos Aires, Paraguay 2155, Buenos Aires, Republica Argentina

R. J. Reiter — Department of Anatomy, School of Medicine and Dentistry, The University of Rochester, 260 Crittenden Boulevard, Rochester, New York 14620, U.S.A.

H. M. Shein — Department of Psychiatry, Harvard Medical School, Belmont, Massachusetts 02178, U.S.A.

Bertha Singer — Department of Physiology, The Medical School, University of Birmingham, Birmingham, 15

R. J. Wurtman — Department of Nutrition and Food Science, Massachusetts Institute of Technology, Cambridge, Massachusetts 02139, U.S.A.

Preface

At the Third International Congress of Endocrinology in Mexico City in 1968, Professor R. J. Wurtman approached the Director of the Ciba Foundation, Dr Wolstenholme, to suggest that one of the Foundation's small international symposia should be held to discuss recent progress in research on the pineal gland. There was a certain nobility about this proposal, in that *The Pineal* (Academic Press, 1968), the excellent and comprehensive review by Professor Wurtman, Dr J. Axelrod and Professor D. E. Kelly, was in press at the time. It was already obvious, however, that research on the pineal was going so well that there was much promise of a useful symposium in two years' time. Further talks were held in Stresa, Italy, in 1969 between Professor Wurtman, Professor L. Martini, Professor J. Ariëns Kappers and Dr Wolstenholme, which helped to decide the scope and membership of the Foundation's symposium, and in the event, in June 1970, the wealth of new material with all its interesting potentialities surprised even those most closely involved in this area of research.

The pineal gland may well be about to attract the same limelight as the adrenal cortex some twenty years ago, with an equal impact on the better understanding of human functioning and behaviour, in health and disease.

The editors are indebted to all contributors, particularly those named above, for unstinted and enthusiastic cooperation in the preparation of this book.

The Ciba Foundation

The Ciba Foundation was opened in 1949 to promote international cooperation in medical and chemical research. It owes its existence to the generosity of CIBA Ltd, Basle (now CIBA-GEIGY Ltd), who, recognizing the obstacles to scientific communication created by war, man's natural secretiveness, disciplinary divisions, academic prejudices, distance, and differences of language, decided to set up a philanthropic institution whose aim would be to overcome such barriers. London was chosen as its site for reasons dictated by the special advantages of English charitable trust law (ensuring the independence of its actions), as well as those of language and geography.

The Foundation's house at 41 Portland Place, London, has become well known to workers in many fields of science. Every year the Foundation organizes six to ten three-day symposia and three or four shorter study groups, all of which are published in book form. Many other scientific meetings are held, organized either by the Foundation or by other groups in need of a meeting place. Accommodation is also provided for scientists visiting London, whether or not they are attending a meeting in the house.

The Foundation's many activities are controlled by a small group of distinguished trustees. Within the general framework of biological science, interpreted in its broadest sense, these activities are well summed up by the motto of the Ciba Foundation: *Consocient Gentes*—let the peoples come together.

CHAIRMAN'S INTRODUCTION

Professor L. Martini

The first thing I want to say is that all of us must be very grateful to the Ciba Foundation and to Dr Wolstenholme in particular for having arranged this meeting for us. Secondly, I wish to point out a few peculiar things about the pineal gland.

The first peculiarity is that scientists have not been really interested in this gland until very recently. I believe one of the reasons why this happened is that the pineal gland has interested the philosophers for a long time; it is possible that endocrinologists do not have much respect for philosophers. Another possible reason is that animals normally survive pinealectomy (provided the surgeon is a good one); this puts the pineal gland in a kind of second rank among endocrine structures. In addition, the effects of pinealectomy are apparent for some time, but later on pinealectomized animals recover and become perfectly normal again.

A second peculiarity of the pineal gland is that you cannot bring back a pinealectomized animal to its normal status by administering systemically crude pineal extracts or the more refined compounds which have recently been isolated from the gland. Transplants of pineal tissue are also ineffective (Reiter and Fraschini 1969). The reason why you cannot reverse the effects of pinealectomy by transplanting the pineal gland is now apparent. Thanks to studies which will be reviewed at this meeting we now know that the pineal gland has a peculiar sympathetic innervation which is essential to its function; a transplanted pineal gland cannot be re-innervated in the same way (Wurtman, Axelrod and Kelly 1968). This brings me to a third peculiarity of the pineal gland: this gland is located in strict contact with the brain; however, its innervation does not originate from the nervous structures which are close to the gland.

Another peculiarity of the pineal gland is the fact that the receptors sensitive to its hormones are localized almost exclusively in the brain. Published evidence for a nervous site of action of pineal hormones includes (a) the studies by Wurtman and his co-workers (Antón-Tay and Wurtman 1969) indicating that exogenous melatonin is concentrated by nervous structures; (b) the observation that melatonin may modify some biochemical processes taking place in the brain (as, for instance, the metabolism of serotonin) (Antón-Tay et al. 1968); and (c) the data obtained in my laboratory showing that brain implants of melatonin, but not intra-pituitary ones, may reduce gonadotropin secretion (Fraschini, Mess and Martini 1968). I am sure that additional data along these lines will be presented at this meeting.

The final peculiar thing about the pineal gland is indicated by the type of scientists who have become interested in it. A general pattern is usually seen in science. A scientist normally wants to make a reputation for him-self and, in order to do so, he picks up a respected topic and devotes himself fully to it. Exactly the reverse happened in the case of the pineal gland. A group of distinguished and already recognized scientists decided to make this gland fully and, we hope, definitely respectable.

REFERENCES

ANTÓN-TAY, F., CHOU, C., ANTON, S. and WURTMAN, R. J. (1968) *Science* **162**, 277–278.
ANTÓN-TAY, F. and WURTMAN, R. J. (1969) *Nature, Lond.* **221**, 474–475.
FRASCHINI, F., MESS, B. and MARTINI, L. (1968) *Endocrinology* **82**, 919–924.
REITER, R. J. and FRASCHINI, F. (1969) *Neuroendocrinology* **5**, 219–255.
WURTMAN, R. J., AXELROD, J. and KELLY, D. E. (1968) *The Pineal*. New York and London: Academic Press.

THE PINEAL ORGAN: AN INTRODUCTION

J. Ariëns Kappers

The Netherlands Central Institute for Brain Research, Amsterdam

RESEARCH on the pineal organ in various vertebrates has now so much intensified that it is impossible to offer a comprehensive survey of all its different aspects as an introduction to this symposium. In the present paper, therefore, I shall deal with a limited number of subjects, drawing your attention to some problems still to be solved.

First and foremost I shall deal with the phylogenetic development of the pineal. I am sure that Dr Collin and Professor Oksche will give more details (see pp. 79 and 127).

Far from being a new acquisition in mammals, the pineal has a long and interesting evolution during which it shows a striking transformation in structure, function and innervation pattern. It is increasingly clear, however, that the way in which the mammalian pineal functions has very old phylogenetic roots.

PINEAL ORGAN IN ANAMNIOTES

In fishes and amphibians the development and structure of the epiphysis is, in principle, very similar to that of the retina of the eye, although some differences exist (Kappers 1965). In the epiphysial epithelium three cell types can be distinguished: (1) neurosensory photoreceptor cells of a ciliary type, (2) supportive elements which may show certain specializations, and (3) sensory nerve cells. All the cells mentioned derive from the embryonic neuroepithelium which forms, in every vertebrate, the primary anlage of the organ.

The pineal photoreceptor elements are neurosensory or primary sensory cells, not neurons. They are sensitive to photic stimuli and convey the transduced photic impulse to the next element, the sensory neuron. The outer segment of the photoreceptor cell, which shows a complicated structure, is sensitive to photic stimuli and can be termed the photic pole of the cell. The basal process of the cell is directed toward the basement membrane of the pineal epithelium. Its terminal ending which, in fishes and amphibians, does not generally reach the basement membrane, is in

synaptic contact with either the dendrites or the soma of the intraepithelial
sensory nerve cells. These neurons are the homologues of the large nerve
cells of the inner layer of the retina of the eye, the axons of which constitute
the optic nerve. In the pineal, the axons of these cells constitute the pineal
tract which runs to the epithalamic region of the brain. The synaptic
ending of the basal process of the photoreceptor cell contains clear vesicles
(Oksche and Vaupel-von Harnack 1963 and Ueck 1968a, b in anuran
amphibians; Rüdeberg 1966, 1968, 1969 in fish), but often also synaptic
ribbons or "vesicle-crowned rodlets" (e.g. Collin 1969b in lamprey; Kelly
1967 in newt). The synaptic ribbons recall similar organelles present in
the presynaptic endings of photoreceptor cells in the retina.

After reaching the epithalamus the sensory pineal fibres mostly join
those of the posterior commissure, spreading in a lateral and ventral direction (Kappers 1965 in fish; Ueck 1968b in anuran amphibians). It is
uncertain whether some join the fibres of the habenular commissure. It is
a serious handicap to our understanding of the function of this direct
photosensory pineal pathway in lower vertebrates that the site of termination of these fibres in the brain is not known with certainty (see Kappers
1965 for references).

In summary, it appears that the direct photosensory function of the
organ depends on two types of cells which are synaptically connected,
namely the neurosensory photoreceptor cell and the sensory neuron.
Evidently, this function will be impaired if the photoreceptor cell loses its
photosensitivity or if the nerve cells are lost. Loss of the nerve cells is a very
crucial point because the basal processes of the photoreceptor cells are not
connected directly with the brain.

The direct photosensitivity of the pineal of fishes and amphibians has
also been demonstrated electrophysiologically. It was shown (Morita
1966a) that the constant train of impulses fired normally by the pineal nerve
cells of trout decreases when the organ is illuminated. A sustained discharge of action potentials was also recorded from the pineal stalk of
anuran amphibians in the dark. This activity was likewise inhibited by
direct illumination (Morita 1965; Morita and Dodt 1965). For details of
the light response of the anuran pineal, see the papers by Dodt and Jacobson
(1963), Dodt and Morita (1964) and Morita (1969).

Formerly, it was generally held that the pineal of fishes and amphibians
has a photosensory function only, but there is increasing evidence for a
second, secretory function. Dense-cored vesicles, measuring about 100 nm
(1000 Å) in diameter, have been observed to originate in the Golgi zone of
the photoreceptor cells and to accumulate in the basal process (Rüdeberg
1969 in dogfish; Collin 1969b, c in lamprey; Oksche and Vaupel-von

Harnack 1963, Ueck 1968a, b and Charlton 1968 in anuran amphibians). Their chemical composition is so far unknown. ^{14}C-labelled 5-hydroxy-tryptamine and methyl methionine, precursors of melatonin, were shown to be selectively incorporated in the epiphysis of *Xenopus* (Charlton 1964, 1966b) and the enzyme hydroxyindole-O-methyltransferase was also demonstrated in the amphibian pineal region (Axelrod, Quay and Baker 1965; Quay 1965). This is indirect proof of the synthesis of melatonin, which was also directly demonstrated in the *Xenopus* pineal by a special fluorescence technique (Van de Veerdonk 1965, 1967; Balemans and Van de Veerdonk 1967; Balemans, Van de Veerdonk and Van de Kamer 1967) after an earlier failure to demonstrate 5-hydroxy- and 5-methoxyindoles in the pineal of *Hyla* (Eakin, Quay and Westfall 1963) by spectrofluoro-metry. On the ground of comparative structural and functional con-siderations it can be assumed that the compound is produced by the photoreceptor elements which therefore show both a photosensory and a secretory function.

The uptake of labelled precursors of melatonin by the pineal of *Xenopus* depends upon the colour of the background on which the animals are kept after injection (Charlton 1966b), while the organ may directly control the primary response to colour change in eyeless *Xenopus* (Charlton 1966a). This suggests that production of melatonin by the photoreceptor cells may depend on photic stimuli directly received by these same cells. Much work has been done on pigment regulation in lower vertebrates in relation to the function of the pineal (see Bagnara 1965 and Kappers 1969b for references).

No difference was found in thyroid and interrenal gland activity in pinealectomized goldfish from that of controls (Peter 1968), while the gonadosomatic index also remained unchanged. Recently, however, mela-tonin was identified by thin-layer chromatography in the pineal of the Pacific salmon (Fenwick 1970). The amount stored in the pineal was approximately six times as great in immature salmon as in mature fish, suggesting that the pineal melatonin store is related to gonadal function. Intraperitoneal injections of melatonin into goldfish inhibited the increase in gonadal size which accompanied increased daily light exposure in those animals which received placebo injections. The melatonin-treated fish also showed larger pituitary gonadotropic cells. This points to a light-dependent effect of pineal melatonin on the hypophysio-gonadal axis in a fish.

Because, in the mammalian pineal, the function of the pinealocytes is known to depend, at least partly, on the sympathetic innervation of the organ, it is of interest whether the pineal of anamniotes also shows such an innervation. Oksche and Vaupel-von Harnack (1963, 1965a) postulated the autonomic origin of unmyelinated fibres containing dense-cored vesicles and running in the pineal tract as well as in the pineal perivascular spaces in *Rana*. Similar fibres were demonstrated by Ueck (1968a) in the perivascular spaces and in the epithelium of anuran pineals. No membrane thickenings pointing to true synaptic contacts between terminals of autonomic fibres and photoreceptor cells were observed. By fluorescence histochemistry, pinealo-petal catecholamine-containing nerve fibres have also been described in *Bufo* (Iturizza 1967). Neither the exact origin nor the function of these fibres is, as yet, known.

PINEAL ORGAN IN REPTILES

Among reptiles, lacertilians and turtles show an interesting evolutionary transformation of the pineal organ. The lacertilian pineal photoreceptor cell rarely shows a normally developed outer segment (Oksche and Kirschstein 1968; Wartenberg and Baumgarten 1968; Petit 1969a; Collin 1967b, 1969b). Many are rudimentarily developed or modified by disorganization or disintegration. In general, the basal processes are not in synaptic contact with sensory neurons, but end on the basement membrane of the epithelium. The number of sensory nerve cells is decreased (Kappers 1967). They can be demonstrated only with difficulty in electron micrographs (Petit 1969a; Collin 1969b). Accordingly, the number of sensory fibres running in the pineal tract is also reduced (see Kappers 1967 and Petit 1969a for their interepithalamic course).

Notwithstanding the tendency to regression of the photosensory apparatus of the lacertilian pineal, electrophysiological investigations have corroborated the morphological evidence that this function is not altogether lost. The lizard pineal, for example, shows spontaneous electrical activity which is inhibited by illumination of the organ. Increasing illumination causes increasing inhibition until there is a complete cessation of firing for the duration of the stimulus (Hamasaki and Dodt 1969).

The well-developed Golgi zone of the chief cells produces dense-cored vesicles of about 100 nm (1000 Å) in diameter (see e.g. Collin 1967b, 1969b; Collin and Kappers 1968; Petit 1969a). Small and larger clear vesicles have also been observed. The vesicles migrate to the basal processes of the cells and their content is released into the pericapillary spaces, while the capillary endothelium can be fenestrated (Petit 1969a; Wartenberg and Baumgarten 1969a). These facts suggest a secretory function of the chief pineal cells, which have been termed secretory rudimentary photoreceptor cells by Collin.

Indoleamine, probably 5-hydroxytryptamine (5-HT), was histochemically demonstrated in the pineal of *Lacerta* (Collin 1967a, 1969a), the reaction being strongest in those cell zones in which the dense-cored vesicles are observed. By fluorescence histochemistry a yellow compound, probably 5-HT, was also demonstrated (Kappers 1967; Quay, Jongkind and Kappers 1967; Collin 1968a, 1969b; Wartenberg and Baumgarten 1969a). Fluorescence is not always localized in granules but more often diffusely spread throughout the cell. Possibly there are two pools of 5-HT in the pinealocytes, an intravesicular, relatively stable one which is resistant to reserpine treatment, and an easily available extravesicular pool (Wartenberg and Baumgarten 1969a). 5-HT has also been demonstrated biochemically in the lacertilian pineal (Quay and Wilhoft 1964) as well as a considerable amount of hydroxyindole-O-methyltransferase (Quay 1965). All these facts suggest the synthesis of melatonin in the lizard pineal.

The pineal pericapillary spaces contain some, probably sensory myelinated nerve fibres (Collin and Kappers 1968) and bundles of unmyelinated fibres the endings of which contain the three types of vesicles characteristic of noradrenergic nerve terminals (Collin and Kappers 1968; Oksche and Kirschstein 1968; Wartenberg and Baumgarten 1968, 1969b; Petit 1969a). Autonomic nerve endings in the pineal epithelium are rare and they do not make true synaptic contacts with the secretory cells (Collin and Kappers 1968; Wartenberg and Baumgarten 1969b). As the exact function of the sympathetic innervation is not known, it can only be surmised that it is involved in the regulation of the production and/or the excretion of pineal cell compounds.

In principle, the pineal of Chelonia (turtles) shows the same structural features (Vivien 1964b; Lutz and Collin 1967; Mehring 1970; Vivien and Roels 1967, 1968; Vivien-Roels 1969; Collin 1969b). The outer segments of the chief cells are rudimentarily developed and the basal processes either reach the basement membrane of the pineal epithelium, showing a so-called vascular polarity, or end on the membranes limiting the intercellular spaces which are extensions of the pericapillary spaces (Mehring 1970). No secretory granules were observed in *Testudo hermanni* during the winter (Lutz and Collin 1967) but they are present in animals living under conditions of artificial lighting (Mehring 1970). Seasonal variations in secretory activity may, therefore, be present. In most chelonians pineal secretory activity is obvious. Endothelial pores can be present (Vivien-Roels 1969).

Features pointing to a direct photosensory function, such as sensory nerve cells, some rare synaptic contacts between basal processes and nerve cells (Vivien-Roels 1969), and a pineal tract are still present but vary according to species. In *Testudo hermanni* the sensory neurons show signs of degeneration in the adult, as do their axons which are in part myelinated (Mehring 1970). In *Pseudemys*, the tract is better developed than in *Testudo*.

Adrenergic fibres and their endings are present in the perivascular spaces as well as within the pineal epithelium (Mehring 1970). The intraepithelial endings form simple appositional contacts with the secretory cells. In summary, it appears that the pineal of Chelonia, like that of Lacertilia, shows a varying tendency to regression of its direct photosensory function, a distinct secretory function and a sympathetic innervation.

In Crocodilia even the anlage of the pineal organ is missing. In Ophidia (snakes) the epiphysis is solid and parenchymatous. In *Tropidonotus*, the Golgi zone of the chief cells produces secretory granules which are emptied into the pericapillary spaces (Petit 1969*b*). Sympathetic fibres run in these spaces as well as in the pineal parenchyma. Here they show close appositional contacts with the basement membrane as well as with the basal processes of the secretory chief cells (Vivien 1964*a*, 1965). The observation of green-fluorescing nerve fibres (Quay, Kappers and Jongkind 1968) corroborates the findings of sympathetic fibres by other methods. So far, no clear proof of a pineal photosensory function has been found in snakes.

A distinct development of ergastoplasm and Golgi zone in *Tropidonotus* pinealocytes and a nearly complete disappearance of secretory granules, by comparison with normal animals, was observed in adults injected with chorionic gonadotropin (Vivien 1965). The secretory as well as the excretory function of the cells would be stimulated by the injections. The presence of a pinealo-petal nerve tract in *Tropidonotus* running along the stalk and originating from cells in the hypendyma of the subcommissural organ (Petit 1969*b*) needs corroboration.

PINEAL ORGAN IN BIRDS

Although the structure of the avian pineal varies widely, most authors agree that the outer segments of the chief cells are rudimentary, regressed or disintegrated (Oksche and Vaupel-von Harnack 1965*b*, 1966; Collin 1966*a*, *b*, 1967*c*, 1969*a*, *b*; Oksche and Kirschstein 1969; Bischoff 1969; Oksche, Morita and Vaupel-von Harnack 1969; Ueck 1970). The basal process reaches the basement membrane of the epithelium and may invaginate into the pericapillary space. Here it is sometimes devoid of its basement membrane covering (Collin 1969*a*, *b*). Again, secretory granules measuring 70–100 nm (700–1000 Å) in diameter and originating in the Golgi zone accumulate in the terminal buds of the basal processes. Synaptic ribbons have been observed in these buds and in the somata of the cells but they are not associated with synaptic contacts (Collin 1968*b*, 1969*a*, *b*; Ueck 1970).

Pineal tract fibres have been found (unpublished observation by the present author; Quay and Renzoni 1963, 1967; Oksche and Kirschstein 1969; Oksche, Morita and Vaupel-von Harnack 1969; Ueck 1970), while rare nerve cells and synaptic junctions between receptor elements and nerve cells have been demonstrated by electron microscopy in *Passer* (Ueck 1970). In some birds at least, a rudimentary pineal photosensory function still exists, although the photic poles of the chief cells are practically absent. In the basal part of the pineal, which is continuous with the stalk, sustained, low-amplitude spikes can be recorded which are not influenced by light (Morita 1966*b*, and Oksche, Morita and Vaupel-von Harnack 1969 in the pigeon; Ralph and Dawson 1968 in *Coturnix* and *Passer*). Pineal electrical activity could not be elicited either by direct illumination of the organ or by photic stimulation of the eyes. Nevertheless the avian pineal plays a role in the effect exerted by light on the reproductive system, as will be shown later.

The avian organ is innervated by noradrenergic fibres (Bischoff and Richter 1966; Gonzalez and Hidalgo 1966; Collin 1969*a*, *b*, also for references; Oksche and Kirschstein 1969; Oksche, Morita and Vaupel-von Harnack 1969; Hedlund 1970; Ueck 1970). Nerve fibre trunks extend dorsally along the venous sinuses and pierce the pineal capsule to enter the organ (Quay and Renzoni 1963; Oksche and Kirschstein 1969). Some rare adrenergic fibres were observed in the nerve bundle accompanying the pineal stalk (Oksche and Kirschstein 1969). The fibres, which have also been demonstrated by fluorescence histochemistry, run in the interlobular connective tissue strands along the blood vessels in the perivascular spaces. They either penetrate the basement membrane of the epithelium to enter the parenchymal compartment (Bischoff and Richter 1966; Gonzalez and Hidalgo 1966; Collin 1969*a*, *b*; Hedlund 1970) or not (Ueck 1970; Hedlund 1970), probably according to species. Bilateral superior cervical ganglio-nectomy proved that the avian sympathetic fibres originate primarily if not exclusively in these ganglia (Hedlund 1970).

A yellow fluorescence (Fuxe and Ljunggren 1965; Hedlund 1970; Ueck 1970) pointing to the presence of 5-HT is equally distributed over the entire parenchyma and does not seem to be bound specifically to granular material (Ueck 1970). Considerable amounts of 5-HT as well as other hydroxy- and methoxyindoles have been found biochemically in the pigeon pineal (Quay 1966). A daily rhythm in pineal 5-HT content can be triggered partly by light and darkness although its regulation appears to be basically endogenous. Hydroxyindole-O-methyltransferase activity is at least 200 times higher in the chick than in the rat pineal, but, in contrast to the condition in the rat pineal, this activity increases in light and decreases in darkness (Axelrod and Wurtman 1964). Neither bilateral enucleation of the eyes nor pineal sympathetic denervation prevented the elevation of enzyme activity induced by light (Lauber, Boyd and Axelrod 1968). Evidently, in contrast to the mammalian pineal gland, neither the retinas nor an intact pineal sympathetic innervation are essential for environmental control of melatonin production in the chick pineal. This casts some doubt on the regulation of biochemical processes in avian pinealocytes by the sympathetic system, or at least on its exclusive role in this regulation. It has been suggested that the thin avian skull allows light to penetrate and reach the organ directly. This idea is supported by recent experiments in the canary (Munns 1970). It was demonstrated that birds in constant light without an opaque covering of the pineal region by a black polyester resin layer had more than a two-fold elevation in pineal HIOMT activity when compared to birds either in constant darkness or with opaque coverings over the pineal region. Moreover, these birds showed reduced spermatogenesis. It may be that, in birds, the chief pineal cells are directly affected by light, the photic stimuli regulating the synthesis of compounds present in the same cells. In contrast, the functioning of the mammalian pinealocyte is regulated by light transmitted by way of the eyes and the sympathetic innervation.

That the sympathetic pineal innervation in birds is not without any function, however, follows from the observation that bilateral superior ganglionectomy in quail is followed by a decrease in egg production (McFarland, Homma and Wilson 1968; Sayler and Wolfson 1968). After a time the birds regain their preoperative level of egg production. Bilateral ganglionectomy in immature quail results in a delay of the onset of egg laying. Both ganglionectomy and pinealectomy delay the onset of laying and both effects are transitory (Sayler and Wolfson 1967). Evidently, pineal sympathetic innervation in quail is somehow involved in the functioning of the reproductive system, but whether photic stimuli are transmitted to the organ by this innervation is not clear from these experiments. Although a number of papers claim that the avian pineal is involved in the reproductive process, pinealectomy was found ineffective in preventing gonadal inhibition or atrophy in immature and in mature quail in non-stimulatory photoperiods (Arrington, Ringer and Wolford 1969). The rate of sexual maturation of 8-week-old females given stimulatory photoperiods was not affected by pinealectomy and there was only a trend in the results indicating that pinealectomy reduced or delayed gonadal atrophy in sexually mature males when put under non-stimulatory photoperiods—that is, in increasing periods of darkness. It may be that pinealectomy or pineal denervation exerts an influence on the reproductive system only in normal illumination or in stimulatory photoperiods.

For a discussion of the circadian rhythm and photoperiodism in connexion with extraretinal light perception in birds, as postulated by Menaker, see a paper by Oksche and Kirschstein (1969) and the contribution by Professor Oksche to this symposium (p. 127).

PINEAL ORGAN IN MAMMALS

In the pineal organ of mammals the specific cell is the pinealocyte which, in its adult state, shows no vestiges of an outer segment. Remnants of a ciliary apparatus may, however, be present. The cells show one or more long processes which end in terminal buds. For an excellent survey of the microscopic anatomy and cytology of the mammalian pineal, see Bargmann's (1943) extensive paper (see also Kappers 1969a).

Although the pineal gland of mammals is part of the brain it does not show either afferent or efferent nervous connexions with the brain proper. Fibres of the habenula and posterior commissure may intermingle with the pineal parenchyma but, so far, it has not been demonstrated by anatomical or by physiological methods that they play a functional role in pineal innervation.

It is agreed that the mammalian pineal is exclusively innervated by the peripheral autonomic nervous system (Kappers 1960, 1965, also for references; Kenny 1965) which forms a rich network of fibres, associated with lemmocytes, except in a few species (Owman, 1965). In most mammals these fibres are sympathetic postganglionic fibres originating in the superior cervical ganglia. This means that the gland is an end organ of the peripheral sympathetic system, which is of great consequence for its function.

The fibres can enter the organ by two ways: (1) all along its surface, either in association with the pineal blood vessels or not, and (2) by way of the nervi conarii. It follows that total denervation of the gland can only be achieved by bilateral superior ganglionectomy and not by cutting the nervi conarii alone, if this were technically feasible.

In the macaque monkey, preganglionic parasympathetic fibres coursing in the greater superior petrosal nerves enter the pineal and synapse with intrapineal nerve cells (Kenny 1961). This may mean that parasympathetic cholinergic fibres contribute considerably to the pineal innervation in primates.

Intrapineal nerve cells (autonomic intramural ganglion cells) constantly occur in the pineals of primates including man. They have also been observed in the pineals of many non-primates (see Kappers 1960, 1965 for references). Recently, such cells were demonstrated in the rabbit pineal by my co-worker H. Romijn (unpublished) and by Trueman and Herbert (1970) in the ferret pineal. The latter authors showed that these cells did not contain monoamines but that acetylcholinesterase was present. Arvy (1961) was probably the first to observe a few acetylcholinesterase-positive fibres in the pineal of cattle, sheep and pig. They have also been demonstrated in the rat pineal (Kappers, unpublished; Machado and Lemos 1970). Penetrating from the capsule into the gland in 36–48-hour-old rats, they form a network associated with pineal vessels. Fibres were also seen in close topographical relationship with pinealocytes. All these fibres disappear after bilateral superior ganglionectomy, which suggests their sympathetic origin (Machado and Lemos 1970).

So far, acetylcholinesterase-positive pineal nerve fibres, which are probably cholinergic, have been detected only by histochemical methods and light microscopy. In electron micrographs some nerve endings of fibres running in the pericapillary spaces of the rabbit pineal show exclusively accumulations of clear vesicles measuring about 50 nm (500 Å) in diameter and some few dense-cored vesicles of the large type while, on the other hand, most endings show small clear as well as dense-cored vesicles next to large dense-cored vesicles (H. Romijn, unpublished). Possibly the endings containing small clear vesicles exclusively belong to the acetylcholinesterase-positive fibres. Further electron microscopic studies using different fixation methods are needed to prove this hypothesis. In view of the experimental evidence of a parasympathetic innervation of the monkey pineal mentioned above, it would be especially worthwhile to look for cholinergic fibres in the pineals of primates.

Autonomic fibre bundles coursing in the pericapillary spaces and in the pineal parenchyma can be readily observed by electron microscopy. The latter bundles can reach the parenchyma in two ways: (1) by leaving the perivascular space and penetrating the basement membrane of the pineal parenchyma which is also the external limiting membrane of that space, or (2) directly, without having first accompanied the vessels. Penetration of fibres from the perivascular space into the parenchyma is supposed to occur rather often although it has been demonstrated only once in a mammalian pineal (Wartenberg 1968). A much larger number of sympathetic fibres can certainly reach the parenchyma directly by the second way—that is, either along the nervi conarii or along the entire surface of the gland.

Sympathetic fibres coursing in the pericapillary spaces often end in these spaces. The endings show the usual characteristics of noradrenergic fibres.

As the structure and function of varicosities occurring along the pre-terminal part of such fibres is quite similar to that of their terminals, some of the structures hitherto described as nerve endings may have been varicosities.

The neurotransmitter, most probably noradrenaline, released from these varicosities and endings will stimulate the pinealocytes by diffusing through the basement membrane lining the pineal parenchyma. The neurotransmitter can reach the terminal buds even more easily if they are invaginated into the pericapillary space and devoid of their basement membrane covering. This mode of transmission of autonomic impulses is rather similar to that generally occurring in the stimulation of, for instance, smooth muscle cells by autonomic fibres. In that case also the fibre terminals are often separated by a considerable distance and a basement membrane from their effector cells.

The intraparenchymal sympathetic fibres end in close appositional contact with processes of pinealocytes and their terminal buds but never on the somata of these cells. The nature of this contact was first dealt with by Wolfe (1965; for a discussion on this subject see also Kappers 1969a). In general, no morphological characteristics of true synaptic junctions are observed. True synaptic contacts between endings of noradrenergic intra-parenchymal fibres and pinealocytes have been illustrated only by Wartenberg (see Kelly 1967) and by the present author (Kappers 1969a) in, respectively, the cat and the rat pineal. Here, pre- and postsynaptic membrane thickenings, a subsynaptic web and electron-dense material in the synaptic cleft were present.

Considering that these are terminals of sympathetic postganglionic fibres which, in general, never form true synaptic contacts with their effector cells, it is rather remarkable that rare synaptic junctions of this type have been observed at all in the pineal gland. The transmitter released at intraparenchymal nerve endings can certainly reach the pinealocytes quicker by diffusion than the transmitter released at the endings in the pericapillary spaces because, in the first case, no basement membrane is interposed between these endings and the effector cells. In the exceptional cases in which true synaptic contacts occur, a still quicker and more specifically directed impulse transmission seems warranted. It should be mentioned that, in some cases, rather intimate contacts between axons and smooth muscle cells have been demonstrated by some earlier authors (see Kappers 1964 for references, and Taxi 1965). Recently, membrane specializations have been observed in certain neuromuscular contacts in the vas deferens of the rat (Ivanov 1970). From this it would appear that also in other systems innervated by autonomic fibres, more or less specialized neuroeffector contacts do occur.

The mammalian pinealocyte is a secretory cell which produces, stores and excretes pineal-specific compounds. Storage and possibly also part of the production of secretory substances occurs in the terminal buds of the pinealocyte processes. They contain dense-cored vesicles, varying in number according to species (see Pellegrino de Iraldi 1969, also for references and the nature of their content), clear vesicles and much larger spaces which are membrane-bound and may be part of the smooth endoplasmic reticulum. We shall hear more about these organelles in Dr Arstila's paper (pp. 147–164). Most often the buds terminate either on the basement membrane of the pineal parenchyma or on intercellular spaces which communicate with the pericapillary spaces.

In some species processes of gliocytes intervene between the terminal buds and the basement membrane (Wartenberg 1968) while in others the buds may invaginate into the pericapillary space. In the latter case the bud may even lose its basement membrane covering, then hanging naked in the pericapillary space, as has also been described in birds. As in some Sauropsida the intercellular space sometimes shows an electron-dense content, indicating the presence of extruded secretory products. Extrusion of the content of granules present in the buds has been demonstrated in the rabbit pineal (Leonhardt 1967; H. Romijn, unpublished). In some mammals, such as the rabbit, the pericapillary spaces form long extensions in the parenchyma. These extensions are narrow clefts containing bundles of collagenous fibres. Terminal buds of pinealocytes end on these clefts and it can be assumed that they are receptacula for the pineal secretory substances extruded into them.

In rat (Milofsky 1957) and in mouse (Ito and Matsushima 1968) the pineal capillary endothelium is distinctly fenestrated. If no pores seem to be present, the endothelial wall is often extremely thin locally.

All the structural features mentioned suggest that the pinealocytes extrude their products into the blood circulating in the capillaries via the basement membrane of the pineal parenchyma, the pericapillary spaces, the basement membrane covering the capillary endothelium, and the endothelial wall. In the parenchyma extrusion occurs also into intercellular spaces which are in open communication with the pericapillary spaces.

FUNCTIONAL EVOLUTION OF THE PINEAL

Some general conclusions on the structure, function and innervation of the pineal can be drawn on the basis of its phylogenetic development already described.

(1) The mammalian pinealocyte is phylogenetically derived from the neurosensory photoreceptor element present in the pineal of anamniotes. It is not a modified nerve cell. During its evolution this cell loses its outer segment or photoreceptive pole while its synaptic pole also disappears. Likewise, the nervous apparatus conducting the transduced photic stimuli from the photoreceptor cells to the brain is gradually lost. This means that the pineal loses its capacity to convey photic stimuli to the brain. If some intraepithelial pineal sensory nerve cells are left in any given pineal it can be assumed that this type of direct pineal photosensory function is still intact, however restricted. Very early in pineal phylogeny signs are found of a secretory function of the chief pineal cells. It is quite probable that, in one and the same cell type, a photosensory and a secretory function are combined. Gradually the chief pineal cell loses its photoreceptive capacity and becomes preponderantly a secretory element which, however, possibly remains directly photosensitive or becomes indirectly photosensitive by a circuitous route, via the retinas and a complicated neural pathway to be mentioned later. The transformation described is most clearly shown in the pineal of Sauropsida. In one pineal epithelium the chief cells may show different gradations of the process of transformation, but, in principle, there is only one single cell type. A clear distinction between two basically different types of chief pineal cells cannot be made.

(2) Alongside the gradual loss of the pinealo-fugal sensory innervation pattern there is an increasing development of an autonomic pinealo-petal motor innervation pattern. Already distinct in some fishes and amphibians and very evident in Sauropsida, this type of innervation pattern is the only one present in the mammalian pineal. As is known, the sympathetic fibres innervating the mammalian pineal mediate (among other things) photic stimuli to the organ. It would be reasonable to accept that, because the autonomic pineal innervation regulates the photo-dependent synthesis of compounds in the mammalian pinealocyte, the same will be true for the pineal photoreceptor elements and the secretory rudimentary photoreceptor cells in non-mammalian vertebrates. On the ground of some of the observations cited, however, it cannot be excluded that in nonmammals the production and/or the excretion of pineal substances may be regulated by photic impulses directly received by the same cell which produces the pineal secretory substances. In these cases, the chief pineal cells are directly photosensitive although they may have lost their photoreceptor capacity. As we have seen in birds this does not mean that the sympathetic innervation is of no consequence for the regulation of reproductive processes via the pineal but probably only that in non-mammals

also, other, non-photic impulses may be conveyed to the pineal via its sympathetic innervation which influence its function.

(3) In the phylogenetic development of the autonomic innervation pattern of the pineal a distinct trend toward an ever more extensive and efficient stimulation of the chief cells by autonomic fibres can be observed. Three stages can be distinguished.

Stage (*a*): invasion of the organ by postganglionic fibres along the perivascular spaces. At this stage the fibres end exclusively within these spaces and do not contact chief pineal cells, which can only be reached by the transmitter released at the varicosities and endings of the fibres by diffusion through the basement membrane of the pineal epithelium.

Stage (*b*): the sympathetic fibres may leave the perivascular spaces to enter the pineal cell compartment by penetrating its basement membrane. Appositional contacts with chief cells are made by the endings. In this way a somewhat quicker impulse transmission by diffusion is realized than at stage (*a*).

Stage (*c*): the pineal is invaded by postganglionic fibres entering the organ not by way of the perivascular spaces but via the nervi conarii and all along the surface of the pineal. These fibres can distribute directly in the pineal parenchyma. Their endings make close appositional contacts with the secretory pinealocytes and, in rare cases, even well-developed true synaptic junctions are formed. Preganglionic fibres may also enter the organ, synapsing with intramural autonomic nerve cells which give rise to postganglionic fibres distributing in the pineal parenchyma.

The sympathetic innervation pattern of stage (*a*) is the simplest and theoretically the phylogenetically earliest one. It is possibly realized in lower fishes, as can be seen in an illustration of the structure of a lamprey pineal by Collin (1969*a*). In amphibians and Sauropsida both stages (*a*) and (*b*) are realized. Stage (*c*), side by side with stages (*a*) and (*b*), occurs in the mammalian pineal.

The transformation of photoreceptor cells into pinealocytes is traceable not only in the phylogenetic development of the pineal; it is also evident during its ontogenetic development in mammals. Cilia-bearing bulges of cytoplasm extending into the lumen of the pineal anlage in foetal hamsters and rats recall the rudimentary development of outer segments (Clabough 1970). In adult pinealocytes synaptic ribbons are commonly observed, as are remnants of a ciliary apparatus. The function of the synaptic ribbons is still open to discussion (see Kappers 1969*a*, also for references).

Considering the embryonic neuroepithelial origin of the mammalian pinealocyte, its secretory function, the excretion of its products into the general circulation, and its sensitivity to indirect photic stimulation, the mammalian pineal gland can be termed an indirectly photosensitive neuro-endocrine organ. However, when using this term one should realize that the pinealocytes are not true neurons. All of the morphological character-istics of the organ described are typical for endocrine organs in general (see Kappers 1971 for references). This holds also when comparing the (neuro)-parenchymo-haemal contact area of the pineal gland with the neuro-haemal contact areas of the supraoptico-paraventriculo-hypophysial and the tubero-infundibular neurosecretory systems in the hypothalamus. The endings of the peptidergic and aminergic nerve fibres of these systems terminate on the basement membrane of the nervous parenchyma. This membrane is the external limiting membrane of pericapillary spaces which surround, respectively, the capillaries in the pars nervosa of the hypophysis and those forming the primary hypophysial portal plexus in the median eminence. It is agreed that the contents of these nerve endings are released into the blood circulating in these capillaries via the external limiting mem-brane of the pericapillary space, this space, its internal limiting membrane covering the endothelium, and the capillary endothelium which is fenest-rated. Evidently, the structure of the neuro-haemal contact areas of these neurosecretory systems is similar to that of the parenchymo-haemal contact area in the pineal gland. There is one difference only: the pericapillary spaces in the pineal contain bundles of autonomic nerve fibres whereas those in the pars nervosa of the hypophysis and in the median eminence do not (for seeming exceptions, see Kappers 1971). This difference is explained by the fact that the nervous control of the pineal is exogenous—that is, by peripheral sympathetic fibres invading the organ along perivascular spaces; whereas the nervous control of the hypothalamic neurosecretory systems is endogenous—that is by fibres, cholinergic and aminergic, which originate as well as synapse with the elements of these systems within the central nervous system (Fig. 1).

Wartenberg (1968) rightly argued that neural information is transformed by the pineal into a neurohormonal output, although we prefer to use the term "hormonal output" because, although the organ is part of the brain, the pinealocytes are not true neurons as was held by Wartenberg. This same idea has been recently brought forward by Wurtman and Antón-Tay (1969) who termed the mammalian pineal "a neuroendocrine transducer", meaning by "neuro" the neural input and by "endocrine" the hormonal output. This term can be accepted if it is realized that, in this respect, the pineal is no exception. In a similar way the cells of the hypothalamic neurosecretory systems are neuroendocrine transducers because they produce (neuro)endocrine substances under the regulation of nervous impulses, among other things. It is, moreover, probable that not only is

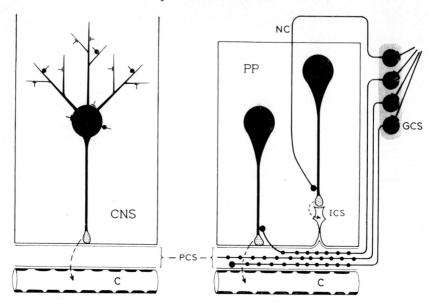

Fig. 1. Diagram comparing the neuro-haemal contact area of a hypothalamo-hypophysial neurosecretory system (*left*) with the parenchymo-
haemal contact area in the mammalian pineal gland (*right*). Endings of
either cholinergic or aminergic nerve fibres associated with terminals of
neurosecretory fibres are not drawn. C, capillary; CNS, central nervous
system; GCS, superior cervical ganglion; ICS, intercellular space; NC,
nervus conarii; PCS, pericapillary space; PP, pineal parenchyma. For
explanation see text.

the mammalian pineal such a "neuroendocrine transducer" but that the
same term may apply to the non-mammalian pineal.

NATURE OF STIMULUS TO THE PINEAL

I shall now deal shortly with the nature of the impulses mediated to the
pinealocytes by their autonomic innervation. It is agreed that photic
stimuli are transmitted to the mammalian pineal by its peripheral sympathetic innervation. The central nervous pathway involved in the mediation
of these stimuli has recently been unravelled (Moore *et al.* 1968). It is now
known that photic stimuli reach the pineal via the retina, the inferior
accessory optic tract coursing in the medial forebrain bundle in the lateral
hypothalamus, a centre in the rostral midbrain tegmentum, a not yet well
analysed, probably scattered fibre bundle in the brain stem, the intermedio-
lateral nucleus in the upper thoracic part of the cord, preganglionic fibres,
the superior cervical ganglia and postganglionic fibres reaching the gland.

Photic stimuli have been shown to regulate HIOMT activity in the gland, among other things. The pineal noradrenaline rhythm also depends on the intactness of the same neural pathway mediating photic stimuli (Wurtman *et al.* 1967).

In the monkey, HIOMT activity in the pineal also depends on conditions of illumination, but, in contrast to the rat, the pineal of monkeys kept in continuous light shows a high enzyme activity and when kept in darkness a low one (Moore 1969). Thus, in this respect, the monkey pineal reacts similarly to the chick pineal. Evidently, light has an opposite effect on pineal HIOMT levels in the nocturnal rat compared to the diurnal monkey and chick. Earlier, I argued (Kappers 1969*a*) that in the rat photic stimuli inhibit pineal activity if the entire neural pathway mediating these stimuli is intact while, on the other hand, the hypothesis that the perception of darkness by the retinas is the adequate stimulus for increased pineal activity is not very tenable. Recently, Wurtman and Antón-Tay (1969) have dealt with the same question. They conclude that the photic control of rat pineal function probably involves either the inhibition of pineal sympathetic tone—and of noradrenaline release—by light or stimulation of this tone by darkness. We should like to support the first alternative on the ground of earlier arguments (Kappers 1969*a*), the more so as a reduction of pineal HIOMT levels has been demonstrated after stimulation of the preganglionic nerve trunks to the superior cervical ganglia in blinded rats or in rats in which the inferior accessory optic tract was cut (Brownstein and Heller 1968). Moreover, light was shown to inhibit the spontaneous tonic level of electrical activity recordable from the nerve terminals in the rat pineal (Taylor and Wilson 1969).

That this problem is more complex, however, appears from the observation mentioned that light affects HIOMT activity in the monkey pineal in an opposite way to the rat pineal. Why should light stimulate pineal activity by way of its innervation in monkey and inhibit pineal activity in rat? A possible but rather speculative way to solve this dilemma is by accepting (1) that in the pineal, as elsewhere, sympathetic fibres act antagonistically to parasympathetic ones and (2) that the monkey pineal may be primarily innervated by parasympathetic cholinergic fibres (see above, p. 11) and the rat pineal primarily although not exclusively by sympathetic noradrenergic fibres. Interestingly, it has been shown that in rats a parasympathetic effector blocker, atropine methyl bromide, inhibits the high level of HIOMT activity normally occurring in darkness while a cholinomimetic compound, oxotremorine oxalate, restores HIOMT activity in darkness. On a normal lighting schedule, rats also showed higher levels of HIOMT activity after receiving injections of the cholinomimetic than after injections of atropine sulphate (Wartman *et al.* 1969). The authors conclude that their experiments indicate that parasympathetic innervation does not contribute significantly to the response of the pineal to the presence of light. On the other hand, facilitation of pineal HIOMT activity in the absence of light would appear to be mediated by the parasympathetic system. From this and the data mentioned above one could conclude that, in the dark, the normal uninhibited tone of the sympathetic and stimulation of the parasympathetic tone would cause high levels of HIOMT activity in the rat pineal. However, in the monkey kept in darkness, the pineal, which may have a much stronger parasympathetic innervation than in rat, shows a low HIOMT activity whereas this activity is high after permanent illumination. It may be that the level is only a relatively high one caused by lack of inhibited sympathetic fibres. However it is not easy to explain the opposite effects of light and darkness, respectively, on the monkey pineal and the rat pineal, and further research should reveal the solution of this problem. The nature of the innervation of the primate pineal is of particular interest.

Very probably, the pineal also responds to other than photic stimuli mediated by its sympathetic innervation. The organ, for instance, was shown to react strongly to stress (Miline 1957; Miline, Krstić and Devečerski 1968). As tegmental centres, which have many afferent neural connexions including with the hypothalamus and the limbic system, project on the intermedio-lateral nucleus in the cord, many types of stimuli set up in very different parts of the central nervous system may alter the tone of the peripheral autonomic fibres ending in the pineal.

There are arguments favouring the idea that the pineal shows a high basic activity which is cyclic under normal circadian conditions of lighting and probably primarily dependent on feedback mechanisms in the *milieu interne*. External stimuli like excessive darkness, but particularly excessive light, act as an accessory regulatory mechanism which is superimposed on the intrinsic regulation set up by internal stimuli. Effects of experimentally produced changes in pineal activity, and therefore in the activity of the reproductive system, show a tendency to disappear. Several authors have demonstrated that, even after pinealectomy, the reproductive system regains its normal activity after some time. Apparently, a new equilibrium is established in the internal regulation of pineal function.

MODE OF SECRETION OF PINEAL PRODUCTS

A final question which has come up lately is whether the mammalian pineal gland releases its secretory products either directly or indirectly into the ventricular cerebrospinal fluid. According to Antón-Tay and Wurtman (1969) it is not quite known whether melatonin is secreted into the blood or into the cerebrospinal fluid, and, on the ground of a close spatial relationship between the suprapineal recess of the third ventricle and the pineal in the hamster, Sheridan, Reiter and Jacobs (1969) suggest that pineal secretory substances could have access to the ventricular system and hence to the hypothalamus and midbrain, which have been shown to take up tritiated melatonin selectively (Antón-Tay and Wurtman 1969).

I do not think there are any arguments in favour of this opinion. Firstly, all data on the fine structure of the gland appear to give overwhelming evidence of its endocrine nature. The pineal secretory products are extruded into the blood circulating in the pineal capillaries which finally drain into the large veins surrounding the organ. Certainly in many mammals a close topographical relationship between the dorsal surface of the gland and the ventral wall of the suprapineal recess, varying in extension, is observed. In most cases, however, the recess covers only part of the dorsal surface of the gland and never its lateral and ventral sides. Moreover, the following facts should be considered.

The pineal is embedded in leptomeningeal tissue forming the septum transversum. A condensation of this tissue constitutes the pineal capsule which varies in thickness but covers the entire organ. At the site where the suprapineal recess covers a smaller or larger part of the dorsal aspect of the pineal, the pineal parenchyma is separated from the ependyma lining this part of the third ventricle by this leptomeningeal pineal capsule as well as by the leptomeningeal covering of the ependyma. In many mammals, moreover, additional loose leptomeningeal tissue is interposed between the coverings mentioned. Within the gland proper a more or less dense superficial limiting glial membrane is also observed. A rather dense glial membrane is, for instance, present all round the pineal of ungulates and primates while it shows a less dense and only local development in the dorsal and caudal border zones of the pineal in lower mammals (Hülsemann 1967, also for further references). On the grounds of these facts I am convinced that pineal secretory products cannot reach the ventricular cerebrospinal fluid, either directly or indirectly.

According to Falck and Owman (1968) the pineal should show signs of its functioning during early prenatal life by way of "ependymosecretion" into the ventricular system. This opinion is based on papers by Olsson (1961) on the development of the subcommissural organ and the pineal in human foetuses, and by Owman (1961) on the pineal of the foetal rat. Following Olsson, subcommissural cells occur in the proliferation of ependymal cells constituting the posterior lobe of the pineal. These cells contain granules which may be of a secretory nature. Olsson is, however, of the opinion that any secretion produced by these cells is discharged into the bloodstream and not by way of the cerebrospinal fluid. Owman (1961) stated that substances produced by the very early ependymal-like pineal cells bordering the pineal recess of the third ventricle are directly depleted into the cerebrospinal fluid. Electron microscopic investigation will have to corroborate these rather suggestive observations. The further embryonic development of the gland (Kappers 1960), however, does not support the idea that pineal substances can reach the ventricle. The ependymal layer constituting the anlage of the organ proliferates and pseudofollicles are formed, the lumina of which do not communicate with the third ventricle and disappear altogether at later stages of development.

SUMMARY

This survey is intended as a general introduction to the symposium. It discusses aspects of the fine structure of the chief pineal cells, which are essentially neurosensory photoreceptor cells in anamniotes and secretory elements in mammals. In reptiles and birds pineal photosensory function is gradually lost, the organ developing an exclusively secretory function. Aspects of pineal innervation, biochemistry and physiology are also dealt with.

During its phylogenetic development the pineal organ shows remarkable and clearly correlated changes in structure, innervation pattern and function. The mammalian pineal gland can be considered an indirectly photosensory neuroendocrine organ with the restriction that its secretory cells are not nerve elements but are phylogenetically transformed neurosensory photoreceptor cells derived from the embryonic neuroepithelium. There are no facts supporting the opinion expressed by some authors that pineal secretory products are extruded directly into the cerebrospinal fluid.

The fact that the mammalian pineal gland is an end organ of the peripheral sympathetic system conveying photic and other stimuli to it, explains the difference between its pattern of neural regulation and that of other neuroendocrine systems (see Fig. 1). Functionally, the mammalian pineal has been rightly characterized as being a "regulator of regulators", the organ never acting directly on peripheral target organs.

REFERENCES

ANTÓN-TAY, F. and WURTMAN, R. J. (1969) Nature, Lond. 221, 474–475.
ARRINGTON, L. C., RINGER, R. K. and WOLFORD, J. H. (1969) Poult. Sci. 48, 454–459.

ARVY, L. (1961) *C. r. hebd. Séanc. Acad. Sci., Paris, Sér. D* **253**, 1361–1363.

AXELROD, J. and WURTMAN, R. J. (1964) *Nature, Lond.* **201**, 1134.

AXELROD, J., QUAY, W. B. and BAKER, P. C. (1965) *Nature, Lond.* **208**, 386.

BAGNARA, J. T. (1965) In *Structure and Function of the Epiphysis Cerebri (Progress in Brain Research* vol. 10), pp. 489–506, ed. Kappers, J. A. and Schadé, J. P. Amsterdam: Elsevier.

BALEMANS, M. G. M. and VAN DE VEERDONK, F. C. G. (1967) *Experientia* **23**, 906.

BALEMANS, M. G. M., VAN DE VEERDONK, F. C. G. and VAN DE KAMER, J. C. (1967) *Gen. comp. Endocr.* **9**, abstract 9.

BARGMANN, W. (1943) In *Handbuch der Mikroskopischen Anatomie des Menschen*, IV/4, ed. Möllendorff, W. von. Berlin: Springer.

BISCHOFF, M. B. (1969) *J. Ultrastruct. Res.* **28**, 16–26.

BISCHOFF, M. B. and RICHTER, W. R. (1966) *Proc. VI Int. Congr. Electron Microscopy, Kyoto*, 1966, pp. 523–524. Tokyo: Maruzen Co Ltd, Nihonbashi.

BROWNSTEIN, M. J. and HELLER, A. (1968) *Science* **162**, 367–368.

CHARLTON, H. M. (1964) *Nature, Lond.* **204**, 1093–1094.

CHARLTON, H. M. (1966a) *Gen. comp. Endocr.* **7**, 384–397.

CHARLTON, H. M. (1966b) *Comp. Biochem. Physiol.* **17**, 777–784.

CHARLTON, H. M. (1968) *Gen. comp. Endocr.* **11**, 465–480.

CLABOUGH, J. W. (1970) *Anat. Rec.* **166**, 291.

COLLIN, J. P. (1966a) *C.r. hebd. Séanc. Acad. Sci., Paris, Sér. D* **263**, 660–663.

COLLIN, J. P. (1966b) *C.r. Séanc. Soc. Biol.* **160**, 1876–1880.

COLLIN, J. P. (1967a) *C.r. hebd. Séanc. Acad. Sci., Paris, Sér. D* **265**, 1827–1830.

COLLIN, J. P. (1967b) *C.r. hebd. Séanc. Acad. Sci., Paris, Sér. D* **264**, 647–650.

COLLIN, J. P. (1967c) *C.r. hebd. Séanc. Acad. Sci., Paris, Sér. D* **265**, 48–51.

COLLIN, J. P. (1968a) *C.r. Séanc. Soc. Biol.* **162**, 1785–1789.

COLLIN, J. P. (1968b) *C.r. hebd. Séanc. Acad. Sci., Paris, Sér. D* **267**, 758–761.

COLLIN, J. P. (1969a) *C.r. Séanc. Soc. Biol.* **163**, 1137.

COLLIN, J. P. (1969b) Thèse, Faculté des Sciences de l'Université de Clermont-Ferrand, 112 Série E, pp. 1–291.

COLLIN, J. P. (1969c) *Archs Anat. microsc. Morph. exp.* **58**, 145–182.

COLLIN, J. P. and KAPPERS, J. A. (1968) *Brain Res.* **11**, 85–106.

DODT, E. and JACOBSON, M. (1963) *J. Neurophysiol.* **26**, 752–758.

DODT, E. and MORITA, Y. (1964) *Vision Res.* **4**, 413–421.

EAKIN, R. M., QUAY, W. B. and WESTFALL, J. A. (1963) *Z. Zellforsch. mikrosk. Anat.* **59**, 663–683.

FALCK, B. and OWMAN, CH. (1968) *Adv.Pharmac.* **6A**, 211–231.

FENWICK, J. C. (1970) *Gen. comp. Endocr.* **14**, 86–97.

FUXE, K. and LJUNGGREN, L. (1965) *J. comp. Neurol.* **125**, 355–382.

GONZALEZ, G. G. and HIDALGO, F. G. (1966) *Trab. Inst. Cajal Invest. biol.* **58**, 55–67.

HAMASAKI, D. I. and DODT, E. (1969) *Pflügers Arch. ges. Physiol.* **313**, 19–29.

HEDLUND, L. (1970) *Anat. Rec.* **166**, 406.

HÜLSEMANN, M. (1967) *Acta anat.* **66**, 249–278.

ITO, T. and MATSUSHIMA, S. (1968) *Hokkaido Univ. Med. Library* Ser. 1, 1–20.

ITURIZZA, F. C. (1967) *J. Histochem. Cytochem.* **15**, 301–303.

IVANOV, D. P. (1970) *J. Neuro-visc. Rel.* **32**, in press.

KAPPERS J. A. (1960) *Z. Zellforsch. mikrosk. Anat.* **52**, 163–215.

KAPPERS, J. A. (1964) *Acta neuroveg.* **26**, 145–171.

KAPPERS, J. A. (1965) In *Structure and Function of the Epiphysis Cerebri (Progress in Brain Research* vol. 10), pp. 87–153, ed. Kappers, J. A. and Schadé, J. P. Amsterdam: Elsevier.

KAPPERS, J. A. (1967) *Z. Zellforsch. mikrosk. Anat.* **81**, 581–618.

KAPPERS, J. A. (1969a) *J. Neuro-visc. Rel.* suppl. 9, 140–184.

KAPPERS, J. A. (1969b) In *Progress in Endocrinology* (*Proc. III Int. Congr. Endocrinology*), pp. 619–626, ed. Gual, C. Excerpta Medica International Congress Series no. 184. Amsterdam: Excerpta Medica Foundation.

KAPPERS, J. A. (1971) In *Symposium on Subcellular Organization and Function in Endocrine Tissues. Mem. Soc. Endocrinology* no. 19, ed. Heller, H. and Lederis, K. London: Cambridge University Press. In press.

KELLY, D. E. (1967) *Anesthesiology* **28**, 6–30.

KENNY, G. C. T. (1961) *J. Neuropath. exp. Neurol.* **20**, 563–570.

KENNY, G. C. T. (1965) *Proc. Australas. Assoc. Neurol.* **3**, 133–141.

LAUBER, J. K., BOYD, J. E. and AXELROD, J. (1968) *Science* **161**, 489–490.

LEONHARDT, H. (1967) *Z. Zellforsch. mikrosk. Anat.* **82**, 307–320.

LUTZ, H. and COLLIN, J. P. (1967) *Bull. Soc. zool. Fr.* **92**, 797–808.

MACHADO, A. B. M. and LEMOS, V. C. J. (1970) *J. Neuro-visc. Rel.* **32**, in press.

McFARLAND, L. Z., HOMMA, K. and WILSON, W. O. (1968) *Experientia* **24**, 245–247.

MEHRING, G. (1970) *Z. Zellforsch. mikrosk. Anat.* in press.

MILINE, R. (1957) *Congr. nat. Sci. méd., Bucarest* (5–11 May, 1957), pp. 421–444. Bucarest: Academy of Science of Rumania.

MILINE, R., KRSTIĆ, R. and DEVEČERSKI, V. (1968) *Acta anat.* **71**, 352–402.

MILOFSKY, A. H. (1957) *Anat. Rec.* **127**, 435–436.

MOORE, R. Y. (1969) *Nature, Lond.* **222**, 781–782.

MOORE, R. Y., HELLER, A., BHATNAGAR, R. K., WURTMAN, R. J. and AXELROD, J. (1968) *Archs Neurol., Chicago* **18**, 208–218.

MORITA, Y. (1965) *Pflügers Arch. ges. Physiol.* **286**, 97–108.

MORITA, Y. (1966a) *Pflügers Arch. ges. Physiol.* **289**, 155–167.

MORITA, Y. (1966b) *Experientia* **22**, 402.

MORITA, Y. (1969) *Experientia* **25**, 1277.

MORITA, Y. and DODT, E. (1965) *Experientia* **21**, 221.

MUNNS, T. W. (1970) *Anat. Rec.* **166**, 352.

OKSCHE, A. and KIRSCHSTEIN, H. (1968) *Z. Zellforsch. mikrosk. Anat.* **87**, 159–192.

OKSCHE, A. and KIRSCHSTEIN, H. (1969) *Z. Zellforsch. mikrosk. Anat.* **102**, 214–241.

OKSCHE, A. and VAUPEL-VON HARNACK, M. (1963) *Z. Zellforsch. mikrosk. Anat.* **59**, 582–614.

OKSCHE, A. and VAUPEL-VON HARNACK, M. (1965a) *Z. Zellforsch. mikrosk. Anat.* **68**, 389–426.

OKSCHE, A. and VAUPEL-VON HARNACK, M. (1965b) *Naturwissenschaften* **24**, 662–663.

OKSCHE, A. and VAUPEL-VON HARNACK, M. (1966) *Z. Zellforsch. mikrosk. Anat.* **69**, 41–60.

OKSCHE, A., MORITA, Y. and VAUPEL-VON HARNACK, M. (1969) *Z. Zellforsch. mikrosk. Anat.* **102**, 1–30.

OLSSON, R. (1961) *Gen. comp. Endocr.* **1**, 117–123.

OWMAN, CH. (1961) *Acta. morph. neerl.-scand.* **3**, 367–394.

OWMAN, CH. (1965) In *Structure and Function of the Epiphysis Cerebri* (*Progress in Brain Research* vol. 10), pp. 423–453, ed. Kappers, J. A. and Schadé, J. P. Amsterdam: Elsevier.

PELLEGRINO DE IRALDI, A. (1969) *Z. Zellforsch. mikrosk. Anat.* **101**, 408–418.

PETER, R. E. (1968) *Gen. comp. Endocr.* **10**, 443–449.

PETIT, A. (1969a) *Z. Zellforsch. mikrosk. Anat.* **96**, 437–465.

PETIT, A. (1969b) *Archs Anat. Histol. Embryol.* **52**, 3–25.

QUAY, W. B. (1965) *Life Sci.* **4**, 983–991.

QUAY, W. B. (1966) *Gen. comp. Endocr.* **6**, 371–377.

QUAY, W. B. and RENZONI, A. (1963) *Riv. Biol.* **56**, 393–407.

QUAY, W. B. and RENZONI, A. (1967) *Riv. Biol.* **60**, 9–75.

QUAY, W. B. and WILHOFT, D. C. (1964) *J. Neurochem.* **11**, 805–811.

QUAY, W. B., JONGKIND, J. F. and KAPPERS, J. A. (1967) *Anat. Rec.* **157**, 304–305.

QUAY, W. B., KAPPERS, J. A. and JONGKIND, J. F. (1968) *J. Neuro-visc. Rel.* **31**, 11–25.
RALPH, C. L. and DAWSON, D. C. (1968) *Experientia* **24**, 147–148.
RÜDEBERG, C. (1966) *Pubbl. Staz. zool. Napoli* **35**, 47–60.
RÜDEBERG, C. (1968) *Z. Zellforsch. mikrosk. Anat.* **84**, 219–237.
RÜDEBERG, C. (1969) *Z. Zellforsch. mikrosk. Anat.* **96**, 548–581.
SAYLER, A. and WOLFSON, A. (1967) *Science* **158**, 1478–1479.
SAYLER, A. and WOLFSON, A. (1968) *Archs Anat. Histol. Embryol.* **51**, 615–626.
SHERIDAN, M. N., REITER, R. J. and JACOBS, J. J. (1969) *J. Endocr.* **45**, 131–132.
TAXI, J. (1965) *Ann. Sci. natur., Zool.* **7**, 413–674.
TAYLOR, A. N. and WILSON, R. (1969) *Anat. Rec.* **163**, 327.
TRUEMAN, T. and HERBERT, J. (1970) *J. Anat.* **106**, 406.
UECK, M. (1968*a*) *Z. Zellforsch. mikrosk. Anat.* **90**, 389–402.
UECK, M. (1968*b*) *Z. Zellforsch. mikrosk. Anat.* **92**, 452–476.
UECK, M. (1970) *Z. Zellforsch. mikrosk. Anat.* **105**, 276–302.
VAN DE VEERDONK, F. C. G. (1965) *Nature, Lond.* **208**, 1324–1325.
VAN DE VEERDONK, F. C. G. (1967) *Curr. Med. Biol.* **1**, 175–177.
VIVIEN, J. H. (1964*a*) *C.r. hebd. Séanc. Acad. Sci., Paris, Sér. D* **258**, 3370–3372.
VIVIEN, J. H. (1964*b*) *C.r. hebd. Séanc. Acad. Sci., Paris, Sér. D* **259**, 899–901.
VIVIEN, J. H. (1965) *C.r. hebd. Séanc. Acad. Sci., Paris, Sér. D* **260**, 5370–5372.
VIVIEN-ROELS, B. (1969) *Z. Zellforsch. mikrosk. Anat.* **94**, 352–390.
VIVIEN, J. H. and ROELS, B. (1967) *C.r. hebd. Séanc. Acad. Sci., Paris, Sér. D* **264**, 1743–1746.
VIVIEN, J. H. and ROELS, B. (1968) *C.r. hebd. Séanc. Acad. Sci., Paris, Sér. D* **266**, 600–603.
WARTENBERG, H. (1968) *Z. Zellforsch. mikrosk. Anat.* **86**, 74–97.
WARTENBERG, H. and BAUMGARTEN, H. G. (1968) *Z. Anat. EntwGesch.* **127**, 99–120.
WARTENBERG, H. and BAUMGARTEN, H. G. (1969*a*) *Z. Anat. EntwGesch.* **128**, 185–210.
WARTENBERG, H. and BAUMGARTEN, H. G. (1969*b*) *Z. Zellforsch. mikrosk. Anat.* **94**, 252–260.
WARTMAN, S. A., BRANCH, B. J., GEORGE, R. and TAYLOR, A. N. (1969) *Life Sci.* **8**, 1263–1270.
WOLFE, D. E. (1965) In *Structure and Function of the Epiphysis Cerebri* (*Progress in Brain Research* vol. 10), pp. 332–376, ed. Kappers, J. A. and Schadé, J. P. Amsterdam: Elsevier.
WURTMAN, R. J., and ANTÓN-TAY, F. (1969) *Recent Prog Horm. Res.* **25**, 493–522.
WURTMAN, R. J., AXELROD, J., SEDVALL, G. and MOORE, R. Y. (1967) *J. Pharmac. exp. Ther.* **157**, 487–492.

DISCUSSION

Wurtman: I would like first to congratulate Professor Ariëns Kappers on a brilliant analysis of the present status of pinealology. It is depressing in one sense, because some of us wrote a book on the subject in 1968 and our hope was that it would continue to be topical for five or six years, but I begin to have second thoughts about its continued topicality (Wurtman, Axelrod and Kelly 1968). The other point that emerges from this paper is that we were very lucky seven years ago at the first gathering of pinealologists, this being the second, to start off on the right interdisciplinary footing. It remains very clear that those of us who don't know much about anatomy must still worry about it, because there are many insights from anatomy that are critically important to those working in physiology, biochemistry and so on. We have all benefited from this interdisciplinary nature of pineal work and I don't see it as something that is about to end.

I would like to abstract one problem from something touched on several times in this paper. That is, what is the minimal evidence that we should require in order to state that the pineal of a given species does make melatonin or serotonin? What are the experimental ways of approaching this? I would like to list five of the many ways that investigators have used to demonstrate melatonin or serotonin synthesis.

The best evidence that a given pineal gland makes melatonin or serotonin is the fact that it contains very large amounts of these indoles. It is of course possible that the gland could store these compounds without synthesizing them, if it concentrated them from the bloodstream. However, if the melatonin content of the pineal is ten thousand times higher than that of any other organ, this is good presumptive evidence that melatonin is in fact made there. One way to confirm this is by giving the animal the precursor for melatonin or serotonin, namely tryptophan, and seeing whether the increment in melatonin in the pineal is very great, and greater than anywhere else in the body. As we all know, it is very difficult to demonstrate melatonin in the pineals of many species. I think this relates to the fact that melatonin is a lipid-soluble compound which apparently is not stored, but is probably made and secreted on demand, and so there's not an enormous reservoir of melatonin in the pineal analogous to the reservoir of adrenaline in the adrenal medulla. This is in the nature of lipid-soluble hormones.

The second way is to show that if you incubate the pineal *in vitro* with the radioactively labelled physiological precursor of melatonin, namely radioactive tryptophan, the pineal can make radioactive melatonin or radioactive serotonin *in vitro*. This indicates that all the enzymes and co-factors that are needed are present in the pineal. Or one can incubate the pineal with very large amounts of non-radioactive tryptophan and show the same kind of conversion to melatonin; this is of course a much less sensitive method. I think it's not adequate to incubate the pineal with 5-hydroxytryptophan, because the conversion of 5-hydroxytryptophan to serotonin involves a relatively non-specific biochemical process (decarboxylation). The enzyme that catalyses this reaction, DOPA decarboxylase, is found in most organs in the body, and so the fact that the pineal can make serotonin from 5-hydroxytryptophan is not especially significant. On the other hand, the fact that the pineal can make melatonin from tryptophan is special.

The third way is also an *in vitro* method and this is to argue that one enzyme, the melatonin-forming enzyme, hydroxyindole-O-methyl-transferase (HIOMT), is the special enzyme for the pineal, and to see whether this enzyme can be demonstrated in pineal homogenates. In mammals it appears, as Dr Axelrod first showed (Axelrod *et al.* 1961), that this enzyme is characteristic only of the pineal gland; it's not found anywhere else, except in pineal tumours and their metastases (Wurtman and Kammer 1966). Studies by Dr David Klein and his associates indicate that another enzyme, the enzyme that acetylates serotonin, while not unique to the pineal may be extremely important in melatonin synthesis, and that there are enormous (ten to thirty-fold) changes in the activity of this enzyme as the lighting environment is changed (Klein, Berg and Weller 1970; Klein *et al.* 1970). So perhaps HIOMT is not the only marker, but it continues to be a very good one in mammals. In lower vertebrates it is not so good a marker; in frogs, for example, HIOMT is not restricted to the pineal; it is also found in the rest of the brain and in the eye.

The fourth experimental system is an *in vivo* method, in which one injects radioactive tryptophan systemically and subsequently demonstrates the presence of retained radioactivity within the pineal, or, in lower vertebrates, within the epithalamic region of the brain. Alternatively, one administers non-radioactive tryptophan and demonstrates the appropriate yellow fluorescence in the pineal. This experimental system is not so good, because demonstrating radioactivity need not mean demonstrating radioactive melatonin or, for that matter, radioactive serotonin. In fact the most likely identity of the radioactivity is not an indole at all, but protein. The same argument can be made against the fluorescence studies; there is some evidence (Björklund and Falck 1969) that the pituitary contains compounds that differ chemically from serotonin but exhibit a fluorescence that resembles that of serotonin. Hence the demonstration of a material in pineals with a yellow fluorescence does not prove that serotonin is present.

Finally, the least satisfactory way is to inject radioactive 5-hydroxytryptophan, or radioactive S-adenosyl methionine or radioactive methionine, and demonstrate radioactivity inside the pineal. This approach is unsatisfactory for several reasons. First, again the most likely chemical nature of the radioactivity is not an indole but a protein. Secondly, even if the pineal region can convert 5-hydroxytryptophan to serotonin, this in no sense proves that it can synthesize the indole from its physiological circulating substrate, tryptophan.

Thus, there are five general categories of evidence for indole synthesis by pineals: the first is to find the non-radioactive compounds naturally present in large amounts, or increase their levels by giving their non-radioactive precursor, tryptophan. The second is to show synthesis *in vitro* of radioactive melatonin from radioactive tryptophan. The third involves identifying characteristic pineal enzymes in homogenates, especially HIOMT. Fourthly is to show *in vivo* the accumulation of radioactivity in the pineal area after giving radioactive tryptophan, the naturally occurring precursor; and fifthly is to show the accumulation of radioactivity after giving methionine or 5-hydroxytryptophan. I hope that as techniques are improved we shall be able to insist on the first marker; that is, it should be possible to demonstrate the concentration of melatonin itself within the pineal, in all species that actually synthesize this compound.

Axelrod: I would also like to congratulate Professor Kappers on a very thorough review. I would like more details on a cholinergic innervation of the pineal. As I understand it, if one denervates the pineal by removing the superior cervical ganglion, all the nerves degenerate. I just wonder what the origin of the cholinergic nerves is?

Kappers: A. B. M. Machado and V. P. J. Lemos (1970) have shown that, in the rat pineal, acetylcholinesterase-positive fibres first appear in nerve trunks present in the capsule of the organ immediately after birth. Some fibres had penetrated the gland at about 36–48 hours after birth and fine branches were observed within the gland by 72 hours, after that time considerably increasing in number. In the adult, a network of these fibres is formed, most of which follow the vessels. Cholinesterase-active fibres, however, could also be traced in relation to the pinealocytes. After removal of both superior cervical ganglia all fibres disappeared completely. It is possible that noradrenergic fibres might also contain acetylcholine. On the other hand it is known that some cholinergic cells are present in sympathetic ganglia. It may be that the preganglionic fibres impinging on these cells are of vagal origin. If I remember correctly, cholinergic nerve cells have also been demonstrated in other paravertebral ganglia; isn't that true, Dr Owman?

Owman: I have no direct information on this, but I agree that both cholinergic and adrenergic fibres may emanate from the superior cervical ganglion.

Arstila: Eränkö and his collaborators (1970) have shown that the sympathetic nerve fibres of the pineal body in the rat, originating from the superior cervical ganglia, contain acetylcholinesterase activity demonstrable by both light and electron microscopy.

Lerner: Is it possible, in addition to elaborating the cholinergic innervation of the pineal, to relate physiological control to various adrenergic fibres and to whether or not stimuli affect alpha and/or beta receptor sites?

Shein: Dr Wurtman and I have some unpublished observations on the effects of alpha and beta adrenergic blocking agents on the capacity of noradrenaline to stimulate melatonin synthesis by adult rat pineal glands *in vitro*. We find that propranolol (a beta blocking agent), but not phenoxybenzamine (an alpha blocking agent), blocks this stimulating effect of noradrenaline. Accordingly, the receptors on the pineal parenchymal cell membrane upon which noradrenaline acts to stimulate melatonin synthesis are probably beta adrenergic receptors.

Lerner: I was wondering if some of the differences in response to light found in various species are associated with differences in the reactiveness of alpha and beta receptor sites and also with the nature of the cholinergic nerve supply to the pineal.

Kappers: I cannot give you information on this point. Personally, I was much interested in the fact that a parasympathetic contribution to pineal innervation may not occur exclusively in primates (Kenny 1961, in the macaque), but also in non-primate mammals. Kenny's investigation should be repeated and it should be examined whether (1) purely noradrenergic fibres originating in the superior cervical ganglia, and (2) cholinergic fibres originating in these same ganglia, contribute to the pineal innervation in the monkey.

Herbert: There may be an alternative to the superior cervical ganglion. The ferret has a very large cholinergic component in the pineal, as I shall be showing later (pp. 303–320). Our preliminary studies indicate that this is not derived from the superior cervical ganglion, because the synapses don't disappear after ganglionectomy. We suspect that they may originate from the habenula, and this raises the possibility that the habenula plays some part in the function of the pineal. The habenula contains large amounts of cholinesterase and, in the ferret, one can sometimes see cholinesterase-positive fibres stretching between the group of cholinergic neurons in the pineal and the habenula itself. Furthermore, under the electron microscope the morphology of the ganglion cells in the pineal corresponds very closely with that of the medial habenular nucleus.

Owman: To add to the confusion about this problem, we have recently found that the habenula in rats receives an adrenergic innervation which disappears after superior cervical ganglionectomy (A. Björklund, Ch. Owman and K. A. West, to be published).

Herbert: We find exactly the same in the ferret—a very remarkable green fluorescence in the walls of the blood vessels of the medial habenular nucleus, but nowhere else (Trueman and Herbert 1970).

Miline: We have heard about the photosensitivity of the pineal gland, but we have not yet mentioned its thermosensitivity. The pineal gland is a thermoreceptor which is engaged in thermoregulation during hibernation

2*

and during adaptation to cold (hypothermal stress). In experiments in bats subjected to auditory stimuli during hibernation and in rats exposed to low temperatures, we showed that the pineal gland is stimulated by external cold; this organ is to be considered as integrated in the regulatory system of hibernation and of adaptation to cold (Miline, Devečerski and Krstić 1969; Miline *et al.* 1970).

The sympathetic innervation of pineal glands has just been mentioned. The superior cervical ganglion gives off a large number of sympathetic fibres to all three parts of the hypophysis, also the hypothalamus (median eminence). We think that the effect of light on the pineal must be interpreted in conjunction with events in the hypophysis. A biological antagonism between epiphysis and hypophysis is evident in this interaction and we think that pineal cells are very sensitive to hormonal influences from the hypophysis. Perhaps the ribbon synapses are involved as hormone receptors? The hypothalamus is a fundamental relay in the correlated activity of the pineal gland and the hypophysis.

Nir: We have some evidence which supports what Dr Miline says about thermosensitivity. We kept female rats at a controlled temperature of 32 ± 1 °C for 20 to 30 days and found that similarly to light, heat has a depressant effect on the nucleic acid and protein content of the pineal.

Martini: What is the evidence that cold and heat are not acting as general stressors?

Nir: We are extending this experiment and measuring the effect of heat on other organs, so we shall know whether this is a specific effect on the pineal or a general, stress effect of heat.

Reiter: Dr Miline, you said that the pineal is stimulated by cold in hibernating species, and I gather that this is also true for non-hibernators?

Miline: We have studied this in a hibernating species, the bat *Rhinolopus ferrum equinum Schr.* In the summer there is a relative depression in the number of nucleoli in the pineal gland and in the activity of the alkaline and acid phosphatases and non-specific esterases. In the winter the pineal gland is hypertrophied, due to hyperplasia of the pinealocytes.

We have exposed rats to cold (temperatures of 3°–10 °C) for 10 days. The supraoptic nucleus of rats with their pineal glands intact shows signs of reduced activity, but in pinealectomized rats the neuroglandular cells of the supraoptic nucleus are hypertrophied, indicating stimulated activity (Miline *et al.* 1969). Thus pinealectomy has provoked an inversion of the behaviour of the supraoptic nuclei under the influence of cold. (See also pp. 372–373.)

Reiter: Are you implying that animals will not hibernate if they do not have a pineal gland?

Miline: I can't say, because we haven't studied hibernation in pineal-ectomized bats.

Owman: With regard to the pituitary system, there is stereotaxic and microspectrofluorometric evidence of a catecholamine innervation (Björklund *et al.* 1970). Dopamine neurons are found in an arcuato-hypophysial system and noradrenaline neurons in a tubero-hypophysial system. Noradrenaline-containing sympathetic nerves are present only around blood vessels; these latter fibres disappear after bilateral removal of the superior cervical ganglia.

Wurtman: Whitby, Axelrod and Weil-Malherbe (1961) showed that the hypothalamus was perhaps unique in that if they administered tritiated noradrenaline to rats intravenously it did not cross the blood-brain barrier anywhere except within this region. E. T. Angelakos has now shown that the uptake of tritiated noradrenaline from the blood into the hypothalamus is lost after superior cervical ganglionectomy (see Angelakos, Irvin and King 1970). Hence it appears that the hypothalamic uptake of circulating noradrenaline is not within brain neurons but is instead within the terminals of sympathetic neurons that travel with the blood vessels.

Martini: A crucial point has been brought up by Dr Kappers: are melatonin and the other pineal principles secreted into the cerebrospinal fluid or into the blood?

Owman: I think it may be difficult to find direct anatomical evidence for the secretion of substances from the pineal to the ventricular system in adult animals. Nevertheless if one perfuses the ventricular system with, for example, bromphenol blue through a cannula in the lateral ventricle, with an extracranial outflow via the cerebral aqueduct (see Feldberg 1963), the pineal becomes completely blue, so substances can pass from the ventricular system into the pineal, and why couldn't the reverse happen? Even though the anatomical pathway may be difficult to find.

Wurtman: In the same sense nobody would suggest that a dopaminergic nerve terminal deep within the caudate nucleus secretes its neurotransmitter for the primary purpose of getting it into the cerebrospinal fluid. Yet Martha Vogt has shown (1969) that if these dopaminergic neurons are stimulated electrically there is an increase in homovanillic acid (the main metabolic product) within the fluid in the lateral ventricles. The situation is analogous because homovanillic acid, like melatonin but unlike dopamine, is *not* an amine, and thus would be expected to gain easy access to the cerebrospinal fluid. What I am suggesting is that the distance from a cell in the pineal or the brain to the cerebrospinal fluid is not the sole determinant of whether or not that cell's secretions reach the cerebrospinal fluid.

Martini: Is there any anatomical route through which blood collected from the pineal gland could reach the choroid plexus and consequently be transformed into cerebrospinal fluid?

Kappers: No, there is no direct way by which blood collected from the the pineal can reach the choroid plexus. As has been demonstrated in mice by von Bartheld and Moll (1954) and in the rabbit by my present co-worker H. Romijn (unpublished), the pineal veins drain directly into the large veins surrounding the organ while these latter veins drain into the confluens sinuum. Thus, the pineal secretory products, extruded into the pineal capillaries, reach the general blood circulation. The arteries of the choroid plexus can, in no way, contain blood directly collected from the pineal.

Oksche: I notice that you used the terms pinealo-fugal and pinealo-petal nerve fibres, Dr Kappers. I am becoming concerned about the different use of the terms "efferent" and "afferent" pineal nerve fibres, explained so clearly in your 1965 review (Kappers 1965). If you take the central nervous system to be the central organ you can say the nerve fibres running from the pineal sense organ to the central nervous system are afferent. But if one thinks of the pineal as an independent organ, one will call fibres leaving the pineal organ efferent fibres (and *vice versa*). I am concerned about the resulting confusion in current publications.

Kappers: I quite agree that there are some terminological problems which may cause confusion. Considering that, ontogenetically, the pineal develops from the brain and on the ground of some similarities in development between the lateral eyes and the pineal, especially obvious in lower vertebrates, I used to call the pineal tract fibres "afferent fibres" because of their origin in the epiphysis and their termination in the brain. These fibres are quite comparable with those of the optic nerve which nobody would call "efferent fibres". "Efferent pineal fibres", then, will be all fibres reaching the pineal and not originating in it. Among these we might think of fibres originating in the brain, especially when we consider that during ontogenesis in many animals the pineal has developed into an organ which is anatomically more or less independent of the brain. So far, however, cerebral fibres coursing to the pineal have not been con-clusively demonstrated. Other "efferent" pineal fibres would be the sympathetic ones. I must confess that, as far as these latter fibres are con-cerned, the term "efferent" is not ideal.

The terms "efferent" and "afferent" have been used in the opposite sense by Dr Collin, the pineal tract fibres being called "efferent" and the sympathetic fibres "afferent". Evidently, Dr Collin's terminology is "pineal-centred".

To avoid confusion in my present paper I used the terms "pinealo-fugal" for the pineal tract sensory fibres which originate in the pineal sensory nerve cells, and "pinealo-petal" for the sympathetic fibres which do not originate in the organ but run to it. If Dr Collin would agree to use these latter terms, no difficulties will be left.

Collin: The terms "pinealo-fugal" or "pinealo-petal" were introduced into the literature by Professor Ariëns Kappers some years ago (1967). In fact, since 1967, I have generally used the terms "afferent", meaning to the pineal ("pinealo-petal"), and efferent, meaning from the pineal ("pinealo-fugal"). If one thinks that the pineal is independent and influences the brain (in its photoreceptive and endocrine functions) this latter nomenclature for the different systems of innervation seems to be correct. Furthermore, from the functional point of view, the cells of the sensory line seem to be of primary importance (Collin 1969) and the different systems of innervation can be considered with respect to these chief cells. Naturally in Professor Kappers' survey (1965) the central nervous system is thought to be central, perhaps on the basis of embryology and anatomy, and so "afferent" and "efferent" are used in the reverse sense. I should myself like the terms "afferent" and "efferent" to be abandoned now; I prefer "pinealo-fugal innervation" (or sensory innervation) and "pinealo-petal innervation" (or autonomic innervation). Furthermore, one cannot ignore the presence of another possible pinealo-petal system, such as for instance a "feedback" system, suggested some years ago by Dr Kelly and Dr Smith (1964).

REFERENCES

ANGELAKOS, E. T., IRVIN, J. D. and KING, M. P. (1970) *Fedn Proc. Fedn Am. Socs exp. Biol.* **29(2),** 416 (abst. 960).

AXELROD, J., MACLEAN, P. D., ALBERS, R. W. and WEISSBACH, H. (1961) In *Regional Neurochemistry*, pp. 307–311, ed. Kety, S. S. and Elkes, J. Oxford: Pergamon Press.

BARTHELD, J. VON and MOLL, J. (1954) *Acta anat.* **22,** 227–235.

BJÖRKLUND, A. and FALCK, B. (1969) *Z. Zellforsch. mikrosk. Anat.* **93,** 254–264.

BJÖRKLUND, A., FALCK, B., HROMEK, F., OWMAN, CH. and WEST, K. A. (1970) *Brain Res.* **17,** 1–23.

COLLIN, J. P. (1969) *Annls Stn Biol. Besse-en-Chandesse* suppl. 1, 1–359.

ERANKÖ, O., RECHARDT, L. and CUNNINGHAM, A. (1970) *Scand. J. Clin. Lab. Invest.* suppl. 113, 82.

FELDBERG, W. (1963) *A Pharmacological Approach to the Brain from its Inner and Outer Surface,* pp. 9–29. London: Arnold.

KAPPERS, J. A. (1965) In *Structure and Function of the Epiphysis Cerebri (Progress in Brain Research* vol. 10), pp. 87–153, ed. Kappers, J. A. and Schadé, J. P. Amsterdam: Elsevier.

KAPPERS, J. A. (1967) *Z. Zellforsch. mikrosk. Anat.* **81,** 581–618.

KELLY, D. E. and SMITH, S. W. (1964) *J. Cell Biol.* **22,** 565–587.

KENNY, G. C. T. (1961) *J. Neuropath. exp. Neurol.* **20,** 563–570.

KLEIN, D. C., BERG, G. R. and WELLER, J. (1970) *Science* **168,** 979–980.

KLEIN, D. C., BERG, G. R., WELLER, J. and GLINSMANN, W. (1970) *Science* **167,** 1738–1740.

MACHADO, A. B. M. and LEMOS, V. P. J. (1970) *J. Neuro-visc. Rel.* **32,** in press.

MILINE, R., DEVEČERSKI, V. and KRSTIĆ, R. (1969) *Acta. anat.* **73,** suppl. 56, 293–300.

MILINE, R., DEVEČERSKI, V., ŠIKAČKI, N. and KRSTIĆ, R. (1970) *Hormones,* in press.

MILINE, R., WERNER, R., ŠĆEPOVIĆ, M., DEVEČERSKI, V. and MILINE, J. (1969) *Bull. Ass. Anat.* **145,** 289–293.

TRUEMAN, T. and HERBERT, J. (1970) *Z. Zellforsch. mikrosk. Anat.* **109,** 83–100.

VOGT, M. (1969) *Br. J. Pharmac.* **37,** 325–337.

WHITBY, L. G., AXELROD, J. and WEIL-MALHERBE, H. (1961) *J. Pharmac. exp. Ther.* **132,** 193–201.

WURTMAN, R. J., AXELROD, J. and KELLY, D. E. (1968) *The Pineal.* New York and London: Academic Press.

WURTMAN, R. J. and KAMMER, H. (1966) *New Engl. J. Med.* **274,** 1233–1237.

NEURAL CONTROL OF INDOLEAMINE
METABOLISM IN THE PINEAL

JULIUS AXELROD

*Laboratory of Clinical Science, National Institute of Mental Health,
Bethesda, Maryland*

DURING the past decade considerable new information about the bio-chemistry of the pineal gland has been obtained. The initial stimulus was the isolation and identification of melatonin (N-acetylmethoxytryptamine) in the bovine pineal gland (Lerner, Case and Heinzelman 1959). This discovery led to the identification of other indoles in the pineal, such as serotonin, 5-hydroxyindole acetic acid, 5-methoxyindole acetic acid, 5-hydroxytryptophol and 5-methoxytryptophol (Giarman and Day 1959; McIsaac *et al*. 1965). In addition, other biogenic amines, noradrenaline, dopamine and histamine, were also found to be highly localized in the mammalian pineal (Pellegrino de Iraldi and Zieher 1966; Machado, Faleiro and DaSilva 1965).

BIOSYNTHESIS OF MELATONIN

The presence of melatonin in the pineal led to a search for the enzyme that makes this compound and the individual steps in its biosynthesis. Hydroxyindole-O-methyltransferase (HIOMT), an enzyme that forms melatonin, was isolated from the pineal (Axelrod and Weissbach 1961) and was found to be highly localized in this organ (Axelrod *et al*. 1961). Like other O-methyltransferases, the melatonin-forming enzyme required S-adenosyl methionine as the methyl donor. Although serotonin and other 5-hydroxyindoles served as methyl acceptors, N-acetylserotonin was about 20 times more active as a substrate. These observations indicated that N-acetylation preceded O-methylation in the formation of melatonin. Studies in pineal organ culture showed that tryptophan and 5-hydroxy-tryptophan could serve as precursors in the formation of serotonin and melatonin (Shein, Wurtman and Axelrod 1967). Thus, the biosynthesis of melatonin in the pineal proceeds as shown in Fig. 1.

The first step is catalysed by the enzyme tryptophan hydroxylase (Lovenberg, Jequier and Sjoerdsma 1967), and the second by aromatic amino acid decarboxylase to form serotonin (Snyder and Axelrod 1964). Part of the serotonin is then acetylated by an acetylating enzyme (Weissbach, Redfield and Axelrod 1960). The final step involves O-methylation to melatonin by hydroxyindole-O-methyltransferase. The enzymes catalysing the formation of melatonin are highly concentrated in the mammalian pineal, while HIOMT is uniquely localized in this organ.

Most of the enzymic steps in the formation of serotonin occur in the parenchymal cells of the pineal (Owman 1965). The serotonin formed in the pineal then undergoes a complex fate (Wurtman, Axelrod and Kelly 1968). Part is N-acetylated to N-acetylserotonin and part is deaminated by

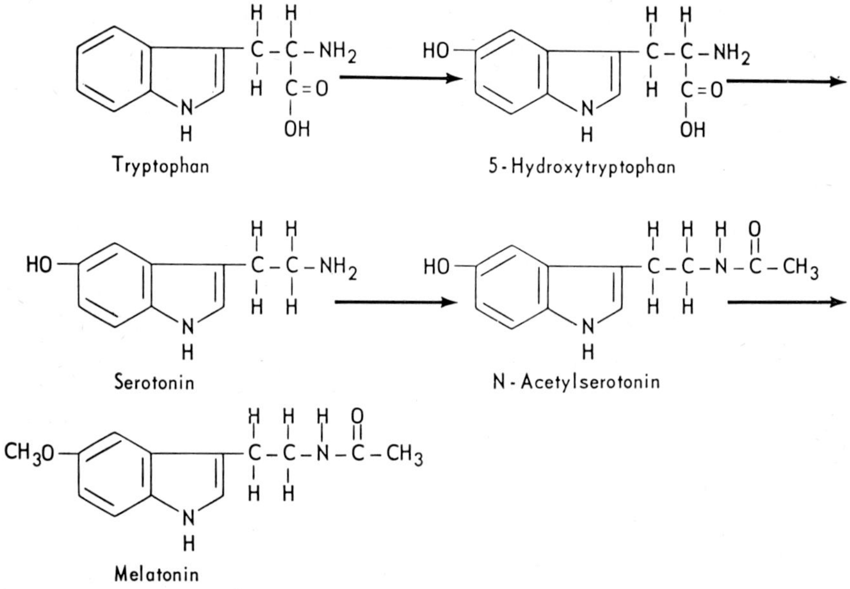

FIG. 1. Biosynthesis of melatonin.

monoamine oxidase to form 5-hydroxyindole acetic acid and 5-hydroxytryptophol. Considerable amounts of serotonin also enter the sympathetic nerve terminals that innervate the pineal parenchymal cells. When the serotonin crosses the neuronal membrane into the axoplasm it is rapidly taken up in a storage granule where it is protected from enzymic destruction.

NEURAL CONTROL OF MELATONIN SYNTHESIS

When female rats are kept in continuous light they undergo persistent oestrus (Fiske, Bryant and Putnam 1960). This can be overcome by

injections of melatonin (Wurtman, Axelrod and Chu 1963). These observations suggested that environmental lighting might influence melatonin
synthesis. To examine this possibility, rats were placed in constant light or
darkness for about one week and the activity of the melatonin-forming
enzyme HIOMT was examined (Wurtman, Axelrod and Phillips 1963).
Under these conditions a marked difference in HIOMT activity was found
(Fig. 2, sham-operated). Animals kept in constant light had about one-half
the enzyme activity of those in continuous darkness. This effect of lighting
appeared to be selective since monoamine oxidase, an enzyme involved in
the metabolism of serotonin, was unaffected by environmental lighting.
It appeared that light suppressed the synthesis of melatonin and thus
increased the incidence of oestrus. The pineal HIOMT activity was
reduced by light intensities from 4 to 8 5-foot candles (Quay 1968). A
photoperiod of 22L:2D was equivalent to continuous light and 14L:10D
was equivalent to continuous darkness.

The effect of lighting on pineal HIOMT was found in immature rats, as
well as in oophorectomized and hypophysectomized animals. These
observations suggested that the response of HIOMT to environmental
lighting did not require the gonads or pituitary gland. Blinding, however,
abolished the effects of lighting on pineal HIOMT in the rat, indicating
that the retina was involved (Wurtman, Axelrod and Fischer 1964). The
innervation of the rat pineal cells by sympathetic nerve terminals arising
from the superior cervical ganglia (Kappers 1960) suggested that information about environmental light reaches the pineal gland by a neural
route. In the following experiment the superior cervical ganglia were
removed bilaterally and the rats were placed in constant light or darkness
(Wurtman, Axelrod and Fischer 1964). This procedure abolished the
effects of environmental lighting (Fig. 2).

The postganglionic sympathetic nerves innervating the pineal contain
both serotonin and noradrenaline. Both of these biogenic amines are
present in the brain and their normal levels are dependent on the integrity of
the medial forebrain bundle passing through the lateral hypothalamus
(Heller and Moore 1965). Lesions in this area of the brain are tantamount
to a denervation of central sympathetic fibres. When the medial forebrain
bundle of the rat was cut bilaterally, environmental lighting no longer had
any effect on pineal HIOMT (Axelrod, Wurtman and Snyder 1965) (Fig.
2). The effects of lesions of the medial forebrain bundle on pineal cells are
mediated across the superior cervical ganglia and probably via several
synapses. Thus there appears to be a central trans-synaptic regulation of a
biochemical event (HIOMT activity in pineal cells) outside the central
nervous system.

To further examine the visual pathway involved in transmission of light messages from the retina to the pineal, the inferior accessory optic tract was transected (Moore *et al.* 1967). This lesion abolished the fall in HIOMT caused by continuous light. In another experiment, lesions were made to remove all light inputs to the terminal nuclei of the primary optic tracts without interference with the inferior accessory optic tract (Moore *et al.* 1968). This operation permitted the characteristic fall in HIOMT in rats kept in continuous light, by comparison with those in constant darkness. A similar accessory optic system was found in monkeys (Moore 1969).

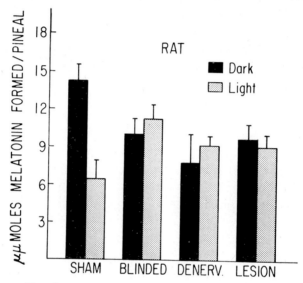

FIG. 2. Neural control of HIOMT activity in rat pineal. Rats were kept in continuous darkness or light 7 to 30 days after blinding, bilateral denervation of superior cervical ganglia (Denerv.) or bilateral lesions in the medial forebrain bundle. Results are expressed as mean ± s.e.m. [14C]-melatonin formed when homogenates of pineal were incubated with [14C]-S-adenosyl methionine and N-acetylserotonin. (Wurtman, Axelrod and Fischer 1964; Axelrod *et al.* 1966.)

These and other observations indicate that information about environmental lighting reaches the pineal via the retina and the inferior accessory optic tract, which then leaves the primary optic projections just behind the optic chiasma to run through the medial forebrain bundle and terminate in the medial terminal nucleus. The light message reaches the preganglionic sympathetic fibres of the spinal cord by an unknown pathway to synapse with the superior cervical ganglia. The postganglionic fibres innervate the parenchymal cells of the pineal by means of numerous varicosities. These sympathetic nerve terminals liberate noradrenaline and possibly serotonin.

The role of the neurotransmitter noradrenaline in mediating the effects of environmental lighting was examined in organ culture. It was found that tryptophan or 5-hydroxytryptophan is transformed to serotonin, N-acetylserotonin, 5-hydroxyindole acetic acid and melatonin in organ culture (Wurtman *et al.* 1968, 1969). Inhibition of protein synthesis by cycloheximide completely suppressed all the intermediate steps in the formation of melatonin from tryptophan. This suggested that the formation of new enzyme protein was involved in the synthesis of melatonin in organ culture. The addition of noradrenaline to pineal organ cultures caused a marked stimulation in the formation of melatonin (Axelrod, Shein and Wurtman 1969), N-acetylserotonin and N-acetyltransferase (Klein and Weller 1970), but not serotonin or HIOMT. Dibutyryl cyclic adenosine monophosphate also stimulated the formation of N-acetylserotonin, N-acetyltransferase (Berg and Klein 1970) and melatonin in pineal organ cultures (Shein and Wurtman 1969; Klein *et al.* 1970). These observations indicate that absence of light stimulates the release of noradrenaline from the sympathetic nerve terminals. The noradrenaline, via cyclic adenosine monophosphate (cyclic AMP), then stimulates the formation of the N-acetyltransferase enzyme which in turn forms more N-acetylserotonin, the substrate for HIOMT. The molecular mechanism whereby light reduces HIOMT activity still remains to be established.

NEURAL CONTROL OF SEROTONIN METABOLISM

Serotonin undergoes a circadian rhythm in the rat pineal gland (Quay 1963). The levels of the indoleamine are highest at midday and fall precipitously at night to a low level at about 11 p.m. Studies on the factors controlling the serotonin rhythm in the pineal showed that it persisted in continuous darkness or when rats were blinded, indicating its endogenous nature (Snyder *et al.* 1965) (Fig. 3). Removal of the ovaries, pituitary, thyroid or adrenal gland had no effect on the pineal serotonin rhythm. However, the rhythm was abolished in the presence of one additional photoperiod (4 hours) of light or constant light (Fig. 3). Reversal of the light period turned the period of the rhythm around by 180°, indicating that the serotonin rhythm is cued by environmental lighting (Snyder, Axelrod and Zweig 1967).

The influence of the nervous system on the pineal serotonin rhythm was examined by ablating the pineal sympathetic nerve supply, by the bilateral removal of the superior cervical ganglia (Snyder *et al.* 1965). Denervation of the pineal abolished the serotonin rhythm midway between the lowest and highest values (Fig. 3). In another experiment the sympathetic nerves were cut preganglionically, thus separating the central nervous system from the pineal. This procedure also suppressed the daily rise and fall of pineal serotonin. Depleting central brain biogenic amines with reserpine prevented this rhythm (Snyder and Axelrod 1965). Preliminary studies also indicated that lesions in the medial forebrain bundle abolished the serotonin rhythm. These observations suggest that the driving mechanism for the pineal serotonin rhythm is localized in the brain and that the neural message is carried by tracts containing biogenic amines.

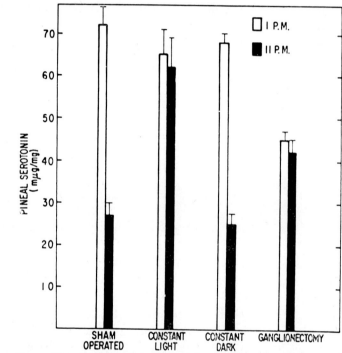

FIG. 3. Neural control of pineal serotonin rhythm. Groups of rats were kept in constant light or dark or under diurnal conditions (12L:12D). Superior cervical ganglia were removed and rats kept in diurnal light for 7 days.

The pineal serotonin rhythm could be due to daily variations in the formation of serotonin from its precursor amino acid, in deamination by monoamine oxidase, or in N-acetylation by the N-acetyltransferase enzyme. Administration of tryptophan or 5-hydroxytryptophan at various periods during a 24-hour day caused no difference in the rate of formation of serotonin (Snyder, Axelrod and Zweig 1967). Pineal monoamine oxidase, the principal enzyme involved in serotonin metabolism, also showed no difference in activity when measured around the clock. However,

N-acetyltransferase, the enzyme that catalyses the conversion of serotonin to N-acetylserotonin (Weissbach, Redfield and Axelrod 1960) showed a marked diurnal change in activity in the rat pineal, the highest activity being present at night (D. C. Klein and G. R. Berg, personal communication). Thus the increased activity of this enzyme during the night would N-acetylate more serotonin, thus reducing the level of this amine in a periodic manner.

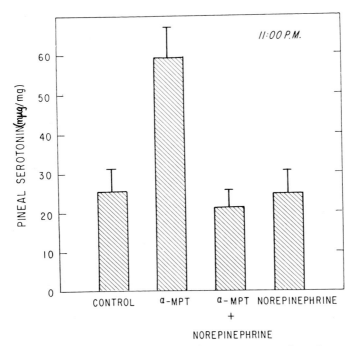

FIG. 4. Reciprocal relationship between pineal serotonin and noradrenaline (norepinephrine). Groups of rats were given 250 mg/kg α-methyl-*p*-tyrosine (αmpt) at noon and/or 5 mg/kg noradrenaline bitartrate at 7 and 9 p.m. and killed at 11 p.m. Results are expressed as mean ± S.E.M. serotonin.

A 24-hour rhythm in the noradrenaline content in the rat pineal has been found (Wurtman *et al.* 1967), maximal activity occurring at night and lowest during the daytime. This rhythm is about 180° out of phase with the serotonin rhythm. The noradrenaline rhythm in the pineal is abolished by continuous lighting, continuous darkness or blinding, indicating its exogenous nature. Information about environmental lighting is transmitted along the inferior accessory optic tract in a way similar to that described earlier.

Since both noradrenaline and serotonin reside within the same nerve terminals innervating the pineal cells, the interrelationship between these two monoamines was examined (Zweig and Axelrod 1969). The noradrenaline content of the pineal was selectively depleted by inhibiting tyrosine hydroxylase with α-methyl-p-tyrosine. The administration of the tyrosine hydroxylase inhibitor caused a small but significant elevation of pineal serotonin at 1 p.m. and a doubling of the serotonin level at 11 p.m. when its normal levels were lowest (Fig. 4). When the α-methyl-p-tyrosine blockade of catecholamine synthesis was bypassed by giving dopamine or noradrenaline, the elevation of the pineal serotonin was abolished. Removal of the sympathetic nerve supply to the pineal by ganglionectomy overcame the effects of α-methyl-p-tyrosine. Thus, a reciprocal relationship between the contents of noradrenaline and serotonin in the sympathetic nerves of the pineal indicates that the daily rise and fall of noradrenaline plays a role in the circadian rhythm in pineal serotonin, by way of regulation of N-acetyltransferase activity as well as by modulating the storage and release of serotonin.

NON-RETINAL PATHWAYS TO THE RAT PINEAL

A study of the development of circadian rhythms in pineal serotonin from birth led to the discovery of an extraretinal pathway to the rat pineal (Zweig, Snyder and Axelrod 1966). Negligible amounts of serotonin were detected in the pineal glands of rats up to three days of age. At six days after birth, small concentrations were measurable in the pineal. Examination of the pineal serotonin content around the clock showed a definite rhythm as early as six days of age. As in the adult rat, the levels of this biogenic amine were two to three times higher at 1 p.m. than at 11 p.m. in darkness (Fig. 5). Exposure to four additional hours of lighting prevented the nocturnal decline, despite the fact that the eyes of the rats were still firmly shut. It was possible that light might penetrate the eyes through the eyelids, or that the response to light by the mother might be communicated to the newborn, or that information about lighting might reach the pineal gland by a pathway that does not require the retina. Eleven-day-old rats and their mothers were therefore blinded and then exposed to diurnal lighting before they were killed at 11 p.m. As in the adult animals, the pineal serotonin rhythm persisted in newborn blinded animals (Fig. 5). However, an additional four-hour lighting period prevented the nocturnal fall in pineal serotonin to daytime levels in blinded rats. This phenomenon did not occur in blinded young (27-day-old) or adult rats, where an additional four-hour photoperiod did not eliminate the nocturnal decline in pineal serotonin. Thus, it appears that light might reach the pineal through the skull. To prevent the light from penetrating the skull, 11-day-old rats were hooded. This resulted in a fall in pineal serotonin in blinded rats when they were exposed to an additional photoperiod of light (Fig. 5). These observations suggested an extraretinal pathway by which information about lighting reaches the pineal gland in newborn rats. The photoeffector mechanism for this appears to be in the brain, since hooding blocks the actions of lighting on pineal serotonin.

Other experiments which were consistent with an extraretinal control of the serotonin rhythm in the pineal of newborn rats were described by Machado, Machado and Wragg (1969; Machado, Wragg and Machado

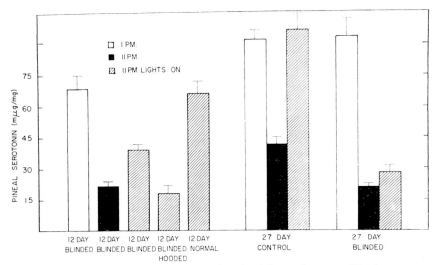

FIG. 5. Non-retinal pathway to the pineal in newborn rats (Zweig, Snyder and Axelrod 1966). Lights were kept on from 7 a.m. to 7 p.m. In groups with an additional photoperiod, lights were kept on from 7 a.m. to 11 p.m.

1969). The pineals of newborn rats were denervated by immunosympathectomy. When the pineal serotonin rhythm was examined in 8-day-old rats it was found to have persisted unchanged. In another experiment the sympathetic innervation to the pineal of newborn rats was removed surgically by bilateral ablation of the superior cervical ganglia. The daily serotonin rhythm still continued in these rats, but a similar denervation in adult rats abolished the rhythm. Thus, in contrast to the adult, the serotonin rhythm in the pineal of the newborn rat does not require a sympathetic innervation.

Recent experiments indicate that the extraretinal receptor in the newborn rat might be localized in the Harderian gland (Wetterberg, Geller and Yuwiler 1970). This gland lies behind and around the vertebrate eye. Its function is unknown but it contains large amounts of protoporphyrin which fluctuate under different lighting conditions. As described above, blinded newborn rats show a fall in pineal serotonin during the dark period of the day. When lights are kept on there is only a partial reduction of pineal serotonin. Removal of the Harderian gland causes a complete fall in the serotonin content of pineals of the newborn rats that were maintained in light and killed at 11 p.m. These experiments gave similar results to those found after hooding of newborn rats. From these observations it appears that the Harderian gland may be an extraretinal receptor in newborn rats that regulates the daily variation in pineal serotonin.

EXTRARETINAL REGULATION OF INDOLE METABOLISM IN BIRD PINEALS

Birds have considerably more HIOMT activity in their pineals than mammals (Axelrod, Wurtman and Winget 1964; Axelrod and Lauber 1968). The HIOMT activity in birds differs from that of mammals with respect to substrate specificity, electrophoretic mobility and kinetic characteristics (Axelrod and Vesell 1970). When male chicks are placed in constant light, HIOMT activity is increased by comparison with those kept in constant darkness (Axelrod, Wurtman and Winget 1964). This phenomenon is the reverse of that observed in rats. To examine the role of the retina and sympathetic nervous system in transmitting information about lighting to the chicken pineal, one group of birds were blinded and in another the pineal glands were denervated by removal of both superior cervical sympathetic ganglia (Lauber, Boyd and Axelrod 1968). The chickens were then kept in continuous light or darkness for about 10 days and the pineals examined for HIOMT activity (Table I).

In confirmation of our previous findings, enzymic activity was about twice as high in birds kept in constant light as in birds in constant darkness.

TABLE I

EFFECT OF ENVIRONMENTAL LIGHTING, BLINDING AND GANGLIONECTOMY ON HYDROXYINDOLE-O-METHYLTRANSFERASE ACTIVITY IN CHICKENS

Procedure	Light	Dark
	Units HIOMT	
Sham operation	$6 \cdot 4 \pm 0 \cdot 45$	$3 \cdot 8 \pm 0 \cdot 32$
Blinding	$6 \cdot 0 \pm 0 \cdot 51$	$3 \cdot 6 \pm 0 \cdot 42$
Ganglionectomy	$5 \cdot 3 \pm 0 \cdot 48$	$3 \cdot 0 \pm 0 \cdot 41$

Groups of six chicks were used in each experiment. Four days after hatching, male White Rock chicks were bilaterally enucleated or ganglionectomized under Combuthal anaesthesia. When they were 4 weeks old chicks were placed in continuous light or darkness for 10 days and their pineal glands were assayed for HIOMT activity. One unit of HIOMT activity equals nmoles (mμmoles) [^{14}C]melatonin formed enzymically per mg pineal from [^{14}C]S-adenosylserotonin. HIOMT in light versus dark, $P < 0 \cdot 001$. (From Lauber, Boyd and Axelrod 1968.)

However, this difference in pineal HIOMT was not abolished in blinded or ganglionectomized birds. Thus, like newborn, but unlike adult rats, the avian pineal gland can respond to environmental lighting in the absence of the retina or the sympathetic nerves. This suggests that the thin skull of the chicken may allow light to penetrate. In addition, the avian pineal gland, or some structure that can influence it, might act as a photoreceptor. Birds have well-developed Harderian glands (Wetterberg, Geller and Yuwiler 1970) and this organ might be a photoreceptor for the avian pineal. It is also possible that the thin skull of birds allows light to reach the brain, and that the hypothalamic region can respond to light. This is indicated by experiments of Benoit and Assenmacher (1959) who found that direct exposure of the hypothalamus to light caused gonadal stimulation in blinded or hooded ducks.

The effect of various wavelengths of light on changes in testes weight and its relationship to the pineal was examined in Japanese quail (Oishi and Kato 1968). A 24-hour day with a long dark period (8L:16D) results in a marked reduction in testes weight. When the heads of the quails were painted with orange-red luminous paint the regression in testicular weight did not occur after the quails were exposed to the 8L:16D period. However, there was a reduction in testicular weight when the birds' heads were covered with green luminous paint. Removal of the pineal caused a reduction in testicular weight even when the quails' heads were painted with red luminous paint and they were exposed to long dark periods.

These results indicate that the pineal gland in the quail serves as a receptor for light of long wavelengths. The pineal gland was also shown to have photoreceptor properties in another bird, the house sparrow (Gaston and Menaker 1968). This species has a circadian locomotor activity which becomes arrhythmic when the pineal gland is removed. It also appears that the circadian locomotor rhythm can persist in blind sparrows, again suggesting the presence of an extraretinal receptor in these species.

SUMMARY

The pineal gland has a considerable capacity to synthesize the indoles serotonin and melatonin. In rats the syntheses of serotonin and the melatonin-forming enzyme are regulated by environmental lighting. Messages about lighting reach the pineal gland via the retina, an accessory optic tract, and sympathetic nerves from the superior cervical ganglia. Environmental light affects indole metabolism in pineals of newborn rats and in birds by non-retinal pathways that do not involve the sympathetic nerves.

REFERENCES

AXELROD, J. and LAUBER, J. (1968) *Biochem. Pharmac.* **17**, 828–830.

AXELROD, J., MACLEAN, P. D., ALBERS, R. W. and WEISSBACH, H. (1961) In *Regional Neurochemistry*, pp. 307–311, ed. Kety, S. S. and Elkes, J. Oxford: Pergamon Press.

AXELROD, J., SHEIN, H. M. and WURTMAN, R. J. (1969) *Proc. natn. Acad. Sci. U.S.A.* **62**, 544–549.

AXELROD, J., SNYDER, S. H., HELLER, A. and MOORE, R. Y. (1966) *Science* **154**, 898–899.

AXELROD, J. and VESELL, E. S. (1970) *Molec. Pharmac.* **6**, 78–84.

AXELROD, J. and WEISSBACH, H. (1961) *J. biol. Chem.* **236**, 211–213.

AXELROD, J., WURTMAN, R. J. and SNYDER, S. H. (1965) *J. biol. Chem.* **240**, 949–954.

AXELROD, J., WURTMAN, R. J. and WINGET, C. M. (1964) *Nature, Lond.* **201**, 1134.

BENOIT, J. and ASSENMACHER, I. (1959) *Recent. Prog. Horm. Res.* **15**, 143–164.

BERG, G. R. and KLEIN, D. C. (1970) *Fedn Proc. Fedn Am. Socs exp. Biol.* **29 (2)**, 615.

FISKE, V. M., BRYANT, G. K. and PUTNAM, J. (1960) *Endocrinology* **66**, 489–491.

GASTON, S. and MENAKER, M. (1968) *Science* **160**, 1125–1127.

GIARMAN, N. J. and DAY, M. (1959) *Biochem. Pharmac.* **1**, 235.

HELLER, A. and MOORE, R. Y. (1965) *J. Pharmac. exp. Ther.* **150**, 1–9.

KAPPERS, J. A. (1960) *Z. Zellforsch. mikrosk. Anat.* **52**, 163–215.

KLEIN, D. C. and WELLER, J. (1970) *Fedn Proc. Fedn Am. Socs exp. Biol.* **29 (2)**, 615.

KLEIN, D. C., BERG, G. R., WELLER, J. and GLINSMANN, W. (1970) *Science* **167**, 1738–1740.

LAUBER, J. K., BOYD, J. E. and AXELROD, J. (1968) *Science* **161**, 489–490.

LERNER, A. B., CASE, J. D. and HEINZELMAN, R. V. (1959) *J. Am. chem. Soc.* **81**, 6084.

LOVENBERG, W., JEQUIER, E. and SJOERDSMA, A. (1967) *Science* **155**, 217.

MACHADO, A. B. M., FALEIRO, L. C. M. and DaSILVA, W. D. (1965) *Z. Zellforsch. mikrosk. Anat.* **65**, 521–529.

MACHADO, C. R. S., MACHADO, A. B. M. and WRAGG, G. E. (1969) *Endocrinology* **85**, 846–848.

MACHADO, C. R. S., WRAGG, G. E. and MACHADO, A. B. M. (1969) *Science* **164**, 442.

McISAAC, W. M., FARRELL, G., TABORSKY, R. G. and TAYLOR, A. N. (1965) *Science* **148**, 102–103.

MOORE, R. Y. (1969) *Nature, Lond.* **222**, 781–782.

MOORE, R. Y., HELLER, A., BHATNAGAR, R. K., WURTMAN, R. J. and AXELROD, J. (1968) *Archs Neurol., Chicago* **18**, 208–218.

MOORE, R. Y., HELLER, A., WURTMAN, R. J. and AXELROD, J. (1967) *Science* **155**, 220–223.

OISHI, T. and KATO, M. (1968) *Mem. Fac. Sci. Kyoto Univ. Ser. B* **2**, 12–18.

OWMAN, CH. (1965) In *Structure and Function of the Epiphysis Cerebri (Progress in Brain Research* vol. 10), pp. 423–453, ed. Kappers, J. A. and Schadé, J. P. Amsterdam: Elsevier.

PELLEGRINO DE IRALDI, A. and ZIEHER, L. M. (1966) *Life Sci.* **5**, 155–161.

QUAY, W. B. (1963) *Gen. comp. Endocr.* **3**, 473–479.

QUAY, W. B. (1968) *Extraits Archs Anat. Histol. Embryol.* **51**, 565–571.

SHEIN, H. M. and WURTMAN, R. J. (1969) *Science* **166**, 519–520.

SHEIN, H. M., WURTMAN, R. J. and AXELROD, J. (1967) *Nature, Lond.* **213**, 730–731.

SNYDER, S. H. and AXELROD, J. (1964) *Biochem. Pharmac.* **13**, 805–806.

SNYDER, S. H. and AXELROD, J. (1965) *Science* **149**, 542–544.

SNYDER, S. H., AXELROD, J. and ZWEIG, M. (1967) *J. Pharmac. exp. Ther.* **158**, 206–213.

SNYDER, S. H., ZWEIG, M., AXELROD, J. and FISCHER, J. E. (1965) *Proc. natn. Acad. Sci. U.S.A.* **53**, 301–305.

WEISSBACH, H., REDFIELD, B. G. and AXELROD, J. (1960) *Biochim. biophys. Acta* **43**, 352–353.

WETTERBERG, L., GELLER, E. and YUWILER, A. (1970) *Science* **167**, 884–885.

WURTMAN, R. J., AXELROD, J. and CHU, E. W. (1963) *Science* **141**, 277–278.

WURTMAN, R. J., AXELROD, J. and FISCHER, J. E. (1964) *Science* **143**, 1328–1330.

WURTMAN, R. J., AXELROD, J. and KELLY, D. E. (1968) *The Pineal*, p. 92. New York and
London: Academic Press.
WURTMAN, R. J., AXELROD, J. and PHILLIPS, L. S. (1963) *Science* **142**, 1071–1073.
WURTMAN, R. J., AXELROD, J., SEDVALL, G. and MOORE, R. Y. (1967) *J. Pharmac. exp. Ther.*
157, 487–492.
WURTMAN, R. J., LARIN, F., AXELROD, J., SHEIN, H. M. and ROSASCO, K. (1968) *Nature,
Lond.* **217**, 953–954.
WURTMAN, R. J., SHEIN, H. M., AXELROD, J. and LARIN, F. (1969) *Proc. natn. Acad. Sci.
U.S.A.* **62**, 749–755.
ZWEIG, M. and AXELROD, J. (1969) *J. Neurobiol.* **1**, 87–89.
ZWEIG, M., SNYDER, S. H. and AXELROD, J. (1966) *Proc. natn. Acad. Sci. U.S.A.* **56**, 515–520.

DISCUSSION

Mess: It has always seemed unlikely to me that light can affect blinded animals because although light could evidently penetrate the skull of newborn rats, a raven for example has a thick skull and a black-pigmented skin and feathers, which make it unlikely that light could reach the pineal gland directly. Perhaps the Harderian gland could provide some explanation.

Wurtman: Professor Jay Forrester, an electrical engineer at the Massachusetts Institute of Technology, has introduced an important principle that may apply here: the principle of the counter-intuitive behaviour of complex systems, which means that in general things tend to work out exactly opposite to what you would predict intuitively! One would not imagine that much light would penetrate through opaque skin, much less wool; however, Ganong and his collaborators (1963) were able to show that in the sheep large amounts of sunlight normally penetrate through the wool, as well as through the skull, and into the substance of the brain. Moreover, thousands of babies with neonatal jaundice are now being treated with light to destroy circulating bilirubin. So environmental light can penetrate through the skin into the capillaries and by direct photochemical reaction destroy enough bilirubin so that jaundiced newborn babies no longer require exchange transfusions. This therapy appears to work in infants of all races.

On the question of the role of the Harderian gland, a critical experiment can be done to determine whether this gland does mediate some of the effects of light on the pineal. As far as I know, no one has demonstrated nerve tracts from the Harderian gland to the brain; therefore if the Harderian gland mediates any of the neuroendocrine effects of light it must do so by fluorescence, as Wetterberg, Geller and Yuwiler (1970) have suggested.

The Harderian gland contains large amounts of porphyrins, which have the property of converting ultraviolet light to visible light. It is possible that the Harderian gland transduces ultraviolet light to visible light which then stimulates the rods and cones directly. So one could study the action spectrum of pineal responses to light in normal animals; that is, one could ask, can cycles of ultraviolet light entrain pineal rhythms in normal animals and can they do so in animals from which the Harderian gland has been removed? If ultraviolet light produces neuroendocrine effects in intact animals, it cannot do so by a retinal mechanism (that is, by activating rods or cones), and might very well act via the Harderian gland. Similarly if removing the Harderian gland or experimentally altering its composition of porphyrins blocks pineal responses to ultraviolet light, this would argue in favour of the Harderian gland having a role in mediating these responses.

Axelrod: At about 12–27 days of age there are large changes in the porphyrins in the Harderian gland in the rat (Wetterberg, Geller and Yuwiler 1970). In fact it isn't ultraviolet light that seems to affect the *pineal* gland, but light of long wavelengths (Oishi and Kato 1968).

Wurtman: Those experiments would then also argue against ultraviolet light affecting the Harderian gland.

Reiter: I cannot envisage the porphyrins being very important in the Harderian gland, because of the thirty or so species that have been studied, only six species had porphyrins present in this gland (E. R. Hayes, unpublished). Secondly, in the hamster, where the pineal gland has equally effective reproductive influences in both sexes, porphyrins reportedly are present in the Harderian gland of the female only.

Kordon: Various experiments have been done on the possibility of a direct light supply to the hypothalamus (Benoit 1970; Ganong *et al.* 1963). Professor Benoit has shown, using microphotoelectric cells introduced stereotaxically into the brain, that red radiation can penetrate the bone and the skin *in vivo* in rather high amounts. Furthermore, when light was supplied directly to the brain through chronically implanted optic fibres, gonadotropic responses were only recorded when the tips of the fibres were located in the ventromedial part of the hypothalamus; there were no effects of a direct light supply to dorsal brain structures or to the epithalamic region.

Reiter: Do we know what portion of the retina detects the light that determines pineal rhythms? Adult albino rats in constant light go blind within about 16 days, owing to a complete disappearance of the rods and cones (O'Steen 1970). What is preventing these animals from acting as though they are in constant darkness? We need to know what is the photoreceptor for the pineal.

Martini: Dr Axelrod, you showed that ganglionectomy and blinding eliminate the rhythm in the formation of melatonin; it seems to me that your data also indicated that, in rats kept in the dark, blinding and ganglionectomy reduce the total levels of melatonin being formed. Is this right?

Axelrod: Yes, that is correct. The effect depends on the length of time since one ganglionectomized the rat. The longer the rat is ganglionectomized, the lower the level of hydroxyindole-O-methyltransferase.

Wurtman: The simplest explanation is that for a period of time after ganglionectomy, degenerating sympathetic nerve endings are releasing large amounts of noradrenaline; after a while this process ceases. As far

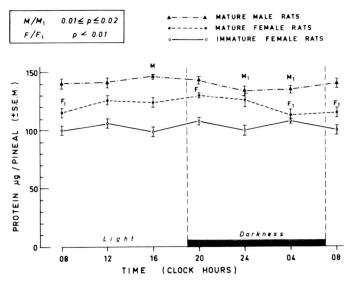

FIG. 1 (Nir). Pineal protein content of adult male and female and immature female rats during a 24-hour period. *P* values represent significance of the difference between mean protein levels for given hours.

as the effects of blinding on HIOMT activity go, one might imagine that the loss of the cyclic light input could have some effect on sympathetic nervous tone.

Reiter: I was initially confused by some of the reports on the effect of ganglionectomy on HIOMT. We repeated some of these experiments and found rather high levels of HIOMT within several days after ganglionectomy, but two weeks later the levels of this enzyme were consistently low. Also, if we immunosympathectomized rats by giving them anti-nerve growth factor shortly after birth, when they became adults we could not find a rhythm in HIOMT.

Axelrod: I think some other mechanism takes over; it appears that like many endocrine effects, nature has a hierarchy of controls and if one is destroyed or damaged another takes over. With immunosympathectomy and ganglionectomy, Machado found that in a newborn rat the serotonin rhythm persists in the pineal, but it is abolished by these procedures in the adult (Machado, Machado and Wragg 1969; Machado, Wragg and Machado 1969).

Nir: We have investigated whether daily fluctuations occur in the metabolism of nucleic acids and protein in the pineal, in an attempt to determine the relationship between circadian changes in environmental

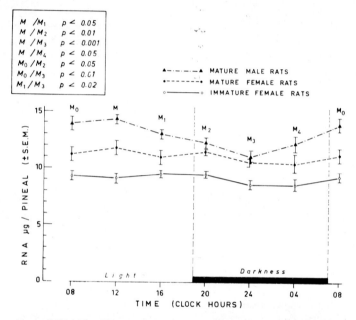

FIG. 2 (Nir). Pineal RNA content of adult male and female and immature female rats during a 24-hour period. *P* values represent significance of the difference between mean RNA levels for given hours.

light and the pineal metabolic rate. Moreover, we wanted to see whether this rate may be associated with that of the gland's synthesis of endocrinologically active compounds.

The daily fluctuations in pineal levels of RNA, DNA and protein were determined in immature (21-day-old) female, and adult (weighing 150 g each) female and male rats. During a 24-hour period, every four hours, animals were killed by neck fracture and their pineals removed and analysed for nucleic acids and protein content. The daily fluctuations in pineal protein are summarized in Fig. 1. It can be seen that in mature male rats a peak level is reached about 4 p.m., preceded by a gradual increase during the period of light and followed by a significant decrease around midnight until the end of darkness. In mature female rats the diurnal rhythm is shifted, the peak and trough being delayed four hours. No such diurnal variations in pineal protein were observed in the immature female animals (some circadian rhythms are known to be absent during early life).

Similarly, marked daily fluctuations in pineal RNA were recorded in mature male rats (Fig. 2), a definite peak occurring at noon and a sharp nadir at midnight. No significant changes were noted in RNA levels of female animals although a similar pattern in their diurnal rhythm is

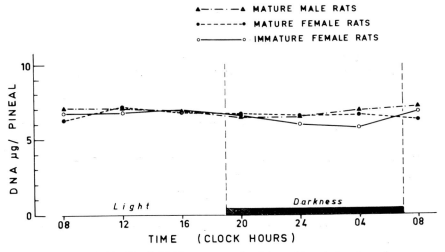

FIG. 3 (Nir). Pineal DNA content of adult male and female and immature female rats during a 24-hour period.

apparent (this may be attributed to metabolic fluctuations brought about by the oestrous cycle and extrinsic factors affecting ovulation).

It is noteworthy that pineal levels of protein and RNA are much higher in mature male than female rats despite their equal body weights.

Diurnal changes in pineal DNA were observed in neither male nor female rats, although a trend towards higher values at midday and lower ones at midnight was characteristic here too (Fig. 3).

In a cytological study a midday peak in the nuclear and nucleolar size in pineal parenchymal cells was found (Quay and Renzoni 1966). We observed greatest protein synthetic activity in pinealocytes during the early afternoon with a peak at about 4 p.m., preceded by an increase in RNA at midday, the hour at which highest nucleolar volumes have been found.

Nucleolar volumes of cells are generally largest during or before the increase in nucleolar RNA, which precedes maximum cytoplasmic protein synthesis. Our results therefore provide metabolic correlates of the nuclear changes and give substance to the assumption that cellular functional activity is indeed related to nuclear size.

Moreover, the diurnal rhythms in the pineal levels of RNA and protein in adult male rats simulate the gland's daily fluctuations of serotonin. The pineal is very rich in and has an exceedingly high turnover of serotonin (Snyder, Axelrod and Zweig 1967). This is consistent with our finding of high metabolic activity of the pineal protein and suggests a relationship between them. Furthermore, it has been shown that actinomycin affects the rat pineal serotonin rhythm, lowering the peak level (Snyder, Axelrod and Zweig 1967). Since puromycin had no effect on pineal serotonin it has been suggested that RNA synthesis may be needed for maintaining high daytime levels of pineal serotonin. Our findings lend support to this theory.

It might be postulated that a diurnal cycle in pineal metabolic activity in the adult rat takes the following course. Towards the end of the period of darkness the gland's noradrenaline content reaches its peak, inducing RNA synthesis most probably at the ribosomal level (perhaps via the adenyl cyclase system). RNA synthesis reaches its peak during the first half of the light period, followed in the second half by a corresponding increase in protein synthesis. The production of specific substances such as melatonin follows, reaching a climax during the first half of the period of darkness.

REFERENCES

BENOIT, J. (1970) In *La photorégulation de la reproduction chez les oiseaux et les mammifères,* pp. 121–149, ed. Benoit, J. and Assenmacher, I. Paris: Centre National de la Recherche Scientifique.

GANONG, W. F., SHEPHERD, M. D., WALL, J. R., VON BRUNT, E. E. and CLEGG, M. T. (1963) *Endocrinology* **72,** 962–963.

MACHADO, C. R. S., MACHADO, A. B. M. and WRAGG, G. E. (1969) *Endocrinology* **85,** 846–848.

MACHADO, C. R. S., WRAGG, G. E. and MACHADO, A. B. M. (1969) *Science* **164,** 442.

OISHI, T. and KATO, M. (1968) *Mem. Fac. Sci. Kyoto Univ. Ser. B.* **2,** 12–18.

O'STEEN, W. K. (1970) *Expl Neurol.* **27,** 294.

QUAY, W. B. and RENZONI, A. (1966) *Growth* **30,** 315–324.

SNYDER, S. H., AXELROD, J. and ZWEIG, M. (1967) *J. Pharmac. exp. Ther.* **158,** 206–213.

WETTERBERG, L., GELLER, E. and YUWILER, A. (1970) *Science* **167,** 884–885.

DEVELOPMENTAL ASPECTS
OF AMPHIBIAN PINEAL SYSTEMS

DOUGLAS E. KELLY

*Department of Biological Structure, University of Miami School of Medicine,
Miami, Florida*

THE main thrust of inquiry on pineal systems has always been aimed toward an eventual understanding of the function of these mysterious organs. This symposium will no doubt emphasize the fact that substantial progress has been made in this direction. To this author it is even more heartening to note that efforts along these lines have embraced a wide variety of organisms, so that an evolutionary insight is also being gained.

This paper will summarize efforts in yet another, not unrelated, direction. Pineal systems, at least in some vertebrates, appear to be valuable cell populations with which to study the patterns and mechanics involved in the shaping of an emerging epithelial organ. From the point of view of simplicity, the pineal system of tailed amphibians has proved most useful; it develops and persists as a single, median dorsal evagination of the diencephalic roof. During late embryonic and early larval life, it is a single hollow vesicle of simple cuboidal to columnar epithelial cells and it is already amply supplied with typical pineal photoreceptor cells. In the West Coast newt *Taricha torosa*, this organ becomes progressively flattened during larval development; throughout post-metamorphic juvenile and adult stages its morphology no longer seems to emphasize photoreceptors (Kelly 1965). A similar pattern is found in the East Coast newt (Flight 1968). In salamanders such as the axolotl (van de Kamer 1949; Slonimski 1947) the vesicle remains as a single saccular organ throughout adult stages, a pattern which is also seen in many fishes. In anuran amphibians, development is more complicated because the initial evagination, the intracranial epiphysis, constricts anteriorly to give rise to a second, smaller, subcutaneous receptor organ, and itself becomes a more lobulated sac (see Eakin and Westfall 1961).

Embryos of *Taricha torosa* are readily available, tolerant to surgical insult, and their saccular pineal organ displays a conveniently small population of cells, a long-term developmental sequence, a high level of morphological differentiation, and an analysable sequence of morphogenetic cell movements and shape changes. This paper summarizes the approaches we have used and what we have learned over the past several years. Some aspects have been published previously. Dr Anita Hendrickson has done the major portion of the more recent radioautographic work and Miss Mary Ann Cahill and Mrs Sandra Kunz have collaborated with Dr Hendrickson and myself in the studies on pineal shape changes and their mechanics.

METHODS AND MATERIALS

For the sake of cytological preservation and resolution in both light and electron microscopy, we have preferred to use specimens embedded in epoxy resin (Luft 1961) and sectioned on an ultramicrotome with a diamond knife. For general purposes the fixatives of choice for young amphibian material are $2 \cdot 5$ per cent osmium tetroxide in chrome saline buffer (Dalton and Felix 1956), or $3 \cdot 0$–$3 \cdot 75$ per cent osmium tetroxide in $0 \cdot 05$ M s-collidine buffer (Bennett and Luft 1959); either agent applied ice-cold for one hour and at a final pH of $7 \cdot 4$. One–two μm sections of this material stained with azure II-methylene blue (Richardson, Jarett and Finke 1960) were used for light microscopical studies. For electron microscopy, much thinner sections were stained with the alkaline lead citrate procedure of Reynolds (1963), often preceded by treatment with half-saturated aqueous uranyl acetate at 55 °C. *En bloc* staining of tissues prior to dehydration and embedding (two hours at room temperature in a $0 \cdot 5$ per cent uranyl acetate solution in veronal acetate buffer) enhances the fine structural visualization of membranous components.

Application of photographic emulsion (Kodak NTB-2) to epoxy-embedded sections for light microscopical radioautography presents difficulties when material fixed with collidine/osmium and stained by the Richardson method must be used. However, these can be overcome by pretreating the sections with $NaOH$–HIO_4 (Hendrickson, Kunz and Kelly 1968) to allow staining at room temperature after exposure and development of the emulsion.

Amphibian embryos and young larvae are resistant to uptake of tritiated thymidine from their aqueous environment, but incorporation of this isotope can be accomplished by micro-injection of $0 \cdot 2$–$0 \cdot 4$ μCi of tritiated thymidine (New England Nuclear, specific activity $1 \cdot 29$ Ci/mM) into the pericardial cavities of animals anaesthetized with MS-222 (Tricaine methane sulphonate, Sandoz Pharmaceuticals). Embryos two weeks before hatching and at hatching age as well as larvae two weeks after hatching were injected by this means and then fixed at times ranging up to 13 days after injection. Radioautographs were prepared as outlined above, and grain counts were done on sagittal sections of the developing pineal organs to determine sources of new cells and routes of cellular migration.

Total and differential pineal cell counts, obtained from serial 1 μm-sections of embryos possessing the earliest manifestation of pineal development and on representative ages to adulthood, yielded added information related to total pineal volume and rates of proliferation for the various pineal cells (Hendrickson and Kelly 1969).

PHOTORECEPTOR DIFFERENTIATION AND OUTER SEGMENT RENEWAL

From the electron microscopical studies of a rapidly increasing number of investigators, the fine structural features of pineal photoreceptors in a wide variety of adult and developing lower vertebrates are now well known. (See e.g. recent reviews such as Collin 1968, 1969; Collin and Kappers 1968; Oksche 1968; Ueck 1969; and Vivien-Roels 1970.) These need not be reiterated here.

In amphibians, it is clear that well-formed photoreceptors are present prior to hatching stages and the assumption of larval life (Eakin and Westfall

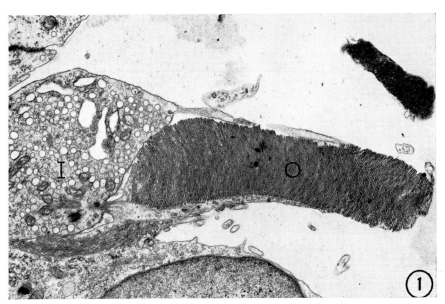

FIG. 1. Electron micrograph showing the outer (O) and inner (I) segments of a photoreceptor cell from the pineal organ of a larval newt. This particular photoreceptor differentiated within a pineal organ that was transplanted as a rudiment from an embryo into the dorsal tail fin of an older host larva and allowed to differentiate there for 55 days. Collidine-osmium fixation, lead and uranyl acetate stained. × 9200.

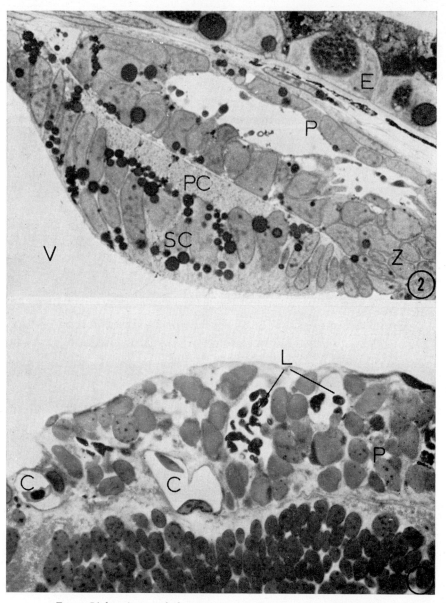

FIG. 2. Light micrograph showing, in sagittal section, most of the pineal vesicle (P) of a two-week-old newt larva. Protruding photoreceptors are visible. E, epidermis; PC, posterior commissure; SC, subcommissural organ; V, third ventricle; Z, proliferation zone. Azure II-methylene blue stained. (Hendrickson and Kelly 1971.) ×480.

FIG. 3. Light micrograph showing, in sagittal section, a small portion of the pineal organ (P) of an adult newt, five years after metamorphosis. Several lumen remnants (L) are found which contain darkly stained photoreceptor outer segment material. Other outer segment material can be seen wedged among pineal cells. Capillaries (C) also occupy parts of the organ. Plastic embedded, Azure II-methylene blue stained. (Hendrickson and Kelly 1971.) ×480.

1961; Kelly 1965) (Fig. 1). In frogs, and probably salamanders, the wide lumen of the intracranial epiphysis contains numerous photoreceptor outer segments during all larval and adult stages. However, in newt species, the progressive flattening of the organ with an attendant closure of a pineal lumen obscures the presence of photoreceptors during later larval and post-metamorphic life (Figs. 2 and 3). Light microscopy of paraffin sections fails to reveal diagnostic images of photoreceptors in the post-metamorphic

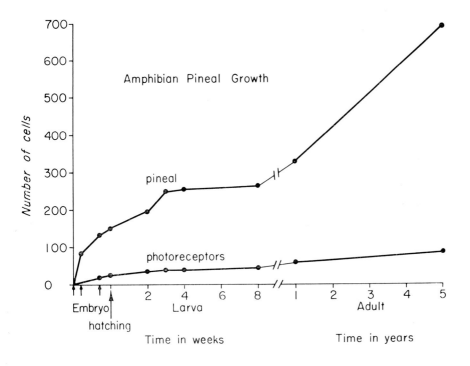

FIG. 4. This graph depicts the increase in total pineal organ cells (upper line) as determined from direct cell counts of both photoreceptors (lower line) plus the combined total of undifferentiated and supportive cells. (Hendrickson and Kelly 1969.)

organ, and electron microscopy discloses only widely separated luminal remnants with quite distorted outer and inner segments. Supportive cells become more prominent and contain aldehyde-fuchsin-stainable accumulations in their cytoplasm. This has led to the conjecture that with maturity, the newt pineal organ may lose its photoreceptive cells and emphasize other, possibly secretory, functions (Kelly 1965).

An intensive study now discloses that this conjecture is not tenable

(Hendrickson and Kelly 1969, 1971). When 1 μm-epoxy embedded serial sections of newt pineal organs are carefully analysed, photoreceptors can be detected and counted by light microscopy at all stages of the life cycle (Fig. 4). The data derived disclose that not only are pineal photoreceptors still present even in fully mature adult animals, but they comprise a constant proportion (14–18 per cent) of the pineal cell population at all larval and post-metamorphic stages. Their obscurity during later stages appears due to their compaction among other cells as the organ is flattened, and their dispersion as the supportive cells increase drastically in individual and collective cytoplasmic volume. This information should be worthwhile to workers such as Adler (1969) who have postulated the presence of extra-retinal photoreceptors, active in the control of circadian behavioural rhythms in adult newts. Until now it was not encouraging to consider the adult pineal organ as a candidate site for such photoreceptors.

With the possible exception of certain lamprey and lizard pineal photoreceptors (Collin 1968, 1969), the outer segments of pineal photoreceptors are not maintained in as orderly an array as is the case with retinal rods and cones (Fig. 5). We (Kelly 1962; Kelly and Smith 1964), as well as others before and since, have interpreted the variety of lamellar configurations in pineal photoreceptor outer segments as evidence for the constant removal and renewal of these membranous components. In newts, these bizarre outer segment configurations are present at all stages in the life cycle during which photoreceptors are found. One must now consider the possibility that outer segment regeneration is occurring throughout the life of the organism. In young larval newts, and in adult amphibians of species which retain widely saccular pineal organs, macrophages are a common occupant of the luminal spaces. Their close spatial relationship to pineal photoreceptor outer segments and, when examined ultrastructurally, their vacuoles which contain abundant whorled membranous material, have led us to postulate that these cells are involved in scavenging and digestion of cast-off outer segments. In the lumen-lacking pineal organs of juvenile and adult newts, similar vacuoles in the supportive cells suggest that these cells perform the phagocytic function (Flight 1968; Hendrickson and Kelly 1971) (Figs. 5 and 6).

Recently means have been devised for labelling retinal photoreceptors with amino acid isotopes. From radioautographs, a progressive movement of the label along the membranous rod outer segment toward its distal tip has been noted (see Young and Droz 1968). There the label seems to be removed by nearby pigment epithelial cells (Young and Bok 1969). These observations suggest that an orderly membrane turnover may be occurring along the outer segment. Using similar techniques, Dr Ann Bunt, working

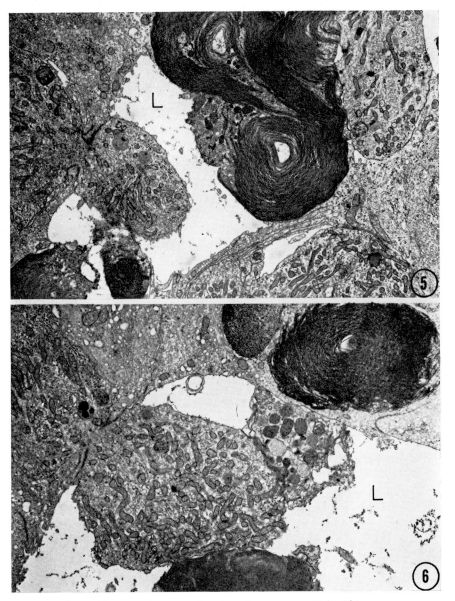

Fig. 5. Electron micrograph showing a lumen remnant (L) within a one year post-metamorphic pineal organ. A greatly distorted photoreceptor outer segment is present in the upper centre of the figure, partly enclosed by surfaces of supportive cells. Many lysosomal vacuoles are seen adjacent to the membrane whorls of this outer segment. Similar vacuoles are present in photoreceptor inner segment profiles at left centre and upper right. Collidine-osmium fixation, lead and uranyl acetate stained. (Hendrickson and Kelly 1971.) ×6400.

Fig. 6. In this section, from the same animal as shown in Fig. 5, a membranous whorl (upper right) appears to be completely surrounded by cytoplasm of a supportive cell. Numerous lysosomes occupy an outer or inner segment remnant in the lumen (L) nearby. Collidine-osmium fixation, lead and uranyl acetate stained. (Hendrickson and Kelly 1971.) ×8800.

in our laboratory, has recently succeeded in labelling frog pineal photo-receptors (Bunt, unpublished data). The label can be detected in the dis-arranged outer segments 25 days after injection, in membranous contents of supportive cell vacuoles after 25 and 60 days, and in similar vacuoles of macrophages after 60 days. Dr Walter Flight (personal communication) now has similar evidence derived from adult East Coast newt pineal organs. Additionally, Dr Bunt has shown that the same macrophage and supporting cell vacuoles are acid phosphatase-rich, as are smaller inclusions in photoreceptor inner segments. This confirms the identification of all these components as members of the lysosome family. Such information strongly reinforces the concept that photoreceptors in amphibian pineal organs utilize an autophagocytic process to shed and renew their outer segments during the adult life of the animal, and that macrophages and/or supportive cells aid in removal of cast-off outer segment material. Incident-ally, it now seems clear that the aldehyde-fuchsin-stainable accumulations seen by light microscopy in supportive cell cytoplasm in newt pineals are not secretory elaborations, but in fact phagocytic vacuoles.

Hence, with respect to the adult newt pineal organ, we must come to the conclusion that in spite of the morphogenetic changes that have flattened its lumen, increased the volume of its supportive cells, and obscured its photoreceptors, morphologically the organ still seems to be a photo-receptor, replete with the usual proportion of photoreceptor cells. We still have no indication of the functional state of the photoreceptors, since no physiological recordings have been made, and no ganglion cells have been identified in the organ.[*] But, on the other hand, evidence for or against a function other than photoreception (for example, endocrine secretion) is lacking.

With this concept of the fine morphology and its dynamics in larval and adult newt pineal organs as background, we have directed our principal inquiry toward developmental mechanics during much earlier periods of the organ's ontogeny.

PROLIFERATION OF PINEAL CELLS

Some years ago we studied the development of the pineal organ of *Taricha torosa* by observing the growth and differentiation of embryonic pineal rudiments when transplanted into the tail fins or anterior ocular chambers of older host larvae (Kelly 1963). An interesting pattern emerged with respect to transplants to the dorsal tail fin region, for when the tiny

---

[*] However, Flight (personal communication) has recently detected a few apparent ganglion cells in serial section electron micrographs of adult East Coast newt pineal organs.

emergent pineal bud alone was transplanted, a smaller than normal, but well-differentiated, pineal vesicle developed (Figs. 1 and 7); on the other hand, when a substantial amount of diencephalic roof tissue was included with the transplant, a normal-sized, differentiated pineal vesicle was

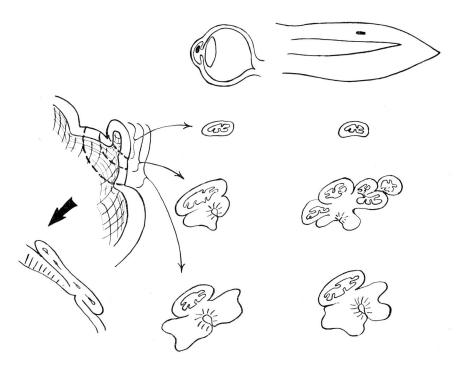

FIG. 7. A diagrammatic summary of pineal transplant experiments. The embryonic pineal bud from the diencephalic roof (left centre) normally develops into a flattened late-larval organ (heavy arrow to lower left). The fine arrows indicate the amount of tissue transplanted from the region into either the anterior ocular chamber (centre vertical row of figures) or dorsal tail fin mesenchyme (right vertical row of figures) of an older host larva. Each small diagram depicts the approximate proportion of pineal and brain tissue which develops from the respective transplant. Note particularly the centre diagram of the right row in which a multi-lobed mass having a higher than normal volume of differentiated pineal tissue has developed. See text for explanation of these growth patterns. (Kelly 1963.)

obtained. More remarkably, if but a moderate amount of diencephalic tissue in the immediate vicinity of the pineal bud was included, a multi-lobed mass of well-differentiated pineal tissue having larger than normal volume often developed. Similar types of transplants to the anterior ocular chamber always produced pineal organs of normal or smaller than normal

3*

dimensions. Since mitotic figures are commonly observed in the diencephalic roof region near the pineal primordium both during normal development and in cases of pineal regeneration after surgical extirpation (Cintron 1963), it seemed logical that we were dealing with the development of an organ whose supply of new cells is localized and is potentially greater than is utilized during normal development *in situ*. Not only does the diencephalic roof appear to be the supply of new cells, but when present in massive amounts, diencephalic tissues (including the optic cup) appear capable of restricting pineal proliferation to normal proportions.

In the years since, we have sought ways of accurately defining the extent and propensities of the diencephalic roof proliferative zone which gives rise to pineal cells. The use of tritiated thymidine radioautography over several newt breeding seasons has provided information on rather specific parameters of pineal growth in this animal (Hendrickson and Kelly 1969).

Embryos injected two weeks before hatching (at which time the pineal bud is just emerging) display a grain distribution pattern which confirms the presence of a proliferation zone in the diencephalic roof immediately adjacent to the neck of the developing organ. Larvae injected at hatching or two weeks after hatching display a discrete pulse label pattern from which the extent of the proliferation zone can be determined and the direction of migration of cells from the proliferation zone into the developing pineal organ observed as well (Fig. 8). Examination of radioautographic sections at different intervals after injection of label discloses that before the hatching stages, daughter cells emerging from the pineal proliferation zone migrate predominantly in a posterior direction to form a diverticulum which bulges over the developing underlying posterior commissure and subcommissural organ. Cells in the posterior pole of this bulge show the earliest signs of differentiation into photoreceptors (Kelly 1965; Hendrickson and Kelly 1971). After hatching, a shift in the migratory flow of new cells results in the anterior expansion of the organ. The roof of the pineal vesicle thus formed displays relatively less evidence of cellular differentiation, becoming increasingly more squamous in appearance. Both photoreceptors and supportive cells of the pineal arise through this proliferative pattern; labelled cells of both types were found after all series of injections. However, fewer total numbers of cells were found to arise the later the injection was performed.

As a result of these studies it can now be said with confidence that the proliferation zone is virtually the sole (soul?) source of new cells for the developing pineal organ. Most of the animals were examined by radioautography applied to serial or nearly adjacent section groups, and in only one or two cases was a heavily labelled cell found which could be interpreted to suggest any mitotic potential outside the proliferation zone. Moreover, it is also apparent that the proliferation zone provides a significant quantity of new cells to the anterior margin of the lengthening subcommissural organ just behind it in the diencephalic roof.

The overall pattern (summarized in Fig. 8) is one in which the proliferation zone occupies the neck of the enlarging pineal organ and the diencephalic roof immediately adjacent to the neck. This centre of mitotic

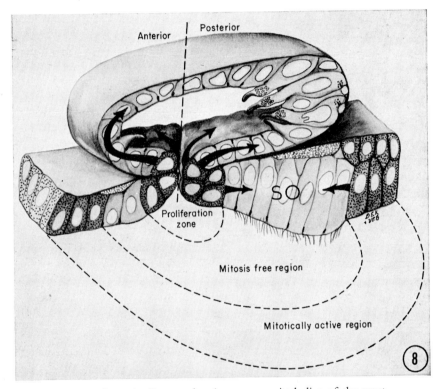

Fig. 8. Schematic diagram showing a parasagittal slice of the newt pineal vesicle and underlying diencephalic roof shortly after the hatching stage. The lumen of the hollow organ is continuous with the third ventricle via an orifice (bottom of vertical dotted line). Stippled cells occupy areas of mitotic activity, as determined from their capacity for incorporating tritiated thymidine. The neck of mitotic cells surrounding the orifice constitutes the proliferation zone which provides new cells to the enlarging pineal vesicle, and also to the anterior aspect of the subcommissural organ (SO). Note that the proliferation zone is surrounded in the diencephalic roof and in the floor of the vesicle by a mitosis-free region in which cells are differentiating and assuming specific shapes. See text for a discussion of factors which control their morphogenesis. Note also that the earliest photoreceptors to reach full differentiation are located in the posterior pole of the pineal organ. (Hendrickson and Kelly 1969.)

activity is surrounded, in the floor of the organ as well as in the diencephalic roof, by a ring of cells in which mitosis is absent and in which daughter cells are undergoing cellular differentiation. The basis for the characteristic patterns of growth observed in the various transplanted pineal rudiments now seems quite obvious; the volume of pineal cells produced is an expression of whether or not the proliferation zone has been included in the transplant. However, even if the proliferation zone has been included, its capacity to produce excessively large numbers of pineal cells appears limited or controlled by an influence emanating from adjacent diencephalic tissues. The nature or source of this influence is not understood at present.

MORPHOGENETIC SHAPING OF THE PINEAL ORGAN

For many years embryologists have theorized about the mechanisms which control the shapes of cells and organs as they develop. However, only recently has it been possible to ascribe cell asymmetries to the action of specific organelles. Among other examples, it can be shown that dramatic shape changes of certain epithelial cells (Cloney 1966) or invaginating cells of the neural groove (Baker and Schroeder 1967), and the development of furrows in symmetrically and asymmetrically cleaving eggs (Szollosi 1970) can all be ascribed to appropriately positioned intracytoplasmic populations of fine filaments. Since Ishikawa, Bischoff and Holtzer (1969) have been able to isolate these filament populations and demonstrate their ability to react with heavy meromyosin, it appears more than likely that they are actin-like, and produce cell shape changes as a result of contractile propensities.

Recently the epithelial buds of embryonic pancreas, lung and lens have been analysed with regard to mitotic patterns and intracellular filament populations that might influence their initial and subsequent shaping (Wessells and Cohen 1968; Wessells and Evans 1968; Wrenn and Wessells 1969). In each of these cases, *no localized* population of cells incorporating tritiated thymidine is found in the forming diverticulum (that is, mitosis is widely scattered), and cytoplasmic filaments located in the apices of the first cells to invaginate seem responsible for starting the diverticulation process. The lens develops as a single vesicle, the pancreas forms a system of terminal acini, and the lung primordia ultimately undergo more extensively branching diverticulations which can be shown not to occur in the absence of collagen.

The newt pineal organ develops as a single vesicle, and its proliferative pattern is much different. Nearly all of its cells are supplied from one,

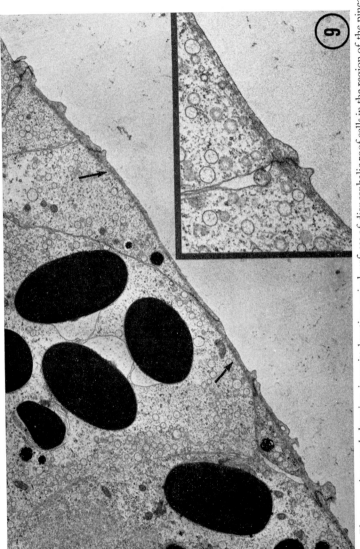

FIG. 9. Electron micrograph showing, in sagittal section, apical surfaces of diencephalic roof cells in the region of the pineal primordium, before the actual appearance of a pineal bud. The cells of this area have been mitotically active and possess a smooth ventricular surface underlain by a web of fine filaments (arrows) which appear to anchor at circumapical intercellular intermediate junctions. The inset shows the filamentous web and one junctional region at higher magnification. Collidine-osmium fixation, lead and uranyl acetate stained. ×6400. (inset ×12 000.)

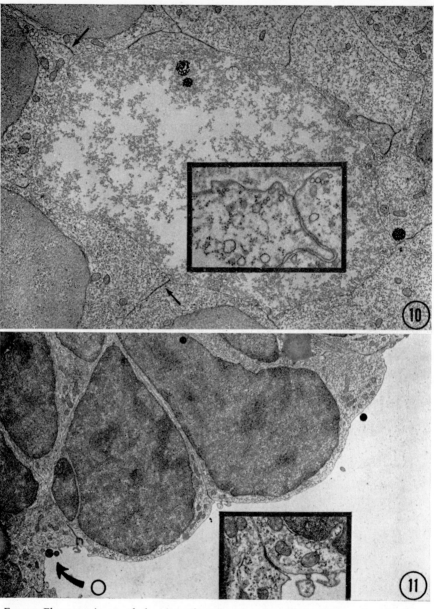

FIG. 10. Electron micrograph showing a frontal section through the orifice and neck of the pineal vesicle of a newt at hatching age. The orifice, containing a flocculent precipitate, occupies the centre of the picture. It is surrounded by cells which are capable of mitosis and which display smooth apical surfaces and intermediate junctions (arrows and inset). The apical cell membranes are underlain by a very scant web of fine filaments. Collidine-osmium fixation, lead and uranyl acetate stained. × 5920. (inset × 26 000.)

FIG. 11. Cells of the proliferation zone of a hatching-stage newt, seen in parasagittal section. The level of the orifice is indicated by (O). The same features noted in Fig. 10 are apparent along the ventricle-facing surfaces of these mitotically capable cells. Chromate-osmium fixation, lead and uranyl acetate stained. × 3360. (inset × 7360.)

localized proliferation zone located in the neck of the organ and the under-lying diencephalic roof. But, in spite of this difference, the pattern of filaments and attachments which may exert contraction and morphogenetic shape changes turns out to be strikingly similar.

The diencephalic roof originates as a simple epithelium which is apparent about two weeks before hatching. At this time the pineal primordium begins its initial appearance as a focal evagination of the roof. Although mitotically active, the cells of the area display zonular (belt-like) cir-cumapical junctions which attach them to their neighbours (Fig. 9). The junctions can best be classified as intermediate junctions (zonulae adhaer-entes), and each one will serve as the insertion for fine (3–5 nm, 30–50 Å) filaments which will bridge or encircle the apical cytoplasm. These are the filaments that form the "terminal web" of many epithelia, and which, in the above-named instances, are suspected of contractile action related to cell-shape changes. During subsequent development, diencephalic roof-derived cells which retain exposure to the pineal lumen, its orifice, or the third ventricle, display this characteristic set of fine filaments and the associated zonular intermediate junctions.

As with the evaginating pancreatic bud (Wessells and Evans 1968) the invaginating lens placode (Wrenn and Wessells 1969), or the invaginating neural tube (Baker and Schroeder 1967), the initial outward thrust of the pineal bud may be mediated by contracting apical filaments which truncate the shape of a few cells in concert to effect an initial evagination. These are newly divided cells which will ultimately occupy the posterior roof of the pineal vesicle. Evagination (rather than invagination) may also be aided by ventricular fluid pressure, although we have no evidence on this possible factor.

As soon as the bud develops to the point that a rudimentary vesicle and neck are distinguishable, differences in the filament-attachment system of the two regions are more evident. The cells of the neck, some of which are mitotically active, possess only scant filaments which underlie a smooth, expanded and slightly bulging cell surface bordering the orifice (Figs. 10 and 11). Those within the vesicle display more obvious filaments and limited apical exposure, with cell surfaces that are either folded or being constricted, collar-like, to bulge into the lumen as newly-acquired photo-receptor inner segments (Fig. 12). The suggestion derived from the fine morphology is that as new cells are passed from the proliferation zone and neck, their apical borders become protracted (perhaps by filament con-traction) to provide the generally truncated shape characteristic of cells lining a vesicle (see arrows in Fig. 8). Of course, as photoreceptors and supportive cells take on their characteristic ramifying and complex shapes

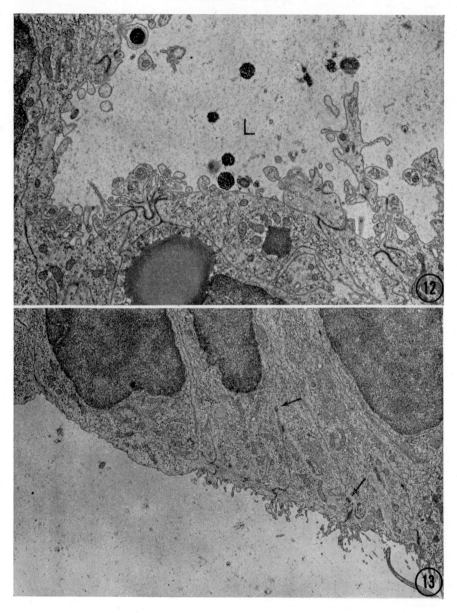

FIG. 12. Sagittal section from the pineal vesicle of the specimen shown in Fig. 11. The cells in this electron micrograph border the pineal lumen (L) just inside the orifice. These cells are no longer mitotically active and are in initial phases of their differentiation into supportive cells and photoreceptors. Their apical surfaces are highly folded, often ramifying into the lumen. Their junctions and attached filaments are more prominent. Chromate-osmium fixation, lead and uranyl acetate stained. × 7520.

in the walls of the differentiating vesicle, the truncation is grossly modified. Nevertheless, once they have left the neck-orifice region, their apices are supported within relatively narrow confines, especially in the extremities of the vesicle, while their basal parts are broader and relatively less populated with shape-altering or maintaining filaments.

The situation is similar on the other, diencephalic roof side of the proliferation zone (lower arrow in Fig. 8). Here cells have moved outward from the neck-orifice to occupy a mitosis-free ring of the diencephalic roof encircling the proliferation zone. Posteriorly this area includes cells of the developing subcommissural organ. This mitosis-free ring also receives new cells from other active areas around its margin. In the ring itself, the cells are generally columnar and display attenuated and folded apical borders (Fig. 13). Their apical filament networks are thick and obvious, especially near the junction areas. Moreover, these cells now display numerous, more highly supportive desmosomal attachments. Collectively, they give the appearance of providing a highly supported, stable ventricular surface. *Like* the cells of the pineal vesicle, this diencephalic roof region can be characterized as one in which cells are differentiating rather than dividing, and in which differentiation includes production of filament patterns concerned with restricting the apical circumference of each cell. But *unlike* cells of the pineal vesicle, the diencephalic roof cells also gain filamentous reinforcement and a degree of attenuation along their basal surfaces. Electron micrographs at various ages and in different planes of section clearly disclose a thin web of cytoplasmic filaments along the basal cell membrane of diencephalic roof cells. This web is not observable along the broader basal surfaces of pineal vesicle cells (Figs. 14 and 15). The fact that the cells of this diencephalic roof area have largely become columnar may also be due to the presumed action of longitudinally oriented microtubules (see Byers and Porter 1964; Wrenn and Wessells 1969), but our study has not been focused on microtubules.

Cells of the proliferation zone, then, from radioautographic and

---

FIG. 13. Sagittal section of the diencephalic roof region of the same animal as in Figs. 11 and 12. The third ventricle occupies the lower part of this electron micrograph. The cells at the extreme left of this picture occupy the edge of the pineal proliferation zone seen in the extreme right of Fig. 11. They display the same smooth, rounded apical surface. The cells in the right of the picture, which occupy the mitosis-free, developing subcommissural organ, have become columnar. Their apical surfaces are folded and underlain by prominent thin filament webs. Intermediate junctions are well developed, as are desmosomes (arrows). Chromate-osmium fixation, lead and uranyl acetate stained. × 4560.

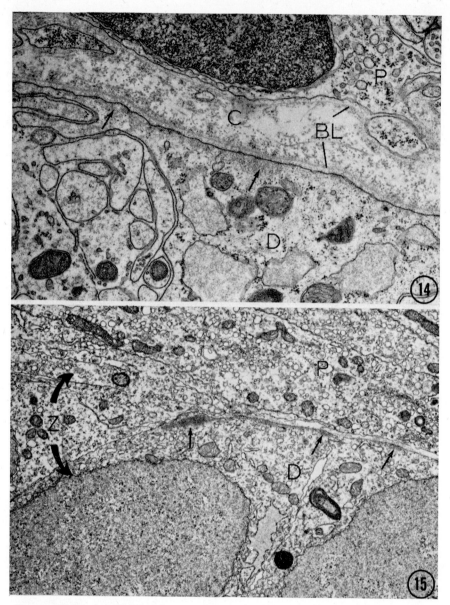

Fig. 14. Higher magnification electron micrograph of the diencephalic roof region in the same animal from which Figs. 11, 12 and 13 were taken. This figure shows a small portion of the region where the pineal vesicle (P) rests upon the diencephalic roof (D). The two components at this stage are separated by basal laminae (BL) which directly enshroud the pineal vesicle and the surface of the diencephalic roof. The intervening connective tissue space between these basal laminae contains collagen fibres (C). The area at (D) is the basal cytoplasm of one of the subcommissural organ cells shown in the right-hand portion of Fig. 13. Note that along its basal surface, a prominent web of fine cytoplasmic filaments (arrows) is present. Such a web is not seen along the basal surfaces of pineal cells in the upper part of the picture. Some of the first axons to develop in the posterior commissure are seen in the lower left corner of the picture. Chromate–osmium fixation, lead and uranyl acetate stained. × 26 560.

morphological evidence, seem to be the least positionally stabilized. One gains the impression that once born, new cells are passively squeezed out of the pineal neck as a consequence of proliferation force, to differentiate and assume the structural stability of the immediately surrounding areas.

At first the pineal bud is not encased by a basal lamina or any visibly detectable collagen. But as it becomes a vesicle, the pineal organ gradually acquires a distinct basal lamina which separates pineal epithelium from surrounding connective tissue. The lamina becomes reinforced by collagen fibres and together these elements form the pineal basement membrane—really the pineal pia mater (Fig. 14). It is interesting that the basal lamina, and ultimately the basement membrane, underlie chiefly those pineal and diencephalic roof cells that are non-mitotic, and which show truncation or a columnar shape. An especially good example can be seen just posterior to the neck. When the pineal is a budding vesicle, no basal lamina is found in the angle formed between the bud and the diencephalic roof. But as the vesicle enlarges, the angle is narrowed so that cells of the vesicle floor and posterior commissural area (both no longer mitotic) approximate each other's basal surface (Fig. 15). They are soon separated by two distinct basal laminae and an intervening connective tissue space in which collagen rapidly accumulates (Fig. 14). At the neck the basal lamina makes a sharp, continuous excursion upward from the diencephalic roof to enshroud the pineal vesicle. Mitotic cells have little or no contact with the lamina; non-mitotic cells of roof and vesicle are probably producing it along their basal surfaces as they differentiate.

Because of its strategic location, and its appearance just after pineal bud formation, it is logical to suspect that the basal lamina and collagen provide added reinforcement in the form of a mechanical collar around the neck,

FIG. 15. An electron micrograph taken in the pineal region of a newt embryo approximately one week before hatching. The basal portions of cells of the diencephalic roof (D) are seen in the lower portion of the picture. In the upper right are basal parts of pineal vesicle cells (P) that have just entered the developing organ. The cellular compartments at the left of the picture (Z) lie at the edge of a pineal proliferation zone. Large arrows indicate the direction of cell movements from the proliferation zone. A narrow extra-cellular angle between pineal vesicle and diencephalic roof is seen running horizontally through the middle of the right-hand part of the picture. Within the extracellular space, basal lamina is just beginning to be deposited by pineal and diencephalic roof cells. Note again the prominent web of fine filaments (small arrows) which occupy the basal surface of diencephalic roof cells, particularly near the apex of the extra-cellular angle. Collidine-osmium fixation, lead and uranyl acetate stained. × 8560.

and that this collar limits further increase in the diameter of the neck. Like the lung (Wessells and Cohen 1968), the pineal diverticulum may depend on collagen for its proper shaping.

It is clear that in achieving and maintaining (for a time) its vesicular shape, the pineal organ of this animal is dependent upon the appropriately timed and controlled interaction of a localized source of new cells, cell adhesion, the likely contraction and support provided by intracellular filament systems, and perhaps also the restraint offered by extracellular products of the same cells.

SUMMARY

As evidenced by their morphological and physiological properties, the pineal organs of amphibians are photoreceptors. Urodeles possess but a single intracranial pineal organ displaying an uncomplicated saccular shape and a high degree of morphological differentiation. In the West Coast newt, *Taricha torosa*, the organ possesses numerous photoreceptor cells and a widely dilated lumen during early larval stages. As development approaches metamorphosis, the organ increases in total size while becoming noticeably flattened. The lumen remains only as scattered isolated compartments. The volume of supportive cells increases significantly and photoreceptor cells are obscured. However, careful counting of cell numbers and types in osmium-fixed, epoxy-embedded serial sections reveals that the photoreceptors are not lost; indeed they remain a constant proportion (14 to 18 per cent) of the total cell population throughout larval, post-metamorphic juvenile and adult life. Their functional state, however, is as yet unknown. There is evidence of loss and renewal of photoreceptor outer segments during all stages. In early larval pineal organs, phagocytosis of outer segment material appears to be mediated by pineal luminal macrophages; by post-metamorphic stages this function is assumed by supportive cells.

Experiments involving pineal transplantation or tritiated thymidine radioautography demonstrate conclusively that during embryonic and larval life, new pineal cells originate from a mitotically active cell population (the "pineal proliferation zone") located in the neck attaching the organ to the diencephalic roof. Daughter cells migrate into the pineal organ, moving into its posterior parts during late embryonic stages while coursing predominantly in an anterior direction after hatching. Both pineal photoreceptors and supportive cells arise in this manner, differentiation of photoreceptors occurring first in those parts of the organ most distant from the proliferation zone. The patterns of adhesion, filament distribution and contraction, and ultimately cytoskeletal support among the cells of this zone and adjacent areas of the pineal organ and underlying brain roof, appear to play important roles in maintaining overall shape during the growth of this organ. These patterns bear both similarities and contrasts when compared with studies by other workers on the development of various saccular epithelial derivatives.

Acknowledgements

The studies reported here have been supported by research grants (GB-20277 and GB-6910) from the National Science Foundation, by a National Institutes of Health grant (HE-02698) for the support of electron microscope facilities at the University of Washington School of Medicine, Seattle, and by a National Institutes of Health General Research Support Grant for electron microscope facilities at the University of Miami School of Medicine. The author is grateful to Dr David Spencer Smith and the Papanicolaou Cancer Research Institute for use of their electron microscope during part of the work.

REFERENCES

ADLER, K. (1969) *Science* **164**, 1290–1291.
BAKER, P. C. and SCHROEDER, T. E. (1967) *Devl Biol.* **15**, 432–450.
BENNETT, H. S. and LUFT, J. H. (1959) *J. Biophys. biochem. Cytol.* **6**, 113–114.
BYERS, B. and PORTER, K. R. (1964) *Proc. natn. Acad. Sci. U.S.A.* **52**, 1091–1099.
CINTRON, C. (1963) Thesis, University of Colorado.
CLONEY, R. A. (1966) *J. Ultrastruct. Res.* **14**, 300–328.
COLLIN, J. P. (1968) *C. r. hebd. Séanc. Acad. Sci., Paris, Sér. D* **267**, 1047–1050.
COLLIN, J. P. (1969) *Archs Anat. microsc. Morph. exp.* **58**, 145–182.
COLLIN, J. P. and KAPPERS, J. A. (1968) *Brain Res.* **11**, 85–106.
DALTON, A. S. and FELIX, M. (1956) *J. biophys. biochem. Cytol. suppl.* 2, 79–81.
EAKIN, R. M. and WESTFALL, J. A. (1961) *Embryologia* 6, 84–98.
FLIGHT, W. F. G. (1968) *Proc. K. ned. Akad. Wet.* **71**, 525–528.
HENDRICKSON, A. and KELLY, D. E. (1969) *Anat. Rec.* **165**, 211–227.
HENDRICKSON, A. and KELLY, D. E. (1971) *Anat. Rec.* in press.
HENDRICKSON, A., KUNZ, S. and KELLY, D. E. (1968) *Stain Technol.* **43**, 175–177.
ISHIKAWA, H., BISCHOFF, R. and HOLTZER, H. (1969) *J. Cell Biol.* **43**, 312–328.
KELLY, D. E. (1962) *Am. Scient.* **50**, 597–625.
KELLY, D. E. (1963) *Z. Zellforsch. mikrosk. Anat.* **58**, 693–713.
KELLY, D. E. (1965) In *Structure and Function of the Epiphysis Cerebri (Progress in Brain Research* vol. 10), pp. 270–287, ed. Kappers, J. A. and Schadé, J. P. Amsterdam: Elsevier.
KELLY, D. E. and SMITH, S. W. (1964) *J. Cell Biol.* **22**, 565–587.
LUFT, J. H. (1961) *J. biophys. biochem. Cytol.* **9**, 409–415.
OKSCHE, A. (1968) *Extraits Archs Anat. Histol. Embryol.* **51**, 497–507.
REYNOLDS, E. S. (1963) *J. Cell Biol.* **17**, 208–213.
RICHARDSON, K. C., JARETT, L. and FINKE, E. H. (1960) *Stain Technol.* **35**, 313–325.
SLONIMSKI, P. (1947) *C. r. Séanc. Soc. Biol.* **141**, 1107–1108.
SZOLLOSI, D. (1970) *J. Cell Biol.* **44**, 192–209.
UECK, M. (1969) *Z. Zellforsch. mikrosk. Anat.* **100**, 560–580.
VAN DE KAMER, J. C. (1949) *Over de Ontwikkeling, de Determinatie en de Betekenis van de Epiphyse en de Paraphyse van de Amphibien.* Arnhem: Van der Wiel.
VIVIEN-ROELS, B. (1970) *Z. Zellforsch. mikrosk. Anat.* **104**, 429–448.

WESSELLS, N. and COHEN, J. (1968) *Devl Biol.* **18**, 294–309.
WESSELLS, N. and EVANS, J. (1968) *Devl Biol.* **17**, 413–446.
WRENN, J. T. and WESSELLS, N. K. (1969) *J. exp. Zool.* **171**, 359.
YOUNG, R. W. and BOK, D. (1969) *J. Cell Biol.* **42**, 392–403.
YOUNG, R. W. and DROZ, B. (1968) *J. Cell Biol.* **38**, 169–184.

DISCUSSION

Miline: We have studied the morphogenesis of the pineal gland of *Rana temporaria* tadpoles kept in darkness. We saw an immigration of mast cells near the subcommissural organ and the pineal gland. Have you made the same observation? Secondly, the maturation of the supraoptic nucleus parallels the development of the pineal gland in this species. Have you found the maturation of these two organs to be parallel or at different rates in the West Coast newt?

Kelly: We have not made parallel observations on the supraoptic nucleus or any of the hypothalamic structures in this species, so I have no information on that aspect.

There are mast cells to be found in the connective tissue spaces around pineal organs in this species (*Taricha torosa*) at all later stages of development. They are rather strange morphologically, by comparison to the mast cells seen in mammalian species, but Japanese workers (Setoguti and Nakamura 1963) have identified such cells as being mast cells. We have never seen them within the pineal parenchyma in newts, nor along ventricular surfaces. As I've indicated, we do find macrophages along pineal luminal and ventricular surfaces during early larval stages.

Axelrod: You mentioned filamentous material in pinealocytes. Barondes (1968) has shown that nerve terminals contain a filamentous material identified as glucosamine. Intercellular recognition is also reported to be mediated by glycoproteins (Crandall and Brock 1968).

Kelly: We may be talking about two separate things here. Extrinsic, cell-coating glycoproteins may well turn out to be involved in cell recognition and attachment. I showed images of filamentous materials that lie *within* the cytoplasm of the cells. Their attachment to cell membranes may also involve glycoprotein vehicles. The evidence that these filaments are contractile is circumstantial, being derived from cases where their specific orientation seems closely associated with very dramatic and rapid changes in cell shape. Ishikawa, Bischoff and Holtzer (1969) have isolated these filaments from a wide variety of epithelial cell types as well as from various mesenchymal cells and their derivatives, and have shown that they react with heavy meromyosin to form the "arrowhead" pattern characteristic of actin filaments reacting with heavy meromyosin. This suggests that these filaments are "actin-like" and produce their effect by a contractile process. I think we now have problems in defining the nature of the action of such filaments; problems which can be related to those that have plagued us with regard to smooth muscle.

Axelrod: I just wonder if these contractile elements are like microtubules of nerves, and whether you have tried specific precipitants of micro-tubular proteins like vinblastin and colchicine?

Kelly: We have not, but several workers are now busy with this kind of analysis of microtubular systems. One can abolish microtubules by appropriate treatment with the agents you mentioned and then analyse developmental changes. Likewise, cytochalasin can be used to destroy selectively the much smaller filament types that I alluded to (see, for example, Wrenn and Wessells 1970), and a similar analysis can be made. According to the earlier work of Byers and Porter (1964), and a number of others since, the 20–25 nm (200–250 Å) diameter microtubules seem to be involved in the *elongation* of cells, not contraction.

In the systems I described here, microtubules are present, predominantly along the long axis of those cells that are becoming columnar. By contrast, the filaments are mainly found paralleling the apical or basal surfaces and seem to be concerned with narrowing either the apex or the base of the cell.

Oksche: The apparent lack of nerve cells in amphibian pineals is a technical problem, I believe, and I think that light microscopic methods are much more helpful here than electron microscopy. It is possible to modify methylene blue and Golgi techniques so that they produce full images of nerve cells in amphibian pineals, with all their processes.

Kelly: I don't doubt this, and although we haven't made a major effort on this problem, I do think that nerve cells are more difficult to discern by any of these techniques in the pineal organ of this species. I'm encouraged by the fact that W. Flight, working on the East Coast newt (personal communication), has been able to detect ganglion cells in the pineal organ but finds very few of them. It may be that in newts this is an organ which just doesn't have a very high complement of nerve cells. While they may easily be detected by certain light microscopical procedures, it may take serial thin sections for electron microscopy, which is what he is doing, to work them out adequately.

Collin: The demonstration of the sensory nerve cells is certainly a difficult technical problem, related to the intrinsic characters of such cells in vertebrates, as several authors have found. But I don't believe that the apparent scarcity of nerve cells in some Anamniota is only due to technical insufficiency: I think the phylogenetic aspects must also be considered. For example, in the lamprey (*Lampetra planeri*) it is very interesting to compare the numbers of ganglion cells in the pineal and in the parapineal. By different methods, in the same animal, ganglion cells are always proportionally numerous in the pineal but scarce in the parapineal. Furthermore, in the pineal, the photoreceptors are typical and numerous. In the parapineal, photoreceptor cells are present, but a great number of them are considered to be rudimentary (Meiniel 1970). Typical synapses of the ribbon type are also more numerous in the pineal. When compared to other pineal organs of Anamniota, the pineal of the lamprey seems to be fully differentiated (see also the comparative study of the pineal tracts in vertebrates, Collin 1969). Dr Meiniel concluded that the parapineal is a photoreceptor but one part of its photoreceptive potential seems to be lost. I think that the famous "rudimentation" of the pineal sensory apparatus in the Amniota, which can be present to a greater or lesser extent and is sometimes complete, is also present in some Anamniota. It is certainly difficult to show this by electrophysiological means, but I think that cytophysiologists can demonstrate this partial "rudimentation".

Dr Kelly, your material is certainly a very interesting one and if one accepts the validity of the few ganglion cells detected, you have perhaps here one proof of the "rudimentation" in the pineal of an Anamniote. Nevertheless, new studies seem needed on the rudimentary character of the outer segments and the connexions between photoreceptor cells and the scarce ganglion cells.

Arstila: Something which seems to be common to all types of photo-receptors is that they are formed of stacks of lamellae, which closely resemble myelin lamellae. I recall that in the rat pineal gland we have sometimes seen pinealocyte processes which contain irregular stacks of closely apposed membranes. Whether these structures have anything to do with the rudimentary photoreceptors, we do not know. A comparative analysis of the development and degeneration of the outer segments in the West Coast newt and these organelles in the rat pinealocyte might be helpful, in order to see whether these organelles display similar fine structural features at any stage of development.

Kelly: Some of our earlier work on adult frogs (*Rana pipiens*) (Kelly and Smith 1964) seems to show that even in the adult pineal organs there are early stages in the development of outer segments: profiles of cilia with membranes beginning to form around them. They closely resemble those seen in eyes and pineal organs during embryonic stages. The implication (now supported by Dr A. Bunt's unpublished work) may be that whole outer segments are constantly being cast off, removed and renewed. An alternative possibility is that only the membranes are being turned over so their material moves gradually from base to distal tip in a way similar to what appears to happen in retinal rods (Young and Droz 1968; Young and Bok 1969).

Dodt: I would like to direct your attention to the exact numbers of receptors and ganglion cells, because this has many implications for the functional aspects of the pineal, such as its capacity to detect small quantities of light.

Kappers: It is quite possible that in the pineals of non-mammalian vertebrates a variable number of basal processes of photoreceptor cells may terminate on pineal sensory nerve cells. So far, however, we are still in the dark about the exact numbers, which may vary considerably in the different classes, orders and even species.

Kelly: In terms of absolute numbers, there are probably fewer than 100 photoreceptors at any one time in the pineal of the West Coast newt during developing or adult stages. As I've indicated, their relation to ganglion cells of the organ is obscure. However, another possibility to be considered is that basal processes of the photoreceptor cells *leave* the organ and find sites of synapse in the diencephalic roof. There is some evidence for this, because Dr A. Hendrickson and I (unpublished data) have found cytoplasmic profiles which contain synaptic ribbons in the posterior commissural region. Those profiles might be either the basal processes of photoreceptors or, by analogy with the situation in the retina, the basal processes of bipolar cells.

REFERENCES

BARONDES, S. H. (1968) *J. Neurochem.* **15**, 699.
BYERS, B. and PORTER, K. (1964) *Proc. natn. Acad. Sci. U.S.A.* **52**, 1091–1099.
COLLIN, J. P. (1969) *Annls Stn Biol. Besse-en-Chandesse* suppl. 1, 1–359.
CRANDALL, M. A. and BROCK, T. D. (1968) *Science* **161**, 473–475.
ISHIKAWA, H., BISCHOFF, R. and HOLTZER, H. (1969) *J. Cell Biol.* **43**, 312–328.
KELLY, D. E. and SMITH, S. W. (1964) *J. Cell Biol.* **22**, 565–587.
MEINIEL, A. (1970) *J. Neuro-visc. Rel.*, in press.
SETOGUTI, T. and NAKAMURA, H. (1963) *Arch Histol. Jap.* **23**, 311–335.
WRENN, J. T. and WESSELS, N. K. (1970) *Proc. natn. Acad. Sci. U.S.A.* **66**, 904–908.
YOUNG, R. W. and BOK, D. (1969) *J. Cell Biol.* **42**, 392–403.
YOUNG, R. W. and DROZ, B. (1968) *J. Cell Biol.* **39**, 169–184.

DIFFERENTIATION AND REGRESSION OF THE CELLS OF THE SENSORY LINE IN THE EPIPHYSIS CEREBRI[*]

Jean-Pierre Collin

Laboratoire de Biologie animale, Université de Clermont-Ferrand, Complexe Scientifique des Cezeaux, Aubière, France

It has been generally accepted for some time that the pineal organ is sensory in lower vertebrates and glandular in higher vertebrates. But in fact the distinction between these two basically different physiological states was still ill-defined until recently, perhaps precisely because this concept needs to be reconsidered.

The transformation of the pineal organ has been considered from the morphological and histological aspects for some time. The electron microscope now enables us to tackle the problem on the level of cellular transformations. This paper deals with the different cell types and with establishing important links in the phylogeny of pineal cells. I have tried, where possible, to infer functional consequences, in agreement with current electrophysiological, biochemical and physiological data.

Several authors agree that the pineal organ of lower vertebrates contains three chief cell types, namely sensory cells, ganglion cells and supportive cells (Fig. 1). If the organ tends to become essentially glandular in the Amniota, how can we explain the well-known morphological and functional transformation ? Two hypotheses may be mentioned. According to the first, the elements involved in the sensory function (photoreceptor cells and ganglion cells whose axons conduct the photic stimuli to the epithalamic part of the brain) disappear and another cell type takes on the function of the pineal—for example the supportive cells (glial cells), which are similar to the Müller cells in the retina of the lateral eyes (Fig. 1a, b). On the other hypothesis, the receptive and conductive elements which were involved in the sensory function in the Anamniota persist throughout the vertebrates (Bargmann 1943) but undergo important transformations (Fig. 1b), or even disappear, in the case of the ganglion cell (Fig. 1b).

[*] In gratitude and with admiration this paper is dedicated to Professor J. Ariëns Kappers on his sixtieth birthday.

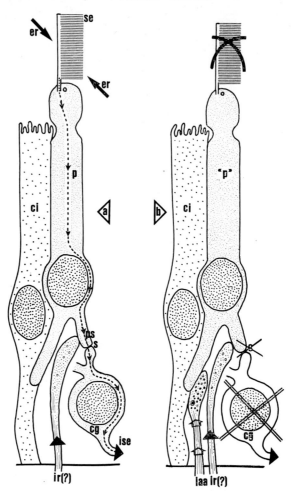

FIG. I. Hypothesis of the continuity of photoreceptor cells in the pineal organs of vertebrates. (*a*) Diagram depicting the cell types of a pineal organ presumed to be photoreceptive. (*b*) Diagram of the three cell types in a pineal organ presumed to have lost the sensory function. Crossed out elements represent the possible transformations, in the sense of a regression. Cg, ganglion cell; ci, supportive cell; er, radiant energy; iaa, autonomic afferent innervation; ir ?, feedback innervation (?); ise, sensory innervation; P and "P", cells of photoreceptor type; ps, synaptic pedicle (neurotransmitter pole); se, outer segment (photoreceptive pole); s, synapse.

In fact, from the most recent investigations it appears that the "photoreceptor" cell is a permanent element in the vertebrate series (Collin 1969*d*), which undergoes important changes during phylogeny so that it is no longer possible, in some groups of vertebrates, to use the term "photoreceptor cell". Although the sensory pinealo-fugal and sympathetic pinealo-petal innervations are closely linked to this subject, on the functional level, I shall not be able to consider them in this paper (Fig. 1); reference should be made to the research and surveys of Kappers (1960–1969), Oksche and co-workers (1962–1969), Collin and co-workers (1966–1969) and Wurtman, Axelrod and Kelly (1968).

DIFFERENTIATION OF PHOTORECEPTOR CELLS IN THE LOWER VERTEBRATES: ELECTRON MICROSCOPIC STUDIES

Petromyzontidae (Lampetra planeri)

The information presented here is a summary of detailed accounts (Collin 1968d, 1969a, b, d; Collin and Meiniel 1968a, b). The photoreceptor cell of *Lampetra*, studied in winter, appears typical (Fig. 2). Like those of the lateral eyes, it is the most differentiated cell type of the pineal retina. It looks like the cone of the lateral eyes and consists of four basic regions: *outer and inner segments* (Figs. 2, 3) joined by a short connecting piece; *a cell body* (Fig. 2) which contains the nucleus; and a *basal pedicle* (Fig. 2) resembling an unmyelinated and branched nerve fibre, which synapses with the dendritic processes (Fig. 2) originating from intraepithelial ganglion cells, as has been shown previously (Collin and Meiniel 1968a, b; Collin 1969b, d).

The outer and inner segments protrude (Fig. 2) into the wide lumen of the pineal organ (the retina is direct). The outer segment (Fig. 3) or photoreceptive pole, a cap-like structure, is derived from the axial centriole (Fig. 4a) and contains a 9 + 0 fibrillar pattern. Striated rootlets (Figs. 3, 4a) extend basally from the centriolar apparatus into the inner segment. Like those of the cones of the lateral eyes, most of the outer segments are composed of many regular disks or sacks (Figs. 3, 5), each of them consisting of a double membrane (Fig. 3). These disks are formed by multiple infoldings of the cell membrane (Fig. 3). Every membrane appears triple-layered (Fig. 4b: the two opaque layers are connected by opaque septa extending across the light middle layer). A similar substructure has also been observed in the membrane elements of the outer segments of retinal receptor cells (Nilsson 1964). Thus the outer segment appears as a stack of varying length made up of very long disks which are often folded (resulting in polymorphism of the outer segments: Figs. 3, 5) and wide open. These observations are quite different from those preliminarily reported by Eakin (1963) in *Petromyzon marinus*. Previously a maximum of 130 disks, approximately 18–23 nm (180–230 Å) thick, had been found. They must be of great importance for the excitation of photoreceptor cells by light, since they appear to offer a large membrane area to the incoming radiant energy.

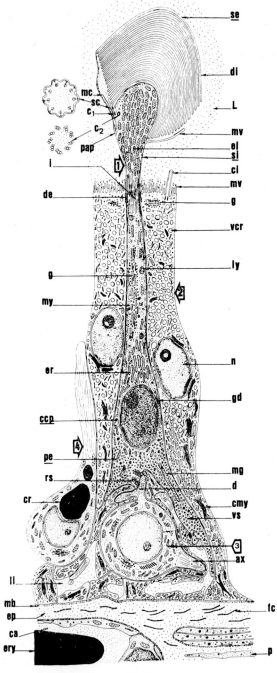

FIG. 2

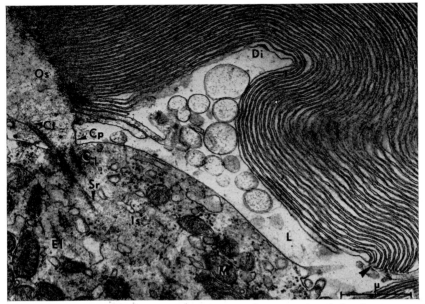

FIG. 3. A photoreceptor cell (pineal organ of *Lampetra planeri*) showing the outer (Os) and inner segments (Is) joined by a connecting piece (Cp). Notice at the arrow that the disks are open to the extracellular space, reminding one of the infoldings of the plasma membrane of the cilium. C_1, axial centriole; Ct, ciliary tubules; Di, disks; El, ellipsoid; L, lumen of the pineal organ; M, mitochondria; Sr, striated rootlets.

The distal part of the inner segment is connected to the proximal part by a neck region, surrounded by a junctional zone (Fig. 2). Numerous microtubules are also found here, running parallel to the axis of the inner segment (Fig. 2). The distal portion of the inner segment contains the centriolar apparatus (Fig. 4*a*) and numerous mitochondria (Fig. 2) with tubular cristae, reminding one of the *ellipsoid* which is supposed to deliver the energy for the activity of receptor cells in the lateral eye (Sjöstrand 1961).

FIG. 2. Schematic representation of cell types found in the retina of the sensory pineal organ of *Lampetra planeri*. (1) Photoreceptor cell. (2) Supportive cell. (3) Ganglion cell. (4) Cell with residual bodies (satellite cells are absent in this diagram). Ax, axon of a ganglion cell; C_1, axial centriole; C_2, oblique centriole; ca, capillary lumen; ccp, cellular body; ci, cilium; cmy, myeloid body; cr, residual body; d, dendritic process; de, junctional zone, desmosome; di, disk or sack; el, ellipsoid; ep, perivascular space; er, granular endoplasmic reticulum; ery, erythrocyte; fc, collagen fibrils; g, Golgi complex; gd, dense granule; i, cellular neck; l, lumen of the pineal organ; li, intercellular space; Ly, lysosome; mb, basement membrane; mc, ciliary club; mg, giant mitochondrion; mv, microvilli; my, myoid; n, nucleus; P, fibroblast; Pap, apical process; pe, synaptic pedicle; rs, synaptic ribbon; sc, connecting piece; se, outer segment; si, inner segment; vcr, crystalline vacuole; vs, synaptic vesicle.

In the proximal portion of the inner segment (the *myoid*), one can recognize lysosomes and a well-developed Golgi complex (Fig. 2) surrounded by numerous vesicles, some of them (mean diameter 100 nm, 1000 Å) having an electron-dense core. Furthermore, a network of the tubular and saccular (rarely agranular) endoplasmic reticulum and free

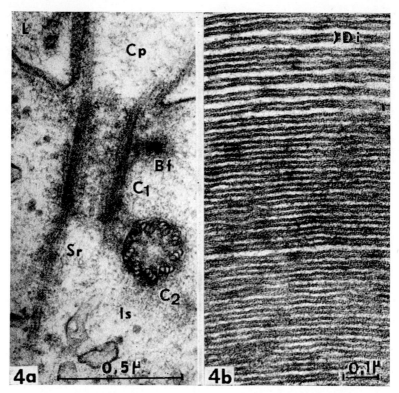

FIG. 4. (*a*) Section of the centriolar apparatus in the inner segment (Is) of a photoreceptor cell in the pineal organ of *Lampetra planeri*. The subunits in the wall of the centriole (C_2) are triple tubular structures. Bf, basal foot; C_1, axial centriole; C_2, oblique centriole; Cp, connecting piece; L, lumen of the pineal organ; Sr, striated rootlet. (*b*) High-power electron micrograph showing profiles of the double-membrane unit disks (Di) of the outer segment of a photoreceptor cell from the pineal organ of *Lampetra planeri*. The fine structure of every membrane is evident in the lower part of the micrograph (see text).

ribosomes surround the nucleus (Fig. 2). The part played by these organelles will be dealt with in a separate section (p. 102).

In the inner segment a typical paraboloid was not found but glycogen particles (energy reserve) are present in all parts of the inner segment. The dilated *cell body* contains a large nucleus and a narrow perikaryon. The *synaptic pedicle* is located in the single ventral plexiform area. This photo-receptor basal process ramifies into several branches. Figs. 6 and 7 show the synaptic zone.

The synaptic pedicle is connected with one or more dendritic processes originating from ganglion cells. In the same way, a dendritic process can be connected with one or more synaptic pedicles (Fig. 6). Synaptic pedicles contain a scanty granular and agranular endoplasmic reticulum, some mitochondria (including one giant mitochondrion), some bundles

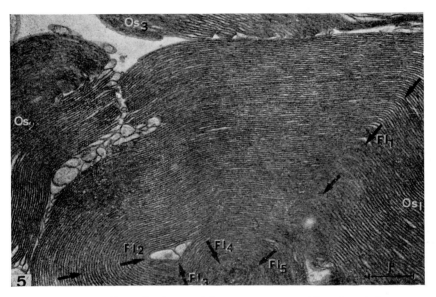

FIG. 5. Small peripheral area of three outer segments (Os_1, Os_2, Os_3) protruding into the lumen of the pineal organ of *Lampetra planeri*. Notice, in inner segment Os_1, the large, regular and curved (Fl_1–Fl_5) disks.

of filaments and electron-dense vesicles originating from the Golgi zone (Fig. 15).

The most striking components involved in synaptic transmission may be mentioned briefly. The terminals of the photoreceptor cells are filled (Fig. 2) with synaptic vesicles (averaging 50 nm, 500 Å in diameter), more or less uniformly distributed throughout the pedicle, although they tend to accumulate near the synaptic ribbons and presynaptic membranes (Fig. 7). The synaptic ribbons (1–7 per branch of pedicle) are confined within the pedicle cytoplasm very close to the presynaptic membrane (Figs. 6, 7), but are not in contact with it. The synaptic vesicles are thought to be the structural elements that contain the neurotransmitter substance.

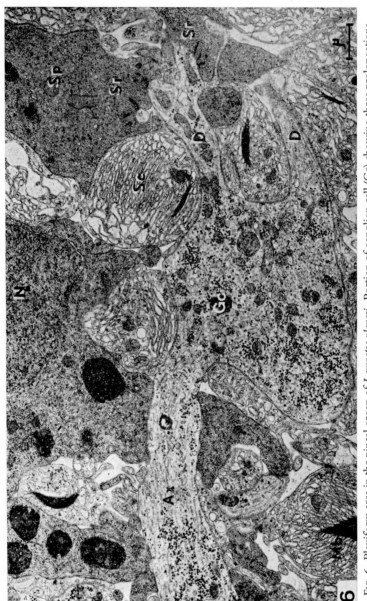

FIG. 6. Plexiform area in the pineal organ of *Lampetra planeri*. Portion of ganglion cell (Gc) showing three prolongations, two dendritic (D) and one axonic (Ax). Synaptic pedicles (Sp) of photoreceptor cells display a dark cytoplasm and numerous synaptic ribbons (Sr) in the vicinity of the dendritic processes (D). Myeloid bodies (Mb) occupy the cytoplasm of support-ive cells (Sc). N, nucleus of a photoreceptive cell.

In the cytoplasm of the synaptic pedicle, between the synaptic ribbons and the presynaptic membrane, is a thin aggregation of dense material (Fig. 7). Such an increase in density is also visible along the postsynaptic membrane (Fig. 7) of the dendritic process, just opposite the synaptic ribbon. Further-more, in the same region, one can recognize transverse filaments or a

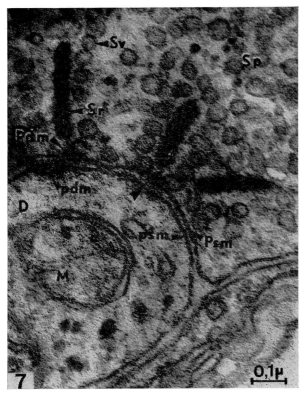

FIG. 7. One synaptic pedicle (Sp) of a photoreceptor cell (pineal organ of *Lampetra planeri*) makes synaptic contact with a dendritic process (D) of a ganglion cell. The synaptic pedicle and the process of the neuron display typical synaptic components: synaptic ribbons (Sr), synaptic vesicles (Sv), an aggregation of dense material (Pdm) just beside the pre-synaptic membrane (Psm). Such an aggregation (pdm) is also present in the dendritic prolongation, just beside the postsynaptic membrane (psm). A longitudinal line, in the synaptic cleft, is indicated by an arrow. M, mitochondrion.

longitudinal line in the synaptic cleft (Fig. 7). All these components of the synaptic membranes appear to be common not only to lateral eye connexions in other vertebrates, but also to chemical synapses.

One of the most striking characteristics of the photoreceptor synapse in the retina of lateral eyes is the fact that dendritic expansions from the bipolar cells penetrate and digitate into the terminal spherule. An important difference appears here: the penetration of the dendritic expansions of ganglion cells (Figs. 2, 6, 7) is not important or quite absent in the pineal, in agreement with the observations of Kelly and Smith (1964) in *Rana*. Moreover, well-developed gutter-shaped depressions, in which are found synaptic ribbons, are quite absent here. What significance all these synaptic components have for the transmission of impulses remains to be ascertained.

Fishes and amphibians

Several ultrastructural investigations were made to gain some understanding of the possible functional significance of the pineal in fishes and amphibians. They indicate a photoreceptive potential of the pineal in these groups. Cone-like photoreceptor cells have been described in the pineal organ of teleosts (Breucker and Horstmann 1965; Rüdeberg 1966, 1968a; Oksche and Kirschstein 1966b, 1967; Omura, Kitoh and Oguri 1969), of dipnoans (Ueck 1969), of chondrichthyes (Rüdeberg 1968b, 1969), of anurans (Oksche and von Harnack 1962; Oksche and Vaupel-von Harnack 1963, 1965a, c; Eakin, Quay and Westfall 1963; Kelly and Smith 1964; Ueck 1968) and of urodele amphibians (Kelly 1965). Cone-like photoreceptor cells resemble those studied in *Lampetra*. Nevertheless, closer attention must be directed to the activity of the Golgi complex and to the connexions between synaptic pedicles and dendritic expansions of ganglion cells.

With electron microscopy, ganglion cells have been found only by Oksche and Vaupel-von Harnack (1963, 1965c) Rüdeberg (1966, 1969) and Ueck (1968). Rüdeberg (1966, 1968a) is doubtful about the presence of synaptic connexions. New studies seem necessary to show the possible relation between the relative scarcity of ganglion cells and synapses and the beginning of the regression of the photosensory function in Anamniota, a fact which is already quite perceptible in Sauropsida (i.e. reptiles and birds).

Lacertilians

The study of the pineal organ in reptiles has been progressing rapidly. Some investigations, such as those made by Steyn (1960), Lierse (1965) and Oksche and Kirschstein (1966a, b, 1968), have reported transformations of the outer segment of sensory cells in several lacertilians, but in all these studies the other regions of the photoreceptor cells, so important for determining their functional significance, are poorly known. Oksche and Kirschstein (1966a, 1968) were sceptical about the photoreceptive function of pineal sensory cells. Wartenberg and Baumgarten (1968) found no evidence of photosensory activity in *Lacerta*.

I have observed specific characteristics of the sensory type of cells which are of primary importance for the functioning of the organ. In *Lacerta muralis* a variety of sensory cells has been found (Fig. 8). Some cone-like photoreceptor cells (Collin 1968*b*, 1969*d*) are still present but the majority of the cells have changed into rudimentary photosensory elements (Collin 1967*a*, *c*, *d*; 1968*b*, *c*; 1969*d*; Collin and Kappers 1968). The cone-like photoreceptors were chiefly found in follicles located in the pars distalis of the pineal organ. Our preliminary investigations (Collin 1968*b*) of the outer (Fig. 9) and inner segments, cell body and basal synaptic pedicle have been completed in our book (Collin 1969*d*).

Only some of the photoreceptor cells (Fig. 8) are well differentiated. These cells resemble those in the parietal eye, with their outer segment and synaptic pedicle (Eakin and Westfall 1959, 1960; Eakin 1963, 1964; Oksche and Kirschstein 1968; Petit 1968; Collin, unpublished results). In *Anguis fragilis* some more or less typical outer segments have been recognized by Oksche and Kirschstein (1968), Collin (1968*a*, 1969*d*) and Petit (1969*b*).

Chelonians

Very recent electron microscopic investigations (Vivien-Roels 1970) on the pineal organ of chelonians have revealed typical morphological features of cone-like photoreceptor cells in *Pseudemys scripta elegans*. They appear to be present only in the posterior wall of the epiphysis cerebri. Like Lutz and Collin (1967) in *Testudo*, Vivien-Roels (1970) was unable to find such typical photoreceptors in the pars distalis and intermedia, where there were only rudimentary photoreceptor cells.

From these recent data it seems to be clear that in lizards and chelonians there is a quantitative regression of typical photoreceptor cells, in agreement with the scarcity of sensory ganglion cells (Kappers 1966, 1967; Collin and Kappers 1968; Collin 1969*d*; Petit 1969*b*; Vivien-Roels 1969, 1970). It is difficult to generalize from this fact to all lizards and chelonians. It is not impossible that a survivor of the secondary era (Mesozoic), such as *Sphenodon*, has retained well-differentiated photoreceptor cells.

THE GRADUAL "RUDIMENTATION" OF SENSORY CELLS: CONCEPT OF MULTIPLICITY OF PHOTORECEPTOR CELLS

Lacertilians

Both reptiles and birds are particularly favourable for the study of the sensory regression of the pineal organ. As has been demonstrated (Collin

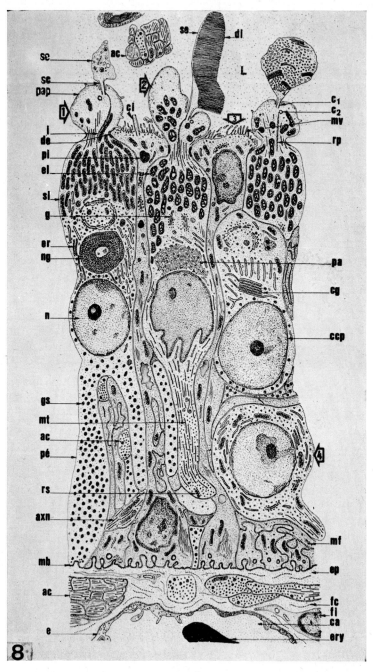

FIG. 8

1967*a, c, d*, 1968*b*, 1969*c, d*; Collin and Kappers 1968; Petit 1969*b*) in *Lacerta viridis* and *muralis*, *Tarentola*, *Chalcides* and *Anguis*, a significant structural regression of the sensory cells occurs. In its general morphological aspects this cell type reminds one of the photoreceptor neurosensory cells, and the four basic regions (see *Lampetra*, p. 81) are still present (Fig. 8). In some structural characteristics, however, this type of element is essentially different, justifying the newly coined term "secretory rudimentary photoreceptor cell" (SRP; Collin 1967–1969).

For example, in *Lacerta muralis*, when compared with the typical conelike photoreceptors (P cells of the same pineal organ), the club-shaped outer segments of SRP cells do not show the regular stacks of disks (Fig. 8). Some outer segments (termed rudimentary: Collin 1967–1969) do not appear to have any organelles. Other rudimentary outer segments show atypical components: clear or dense vesicles, clear vacuoles, dense bodies, multivesicular bodies, and more or less developed concentric membrane structures (Fig. 10). No specific membrane arrangements indicate the presence of a photopigment. Such structures are present in all the lizards studied (see also Oksche and Kirschstein 1968; Petit 1969*b*). This bulbous segment is joined by a connecting piece (9 + 0) to the centriolar apparatus (Fig. 8). In the inner segment, striated rootlets extend from the two centrioles into the basal part (Fig. 8). Another important difference between P and SRP cells concerns the substructure (Fig. 8) of the mitochondria (ellipsoid) and the development and activity of the myoid (ergastoplasm and Golgi complex). Some morphological and functional differences are also found between the glycogenic *nebenkern* of SRP cells and the paraboloid of P cells (see comparative studies and discussion in Collin 1969*d*).

Just below the cell body, the branched asynaptic basal pedicle of the

---

FIG. 8. Pineal organ of *Lacerta muralis*. Diagram illustrating the sensory epithelium. (1) Secretory rudimentary photoreceptor cell (=SRP). (2) Photoreceptor cell (P). (3) Supportive cell. (4) Ganglion cell. Ac: afferent catecholaminergic fibres; Axn, unmyelinated axons; C_1, axial centriole; C_2, oblique centriole; ca, capillary; ccp, cell body of an SRP cell; cg, glycogen body; ci, cilium; de, desmosome; di, disk; e, fenestrated and pinocytotic endothelium; el, ellipsoid; ep, perivascular space; er, granular endoplasmic reticulum; ery, erythrocyte; fc, collagen fibrils; fi, fibroblast; g, Golgi complex; gs, dense granule (50–350 nm, 500–3500 Å); i, cellular neck; L, lumen of the pineal organ; mb, basement membrane; mf, microfilaments; mt, microtubules; mv, microvilli; n, nucleus; ng, glycogen *nebenkern*; pa, paraboloid; pap, apical process of the inner segments of SRP or P cells; pe, synaptic (in P cell) or asynaptic (in SRP cells) pedicle; pi, pigment granule; rp, striated rootlet; rs, synaptic ribbon and vesicles; sc, connecting piece; se, outer segment; si, inner segment.

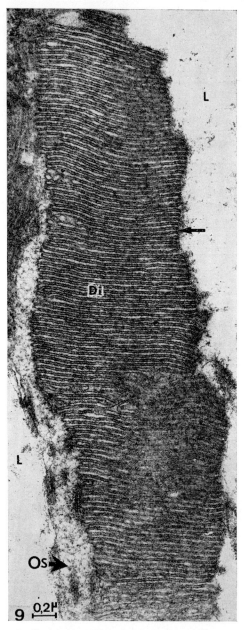

FIG. 9. Longitudinal section through a typical cone-like outer segment
(Os) protruding into the lumen (L) of the pineal organ of *Lacerta
muralis*. The outer segment disks (Di) are connected to the plasma
membrane (arrow).

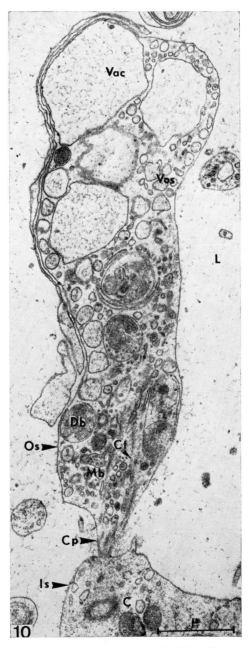

FIG. 10. Rudimentary outer segment (Os) of an SRP cell protruding into
the lumen (L) of the pineal organ of *Lacerta viridis*. Note absence of disks.
Nevertheless, this club-shaped outer segment contains vacuoles (Vac),
vesicles (Vos), dense bodies (Db) and multivesicular bodies (Mb). C,
centriole; Cp, connecting piece; Ct, ciliary tubules; Is, inner segment.

4*

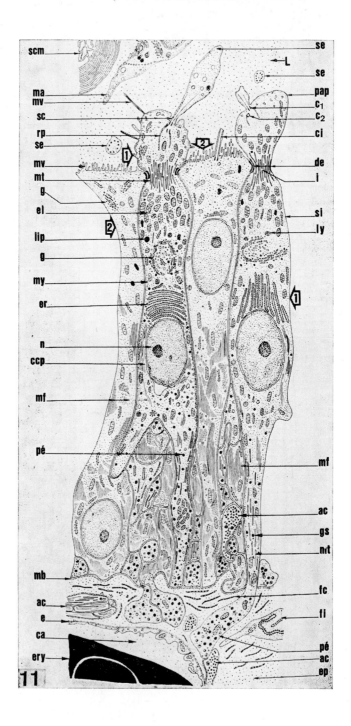

SRP cell is also a very striking characteristic (Fig. 8). At first, typical synaptic connexions were not found (Fig. 8) in the basal processes of SRP cells in many investigations (Collin 1967–1969). Nevertheless, in *Anguis* (Petit 1969*a*, *b*; Collin 1969*d*) and in *Chalcides* (Collin 1969*d*) some atypical structures were found, resembling the vesicle-crowned lamellae of the pineal gland of the rat (Wolfe 1965; Arstila 1967). Their functional significance is still unknown (see discussion in Collin 1969*d*) but we exclude a role in neurotransmission, in the conventional sense. So it is clear that the terminal ending, which originally contained the neurotransmitter substance, is regressive. Furthermore, in numerous cases (Collin 1967*a*, *c*, *d*, 1969*d*; Collin and Kappers 1968; Petit 1969*b*) we have demonstrated that the process makes contact with the basement membrane of the epithelium and in consequence has a vascular polarity (Fig. 8).

From these facts it is clear that SRP cells, with rudimentary outer segments and asynaptic pedicles, have increased, and have then become independent of the ganglion cells (Figs. 8, 21). They represent the majority of "sensory" cells in the pineal organ of the lizards we studied and their photoreceptive function is considered to be lost. But one should not forget that more or less differentiated outer segments also occur (Oksche and Kirschstein 1968; Collin 1967*a*, 1968*b*, 1969*d*; Petit 1969*b*) and that a variety of intermediate cells (P–SRP) are possible between P cells and SRP cells.

All these results and those concerned with innervation explain the qualitative regression of "sensory" cells and in consequence the gradual extinction of the photoreceptive potential in Sauropsida.

Chelonians

In young and adult chelonians many of the photoreceptor cells are also modified. This transformation is morphologically the same as in lacertilians. Thus Vivien and Roels (1967, 1968) and Vivien-Roels (1969, 1970) found rudimentary photoreceptor cells or "pseudosensory cells" in

---

FIG. 11. Cellular types in the follicular epithelium of the pineal organ of the magpie (*Pica pica*). (1) Rudimentary photoreceptor cell. (2) Supportive cell. Ac, autonomic fibres; C_1, axial centriole; C_2, oblique centriole; ca, capillary; ccp, cellular body of a rudimentary photoreceptor cell; ci, cilium; de, desmosome; e, endothelium; el, ellipsoid; ep, perivascular space; er, granular endoplasmic reticulum; ery, erythrocyte; fc, collagen fibrils; fi, fibroblast; G, Golgi apparatus; gs, dense granules (mean diameter 100 nm, 1000 Å); i, cellular neck; lip, lipid droplet; ly, lysosome; ma, macrophage; mb, basement membrane; mf, microfilaments; mt, microtubules; mv, microvilli; my, myoid; n, nucleus; pe, asynaptic pedicle; pap, apical prolongation of the inner segment; ep, striated rootlet; sc, connecting piece; scm, concentric system of membranes; sc, outer segment; si, inner segment.

Pseudemys. In *Testudo*, studied in hibernation, only SRP cells have been seen (Lutz and Collin 1967) in the pars intermedia and distalis of the pineal organ.

Birds

Just as in lacertilians and chelonians, SRP cells in birds do not seem able to respond to a direct light stimulus and in consequence to transmit this response to adjoining neurons. Birds also show an important transformation of the primitively highly specialized photoreceptor cells (Fig. 11).

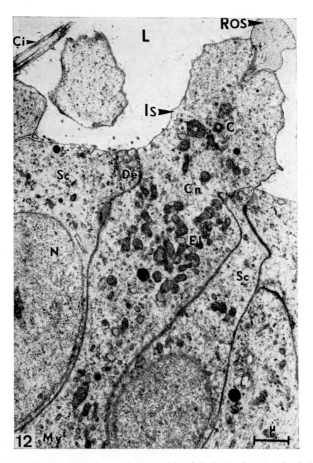

FIG. 12. SRP cell in the epithelium of a follicle in the pineal of the magpie (*Pica pica*). The inner segment (Is) protrudes into the lumen (L) of the follicle. The outer segment is rudimentary (Ros). C, centriole; Ci, cilium of a supportive cell; Cn, cellular neck; De, desmosome; El, ellipsoid; My, region of the myoid; N, nucleus in a supportive cell; Sc, supportive cell.

The functional requirements are met through the newly elaborated segmented organization. The four basic regions still remain, as in lacertilians
and chelonians. Club-like outer segments (Figs. 12 and 13) are present in
embryos and young and adult birds (Collin 1966*a*, *b*, *c*, 1968*a*, 1969*d*; Lutz
and Collin 1967; Oksche 1968; Oksche and Vaupel-von Harnack 1965*b*;

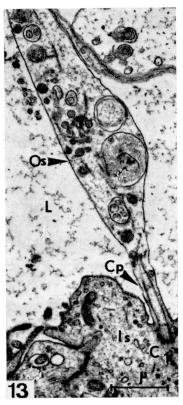

FIG. 13. Rudimentary outer segment (Os) in the pineal of the quail
(young bird). The classical disks are absent but some more or less dense
vacuoles, vesicles and multivesicular bodies are found. C_1, axial centriole;
Cp, connecting piece; Is, inner segment; L, lumen of a follicle.

Oksche, Morita and Vaupel-von Harnack 1969; Quay, Renzoni and Eakin
1968; Bischoff 1969). Sometimes they can be long (several micrometres)
but their internal structures do not consist of regular stacks of flattened
membrane disks. In some cases (Quay, Renzoni and Eakin 1968; Bischoff
1969) the regularly polarized stacks of membranes are not considered to
be typical disks (Oksche and Kirschstein 1969; Collin 1969*d*). The outer
segment is therefore thought to be rudimentary or atypical. The ciliated
connecting structure has lost the two central filaments, as in other sensory

cells, but the nine pairs of circumferential filaments terminate in one of the typical centrioles located with their striated rootlets in the inner segment. The ellipsoid portion (Fig. 12) of the inner segment and the cellular neck (with numerous microtubules) are composed of a more or less dense aggregation of mitochondria, whereas the myoid contains the Golgi

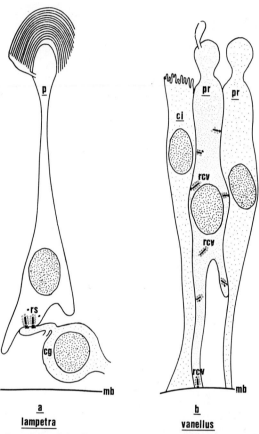

a
lampetra

b
vanellus

FIG. 14. Location of the "synaptic" components in the photoreceptor cells of *Lampetra* and rudimentary photoreceptor cells of the bird *Vanellus*. (a) Somato-dendritic synaptic ribbons (rs) in the photoreceptor cell (p) of *Lampetra*. (b) somato-somatic "vesicle-crowned lamellae" (rcv) (or "ribbons surrounded by vesicles", Collin 1968a) in the rudimentary photoreceptor cells (pr) of *Vanellus*. cg, ganglion cell; ci, supportive cell; mb, basement membrane.

complex—packed vesicular and saccular components with considerable quantities of ribosomes, either free or adhering to the membranes (Fig. 11). The nucleus is located in the broadened cell body (Fig. 11). The branched asynaptic pedicle, attached to the nuclear region (Fig. 11), makes contact with the basement membrane. Furthermore, in the magpie for example, asynaptic pedicles go through the basement membrane (Fig. 11), then extend across the perivascular spaces (vascular polarity). The asynaptic pedicle (Collin 1969c, d) is characterized by a moderate quantity of rough endoplasmic reticulum, mitochondria, systems of microtubules and microfilaments, and dense granules (100 nm, 1000 Å). Numerous clear vesicles, with an average diameter of 50 nm (500 Å) (Vp vesicles of Collin 1969c, d), which are also found in reptiles, are not considered to be "synaptic vesicles". Atypical "synaptic ribbons" or "ribbons surrounded by vesicles" (Collin 1968a, 1969d) are present (Fig. 14) in some species.

Here also, it seems that the SRP cells of the pineal organ of birds have become independent of ganglion cells (Fig. 11). Furthermore, the ganglion cells are scarce. They have been shown recently in electron microscopic studies by Ueck (1970).

In summary, most investigators are unable to find typical sensory cells in birds like the P cells in reptiles. If they are present in some birds, they are certainly rare. Some authors, who have postulated a photoreceptive activity in the bird pineal, have not been able to demonstrate typical cone-like photoreceptors in their electron microscopic studies. Thus a uniform functional scheme, valid for all Sauropsida (reptiles and birds), cannot be established at present.

It is clear that several types of "sensory" cells can be found in the same pineal organ, and this has led to the concept of a multiplicity of "photo-receptor" cells. This idea was assumed by Kappers (1966, 1967) in lacertilians and was demonstrated by Collin (1968–1969). In Anamniota, multiplicity has not yet been established, but it is still a possibility.

In lacertilians and chelonians, typical P cells and SRP cells are present in the same pineal organ but we also think that intermediate cells (P–SRP) are present, perhaps with different degrees of sensory activity. In birds, only rudimentary or atypical "photoreceptor" cells are recognized in the most recent studies. Moreover (Collin 1969d; see also below) the pinealocytes characteristic of snakes and mammals may also be found in Sauropsida.

Ophidians and mammals

It is difficult to find pineal cells resembling sensory cells in snakes or in mammals. Nevertheless, Petit (1969a) and Collin (1969d) found "sensory" cells and pinealocytes in young embryos of *Tropidonotus* and *Vipera*. These cells disappear quickly during ontogeny and in older embryos only pinealocytes are found. In the laboratory rat, Wolfe (1965) found some cells (see discussion in Collin 1969d) with inner segments, reminiscent of those described in the sensory cells of lower vertebrates.

The pinealocyte of ophidians and mammals is now considered to be the chief cell type of the pineal gland in these groups. Studies relating to it are numerous (Wurtman, Axelrod and Kelly 1968; Collin 1969d for references). The pinealocyte does not usually show the segmented organization of photoreceptor cells (Fig. 21), and this can be related to the disappearance of the lumen of the organ. Wartenberg (1968) has discussed the presence of unipolar and multipolar pinealocytes. Pinealocytes make contact with other pinealocytes but processes or pedicles also terminate close to the basement membrane of the epithelium, or enter the perivascular space (vascular polarity). The cytoplasm of the cell body contains the usual organelles (centriolar apparatus, mitochondria, smooth and rough endoplasmic reticulum, Golgi complex, lysosomes, lipid droplets). In *Tropidonotus*, Vivien (1964a) was able to show a 9 + 0 cilium. Anderson (1965), in cattle, also found a bulbous modified cilium. Another cytoplasmic organelle, peculiar to pinealocytes, has been found by several investigators (Wolfe 1965; Arstila 1967; Wartenberg 1968; Collin 1969d). Its overall structure appears (Fig. 21) very similar to the synaptic ribbons of photoreceptor cells, but its functional significance remains obscure. These organelles are called "vesicle-crowned lamellae" and they are an important feature in the evolutionary history of pinealocytes. The pedicles of these cells usually contain mitochondria, microtubules, "vesicle-crowned lamellae", small clear vesicles morphologically equivalent to the synaptic vesicles and dense granules (about 100 nm, 1000 Å in diameter).

In its general aspects the pinealocyte seems quite different from the photoreceptor cell. However, I have suggested why the SRP cells may be considered as the forerunners of pinealocytes (Collin 1969d; see also below).

PHOTORECEPTOR CELLS AND SENSORY FUNCTION IN THE PINEAL ORGAN

Electron microscopic and electrophysiological studies can help to establish the function of any given pineal organ. The epiphysis of the lamprey, *Lampetra planeri*, is characterized by typical cone-like photoreceptor elements. Furthermore, its sensory innervation is relatively well developed (Collin 1968d, 1969b, d). The observations in this paper and those concerning the innervation support the concept that the pineal organ of *Lampetra* is a typically photoreceptive organ, but electrophysiological data are still lacking. Somewhat different conclusions have been drawn for the parapineal organ of the same animal (Meiniel 1970). Presumably the active photopigments are located in the membranes of the disks and phototransductive processes are initiated there, but further biochemical investigations are necessary to demonstrate the photopigment and neurotransmitter substance.

Several electron microscopic (see references above) and electrophysiological findings (Dodt 1963, 1964a, b, c, 1966; Dodt and Heerd 1962; Dodt and Jacobson 1963; Dodt and Morita 1964, 1967; Morita 1965a, b, 1966b, 1969; Morita and Dodt 1965) point to sensory activity in the pineal organ of fishes and amphibians. Since connexions between the cells of the photoreceptor type and ganglion cells have been established to some extent in some species, further anatomical investigation could be important in tracing the possible beginning of regression of some of the sensory elements.

In the lizards a variety of sensory cell types has been found. Cone-like photoreceptors (P cells) are still present but the majority of photoreceptive cells have changed into SRP cells. As far as the pinealo-fugal sensory innervation is concerned, a reduction of the number of sensory cells and of the axons present in the pineal tract occurs (Kappers 1966, 1967; Collin and Kappers 1968; Collin 1969d), in accordance with the regression of the photosensitive function of the sensory cells. In agreement with Kappers (1967), we find (Collin 1969d) that the photosensory function is residual in the pineal organ of some lizards, for instance *Lacerta* and *Anguis*. Recent electrophysiological investigations have been made in *Lacerta* (Hamasaki and Dodt 1969). Photic responses are obtained in *Lacerta*, *Iguana* and *Acanthodactylus*.

It was pointed out earlier that P cells and ganglion cells are only known in the pars proximalis of the pineal organ of chelonians (p. 89). So far, only SRP cells have been observed in other regions. As in *Lacerta*, we consider that a residual photosensory activity is present in these reptiles (Collin 1969d).

Despite many electron microscopic investigations, the presence of fully developed cone-like sensory cells in birds has not been established yet (Oksche 1968; Oksche and Vaupel-von Harnack 1966; Oksche, Morita and Vaupel-von Harnack 1969; Oksche and Kirschstein 1969; Collin 1966a, b, c, 1967b, c, 1968a, 1969c, d; Lutz and Collin 1967; Fujie 1968). The question of the presence of pineal ganglion cells in birds (Quay and Renzoni 1963; Quay, Renzoni and Eakin 1968; Kappers, 1965; Collin 1969d; Ueck 1970) and snakes (Vivien and Roels 1968; Petit 1969a) requires further studies. It is not impossible that some epithalamic components have been incorporated in some pineals of Sauropsida.

The absence of any electrical activity related to the onset or cessation of light in the pineal body of *Coturnix* and *Passer* allows Ralph and Dawson (1968) to conclude: "The negative findings to date are an inadequate sample on which to base conclusions and do not exclude the possibility that some birds may have pineals that are photoreceptive in the conventional sense". However, if we consider the trend of pineal structural and functional evolution and the results of electrophysiological investigations (Morita 1966a; Ralph and Dawson 1968; Oksche, Morita and Vaupel-von Harnack 1969; Hamasaki, cited by Oksche and Kirschstein 1969) it seems likely that much or perhaps all the photoreceptive potential is lost in birds (Collin 1969d). In snakes and mammals the loss of the photoreceptive potential is generally accepted.

To draw final conclusions on the sensory function of the pineal of vertebrates, we can now infer such sensory activity, characterized by achromatic and/or chromatic responses to light stimulation (Dodt, and Dodt and co-workers 1963–1967; Morita and Morita and co-workers 1965–1969; Hamasaki and Dodt 1969), in Anamniota, lacertilians and chelonians. In the different groups different degrees of the photoreceptive potential occur, this potential disappearing gradually as one goes up the vertebrate scale. How the brain uses the information obtained by the light-sensitive cells and transmitted by the pinealo-fugal sensory innervation still remains obscure. Resolution of this important problem depends upon our future knowledge of "the point of impact" of the ganglion cell axonic endings carrying signals to the brain.

SECRETORY ACTIVITY IN SENSORY-TYPE CELLS AND PINEALOCYTES

The pineal is known (more particularly in higher vertebrates) to be very rich in biogenic amines and in the enzymes involved in the synthesis and metabolism of these active compounds (see reviews of Wurtman, Axelrod and Kelly 1968; Kappers 1969). Recent electron microscopic and histochemical data will now be considered in relation to the problem of which cell type is responsible for the synthesis and storage of active compounds.

As with rods and cones of lateral eyes (Young and Droz 1968), the cone-like photoreceptor cells of *Lampetra planeri* (Collin 1968d, 1969a, d) contain a well-developed protein synthetic machinery located in the myoid (Fig. 2). In the same region the Golgi area is evidently responsible for the concentration and packaging of secretory products, because of the close relationship between this apparatus and dense granules having a mean diameter of 100 nm (1000 Å). These dense-cored vesicles, bounded by a membrane 6–7 nm (60–70 Å) in thickness, have a three-layered structure and possess a fine granular appearance which gives them a density varying between moderate and high. A clear zone lies between the matrix and the bounding membrane. However, P cells are not heavily loaded with granules. These

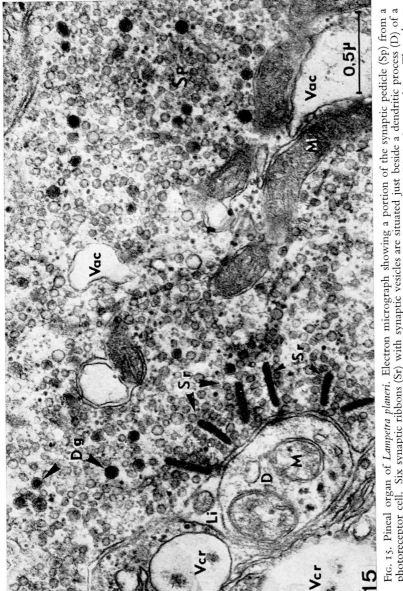

FIG. 15. Pineal organ of *Lampetra planeri*. Electron micrograph showing a portion of the synaptic pedicle (Sp) from a photoreceptor cell. Six synaptic ribbons (Sr) with synaptic vesicles are situated just beside a dendritic process (D) of a ganglion cell. Numerous synaptic vesicles and some dense granules (Dg) are also visible in the cytoplasm. These dense granules, also present in the vicinity of the Golgi complex, migrate into the synaptic pedicle. Li, intercellular space; M, mitochondrion; Vac, vacuole; Vcr, crystalline vacuole.

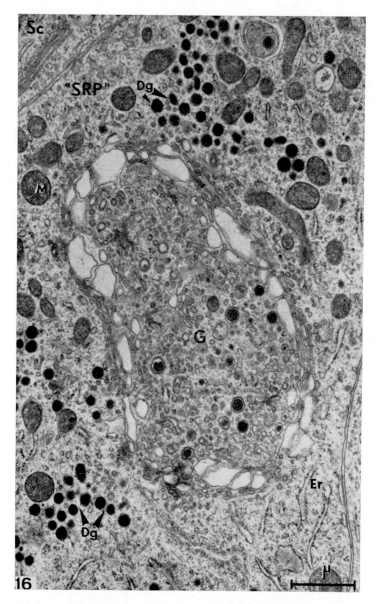

FIG. 16. Electron micrograph of an SRP cell from *Lacerta viridis* illustrating numerous dense granules originating within the Golgi zone (G). These dense granules (Dg) are considered to contain 5-HT. Er, granular endoplasmic reticulum; M, mitochondrion; Sc, supportive cell.

granules are mostly confined to the synaptic pedicles, sometimes just beside the synaptic ribbons or intercellular spaces (Fig. 15). In the same pedicle the presence of all intermediate forms between dense granules and clear vesicles, all of the same diameter, seems to indicate a release mechanism. So far the nature of these granules is unknown, but the possibility that an indoleamine is concentrated here with a protein (?) can be suggested.

In other Anamniota, Collin and Meiniel in *Lampetra* (1968a) and then Ueck (1968) in Pipidae found such granules in the synaptic pedicles of the sensory cells. Thus the observations reported here support the concept that pineal photoreceptor cells can have a functional duality (Collin 1969a, d).

The SRP cells of *Lacerta* show signs of production and storage of the secretory product (Collin 1967a, c, d, 1968c, 1969d; Collin and Kappers 1968). In the region of the myoid, granular endoplasmic reticulum and free ribosomes are well developed (Fig. 8), indicating protein synthesis. In the same region the Golgi complex shows all intermediate forms between Golgi saccules containing small amounts of dense granular material and apparently mature granules filled with a similar substance (Fig. 16). These granules (most of them measuring between 100 and 250 nm—1000 and 2500 Å—in *Lacerta muralis*) are concentrated in special regions (Fig. 8) such as inner segments, cell bodies and asynaptic pedicles often located just beside the perivascular spaces (see Collin 1967c, d, 1968c, 1969d for differences in several lizards). An indoleamine (serotonin, 5-HT) was shown to be important in the pineal epithelium of *Lacerta* (Quay, Jongkind and Kappers 1967; Collin 1967d, 1968c, 1969d; Wartenberg and Baumgarten 1969b). Serotonin (Fig. 17) has been located in SRP cells (Collin 1967d, 1968c, 1969d; Wartenberg and Baumgarten 1969b). After the injection of large doses of reserpine (Collin 1969d) the yellow fluorescence (technique of Falck and Hillarp) disappears completely, but the depletion of granules (Fig. 18a, b) is not so evident (see Collin 1969d). The presence of a storage complex with a protein can therefore be accepted for dense granules. Furthermore, the existence of several possible fractions of 5-HT has been suggested: namely a free serotonin pool and a bound serotonin pool (Collin 1968c, 1969d; Wartenberg and Baumgarten 1969b).

In other lizards, such as *Anguis* (see also Petit 1969b), *Tarentola* and *Chalcides*, a secretory activity is also found in SRP cells (Collin 1967c, 1969d). Granules (mean diameter 100 nm, 1000 Å) are confined to asynaptic pedicles but are scarce in comparison with those studied in *Lacerta* (Collin 1967c, 1969d). Furthermore serotonin is certainly present only in small quantities (Collin 1969d). In *Lacerta*, studied in the winter, I have recently shown (unpublished results) that specimens placed in complete

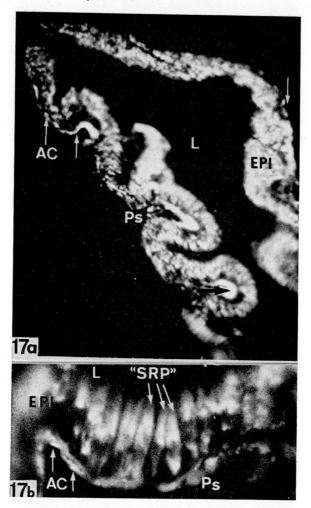

FIG. 17. (*a*) Intensely fluorescent epithelium (EPI) in *Lacerta viridis*, corresponding to the presence of 5-HT (technique of Falck and Hillarp). (*b*) SRP cells emitting an intense yellow fluorescence in the myoid and the synaptic pedicle (technique of Falck and Hillarp). AC, noradrenergic fibres; L, lumen of the pineal organ; Ps, perivascular space.

darkness for several weeks maintain a large store of 5-HT. Evidently in *Lacerta* a fraction of serotonin (probably belonging to the bound pool) does not change immediately in response to darkness.

In the P cells of the pineal organ and of the parietal eye (*Lacerta muralis*) dense-cored vesicles (mean diameter 100 nm, 1000 Å) are observed in the synaptic pedicles. New studies are necessary to ascertain a secretory activity.

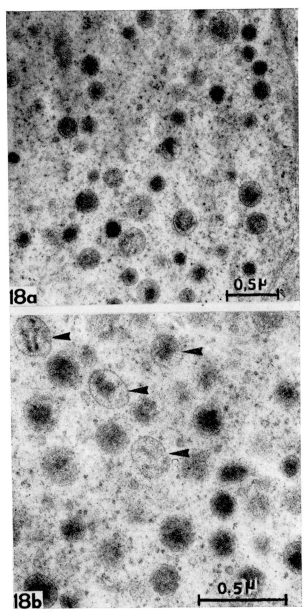

FIG. 18. SRP cells after injection of reserpine, in pineal organs of (a) *Lacerta muralis* and (b) *Lacerta viridis*. Different degrees of depletion of the dense granules are observed (arrows).

The "pseudosensory cells" of the chelonians are known to be of a secretory nature (Vivien and Roels 1967, 1968; Vivien-Roels 1969, 1970; Kappers and co-workers, personal communication 1968). However, in winter, secretory activity was not apparent in total darkness (Lutz and Collin 1967). The presence of 5-HT has also been detected in the epithelium (Kappers and co-workers, and Collin, unpublished results).

Secretory activity of the sensory type of cells (SRP) was established in several birds by Collin (1966c, 1967b, c, 1968a, 1969c, d), then by Fujie (1968), Quay, Renzoni and Eakin (1968) and more recently by Ueck (1970). Mechanisms are similar to those described for reptiles: important activity of the myoid and dense granules (mean diameter 100 nm, 1000 Å) originating in the Golgi zone (Figs. 19 and 20b). At the same time the secretory material is conveyed towards the asynaptic pedicles (Fig. 20a) and accumulates in the vicinity of the basement membrane of follicles or just beside the fenestrated endothelium of capillaries (Fig. 20a). Histochemical techniques enable us to localize the serotonin in the epithelium in some birds (Owman 1964, 1968; Oksche, Morita and Vaupel-von Harnack 1969; Oksche and Kirschstein 1969; Collin, unpublished results), and the possibility that indoleamines (serotonin and melatonin) are synthesized in SRP cells is considered by Collin (1967b, 1969c, d), Fujie (1968) and Ueck (1970).

Vivien (1964a, b, 1965) has shown secretory activity in the pineal organ of the snake epiphysis (Tropidonotus), as indicated by the production of membrane-bounded dense granules in the Golgi apparatus. Vivien also pointed out that pinealocyte processes have a vascular polarity. Lutz and Collin (1967) and Collin (1969d) agree with these preliminary observations of Vivien in studies of embryos and adults of another snake, Vipera. Quay, Jongkind and Kappers (1967) and Quay, Kappers and Jongkind (1968) found 5-HT in the pineal parenchymal cells of Tropidonotus. The mammalian pinealocyte shows, in several cases, a secretory activity identical to that known for snakes (see Collin and Kappers 1968; Collin 1969d; Wurtman, Axelrod and Kelly 1968). It seems quite probable that pinealocytes (=chief cells) are engaged in the production of indoleamines (see also Owman 1965; Arstila 1971).

From recent electron microscopic and histochemical investigations it appears that both sensory cell types and pinealocytes (cells of the sensory line: Collin 1969d) are responsible for the secretory activity and, in some cases, they seem to be involved in the synthesis and storage of active compounds such as indoleamines (5-HT). It is also well known from biochemical and radioautographic studies that serotonin, melatonin and hydroxyindole-O-methyltransferase (HIOMT, which catalyses the last

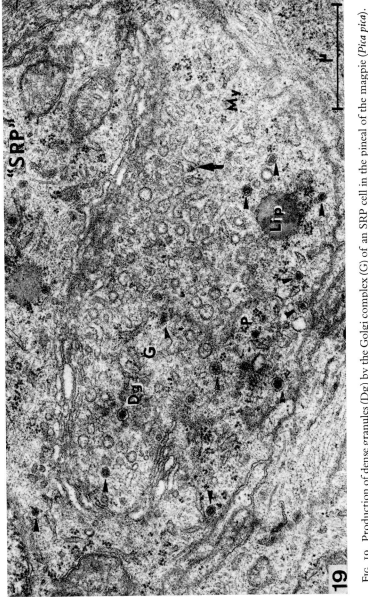

FIG. 19. Production of dense granules (Dg) by the Golgi complex (G) of an SRP cell in the pineal of the magpie (*Pica pica*). Notice at the arrow that membrane-bound granules bud from the Golgi complex. Lip, lipid droplet; My, myoid; P, polysomes.

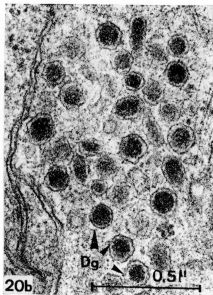

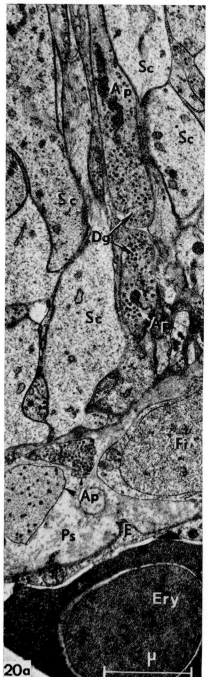

FIG. 20. (*a*) SRP cells from the pineal of the magpie (*Pica pica*) are extending their asynaptic pedicles (Ap) into the basal region of a follicle. In these prolongations numerous dense granules (Dg), originating within the Golgi area, are seen just in the vicinity of the perivascular space (Ps). Some processes of the SRP cells also course within the perivascular space. E, endothelium; Ery, erythrocyte; Fi, fibroblast; Sc, supportive cell. (*b*) Note the typical ultrastructure of the dense granules (Dg) in the asynaptic pedicle of an SRP cell of the magpie. They are bounded by a unit membrane and possess a fine dense granular structure. A clear zone lies between the matrix and the bounding membrane.

step of the transformation of serotonin into melatonin) occur not only in higher vertebrates but in lower vertebrates as well (references in Kappers 1967; Wurtman, Axelrod and Kelly 1968; Collin 1969*d*; Hafeez and Quay 1969). So it does not seem impossible that sensory cells possess a double potential: a photoreceptive and a secretory one.

I shall now turn briefly to the mechanisms of release of the secretory products. Dense granules, invariably produced in the Golgi area of the cells of the sensory line, migrate to the periphery of the cells by means of synaptic or asynaptic pedicles. In *Lampetra, Anguis, Tarentola, Vipera, Tropidonotus, Pica, Coturnix, Vanellus, Turdus* and in mammals, dense granules can be considered to be transient secretory inclusions because of the different stages of evacuation, finally leaving empty vesicles. In synaptic or asynaptic pedicles, the granule contents show a decrease in density: the clear space beneath the membrane increases while the dense contents decrease. Very frequently empty granules or clear vesicles of the same diameter appear in the cytoplasm of the pedicles. Thus the active compounds supposed to be present in such granules pass through the cytoplasm of the pedicle (by diffusion) and out of the cell. The same observations seem valid for mammalian pinealocytes (Collin 1969*d*). So far it has not been possible to postulate such mechanisms of excretion in *Lacerta*, because the different stages are not observed in our material. Different examples of the vascular secretory polarity are given by Collin (1969*d*):

Pedicle→intercellular spaces→basement membrane→perivascular space →capillary endothelium (e.g. *Lampetra*, Fig. 2; *Lacerta*).

Pedicle→basement membrane→perivascular space→capillary endothelium (e.g. *Anguis; Lacerta*, Fig. 8; *Tarentola; Testudo; Vipera; Pica*, Figs. 11, 20*a; Vanellus; Coturnix; Sturnus;* mammals).

Pedicle→perivascular space→capillary endothelium (*Pica*, Figs. 11, 20*a;* mammals).

The vascular system is richly supplied in all cases. Fenestrated capillaries are typical of those found in endocrine glands. Vesicles at the surface and within the endothelium are interpreted as a form of pinocytosis. Thus the endothelial cells seem to be active in capillary exchanges.

In all Amniota in SRP cells and pinealocytes we also found clear vesicles (mean diameter 50 nm, 500 Å) resembling morphologically the synaptic vesicles of P cells. I have termed them Vp (*v*esicles of cells of the *p*hotoreceptor type). They are provisionally not considered to contain a typical neurotransmitter but perhaps(?) a cholinergic substance active in membrane permeability.

We are thus now entitled to think that pineal products are released directly into the bloodstream. The observations reported here do not support the concept that the secretory activity is of an apocrine type, as has been proposed by other investigators.

THE CONCEPT OF THE SENSORY CELL LINE AND
SOME FUNCTIONAL IMPLICATIONS

From the results obtained by us and by other investigators, it is concluded (Collin 1969d) that during phylogenetic development of the epiphysis the sensory photoreceptor cells changed progressively into rudimentary photoreceptor elements, a process which is most pronounced in Sauropsida. In snakes and mammals the rudimentary photoreceptor cells change into pinealocytes or chief pineal cells.

I proposed (Collin 1969d) a definition of the cellular types which form the sensory line: photoreceptor cell (P)—rudimentary photoreceptor cell (RP)—pinealocyte (Pi) (Fig. 21). Of course, this line contains all intermediate cells. A comparative study of the photoreceptor cell and the rudimentary photoreceptor cell (Collin 1969d) establishes the derivation of the latter from the former (Fig. 21). Such a relationship can also be shown (Fig. 21) for the rudimentary photoreceptor cell and the pinealocyte (see Collin 1969d, for further details). These studies place the pinealocyte in its phylogenetic context. In summary, the pinealocyte recalls a rudimentary photoreceptor cell (Collin 1969d) but the segmented organization has largely disappeared. Thus the inner segment seems to have been integrated with the cell body and the polarity of some cytoplasmic organelles disappears (Fig. 21). In its general morphology the pinealocyte is more like a neuronal cell than like a photoreceptor cell (Fig. 21).

At first sight the proposed division (photoreceptor cell, rudimentary photoreceptor cell, pinealocyte) may appear too schematic. As has been mentioned, all the morphologically intermediate cells between these three fundamental cell types can be found (Figs. 8, 21). I have indicated that the photoreceptor cell has a sensory function in the conventional sense, but it must be stressed that the physiological meaning of this function is not clear. For us (Collin 1967b, 1969d) there is no doubt that the rudimentary photoreceptor cell and the pinealocyte, deprived of typical bipolar sensory differentiations, have lost their photoreceptive potential. Between the P and RP cells, which are basically different in their photoreceptive potential, morphological intermediates are likely to exist, though it is not yet possible to establish the different degrees of sensory function. Do the outer segments, poorly equipped with disks, still contain enough active photopigments to keep their original function? When it becomes possible

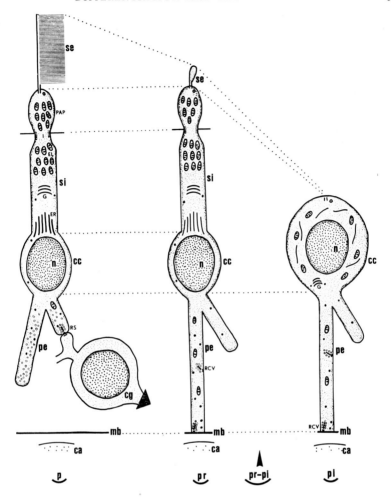

FIG. 21. Diagram illustrating the gradual transformation of the cells of the sensory line. The photoreceptor cell (p) contains four basic regions: se, outer segment; si, inner segment; cc, cellular body; pe, synaptic pedicle. The basal termination (pe) makes synaptic contact with the dendrite of a ganglion cell (cg). The rudimentary photoreceptor cell (pr) also contains the four basic regions but the outer segment (se) is rudimentary and the basal process is asynaptic. This asynaptic pedicle makes contact with the basement membrane (mb). Notice the typical vascular secretory polarity. Some vesicle-crowned lamellae (RCV) are also present. The pr cell is independent of the sensory nerve cells. In its general morphological aspects the pinealocyte (pi) looks like a neuron. The inner segment is incorporated into the cellular body. In pr and pi, the asynaptic pedicles are identical. The pi cell is also independent of sensory nerve cells. All intermediate cells between these three schematic types are supposed to be present. Ca, capillary; EL, ellipsoid; ER, granular endoplasmic reticulum; G, Golgi apparatus; mb, basement membrane; n, nucleus; PAP, apical process of a photoreceptor cell; RS, synaptic ribbon.

to investigate the potential of each intermediate cell type, we expect to find the same scheme, namely the existence of some cells having retained different degrees of photoreceptive potential (=photoreceptor cells) and of others having lost it, such as the rudimentary photoreceptor cell (Collin 1969d); cells intermediate (RP–Pi, Fig. 21) between the rudimentary photoreceptor cells and the pinealocytes are likely to be found too (Collin 1969d). These cells are equally unable to mediate a photoreceptive function.

It seems to be clear now that the rudimentary photoreceptor cell (and its successors, which also become independent of sensory innervation) is the key cell enabling us to interpret the regression and disappearance of the photoreceptive function.

From all these considerations, we have been led to the concept of the multiplicity of the sensory line cells, by which is meant that all the cellular types of the sensory line can be found in the same pineal organ, but according to the degree of differentiation or regression of the organ, one element of the line will be predominant. This concept was developed in the study of reptiles. In lacertilians (Collin 1968b, 1969d) the pineal organ contains elements ranging from the photoreceptor cell to the rudimentary photoreceptor cell (see also Petit 1969a, b). Such variety also occurs in chelonians (Vivien-Roels 1970). In these same groups (and perhaps in some Anamniota) the presence of the pinealocyte (according to our definition: Collin 1966–1969) is quite possible. This allows us to draw a diagram of the phylogeny of sensory pineal elements in vertebrates in which the concept of multiplicity is extended to several groups (Fig. 22). In this scheme the gradual regression of the sensory apparatus and function in the vertebrates is apparent (for further details see Collin 1969d and the legend of Fig. 22). The equally important problem of the regression of the sensory innervation (Kappers 1966, 1967; Collin 1969d; Petit 1969b; Vivien-Roels 1969, 1970) cannot be dealt with here.

The secretory activity, which is more probably of a neurohormonal nature (consisting of the biosynthesis of (1) melatonin from serotonin, which has been histochemically demonstrated in some Sauropsida (Fig. 17) and possibly (2) a protein or (3) a complex protein-indoleamine) in the sensory line cells, indicates that these elements are of primary importance in defining the function of each pineal organ (Collin 1969d). A multiplicity of modes of regulation of the activities of biosynthesis in relationship to the multiplicity of the sensory line cells seems quite possible. Photoperiods are known to be a determining factor in the regulation of synthesis in the pineal. They could have a direct influence in some lower vertebrates, or indirect (via lateral eyes, brainstem centres and peripheral innervation), as

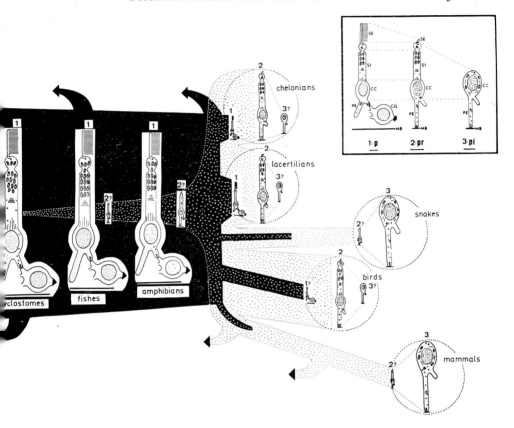

FIG. 22. Phylogeny and possible multiplicities of sensory line cells in the pineal organ of vertebrates (Collin 1969d). In the inset diagram (upper right corner) the three most typical cells of the sensory line are shown: (1) p, photoreceptor cell; (2) pr, rudimentary photoreceptor cell; (3) pi, pinealocyte. The existence of intermediate cells between these three schematic types is assumed. In the main diagram, photoreceptor cells (1) occur in the Anamniota (Petromyzontidae, fishes, amphibians). Their extinction occurs gradually in the Sauropsida, but they are still present in lacertilians (1) and chelonians (1) but are unknown in birds (1 ?). In chelonians (2), lacertilians (2), and birds (2), rudimentary photoreceptor elements are predominant. They are also present in the embryos of ophidians, and their existence is tentatively suggested in adults of ophidians (2 ?) and mammals (2 ?). Possibly they are also present in the pineal organs of fishes (2 ?) and amphibians (2 ?). Pinealocytes are the characteristic elements of the pineal organ of ophidians (3) and mammals (3), but their existence is also assumed in chelonians (3 ?), lacertilians (3 ?) and birds (3 ?). The dark part of the diagram indicates the phylogenetic development and disappearance of photoreceptor cells in the different groups of vertebrates. Dotted regions correspond to the "rudimentation" of sensory cells in Anamniota (2 ?) and the gradual development of rudimentary photoreceptor cells (pr) in Sauropsida. Reversed arrows indicate the disappearance of the pineal organ in some species of vertebrates.

in mammals (see review of Wurtman, Axelrod and Kelly 1968). It should be mentioned here that pinealo-petal autonomic axons have been recently discovered in the Sauropsida by electron microscopy and histochemistry (Collin 1967c, d, 1968a, c, 1969c, d; Collin and Kappers 1968; Oksche 1968; Oksche, Morita and Vaupel-von Harnack 1969; Oksche and Kirschstein 1969; Wartenberg and Baumgarten 1969a; Petit 1969b; Ueck 1970).

The sum of all these data enables us, I think, to revise the concept according to which the epiphysis cerebri is a sensory organ which changed into a gland during phylogeny. It appears rather to be a sensory and endocrine organ which during vertebrate phylogeny gradually loses its sensory activity and retains only its endocrine function in snakes, mammals and most probably in some, if not all, birds. The well-known transformation seems to be in the gradual "rudimentation" of the sensory apparatus (the determination of which will have to be considered) and probably in the mechanisms of regulation of the synthesis of active compounds. Thus we can already think in terms of a multiplicity of types of regulation in relation to the multiplicity of cells of the sensory line.

It seems clear that the pineal organ deserves to be considered as "photo-neuro-endocrine", a term first coined by Scharrer (1964) and since accepted by several authors. Furthermore, it can be specified that the epiphysis cerebri is an indirectly photo-neuro-endocrine organ in some higher vertebrates (for example in mammals) and perhaps (see above) a direct photo-neuro-endocrine organ in some lower vertebrates. So a combined direct and indirect photo-neuro-endocrine organ could be possible in intermediate forms.

I suspect (Collin 1969d) that the *cells* of the *sensory line* (CSL) are responsible for the secretory activity and are of prime importance in determining the function of any given pineal organ. Bearing in mind the neuroepithelial origin of the CSL, it is suggested that the epiphysis cerebri is a "*photo-neuro(CSL)-endocrine organ*".

SUMMARY

Stages in the transformation of photoreceptor cells have been studied in vertebrates. During phylogenetic development of the pineal the *photo-receptor cells* (P; cone-like photoreceptors in Anamniota, Lacertilia, Chelonia) change progressively into *rudimentary photoreceptor elements* (RP), a process which is most pronounced in reptiles and birds. The RP cell is characterized by regression of the photoreceptive outer segment and transformation of the synaptic pedicle, originally containing the neurotransmitter substance. So, "sensory" cells increase their independence from the sensory nerve cells which in photoreceptive pineals conduct the photic stimuli to the epithalamic part of the brain. In snakes and mammals the rudimentary photoreceptor cells change into *pinealocytes* (Pi). In view of the gradual transformation of the cells it is possible that all the types mentioned may be found in the pineals of the same species (concept of multiplicity). These three schematic types of cells (P, RP, Pi) and the intermediate cells constitute *the cells of the sensory line* (CSL). On the basis of electron microscopic and electrophysiological studies, an interpretation is given of the gradual disappearance of the photoreceptive potential in vertebrates.

In regard to the problem of which cell type is responsible for the synthesis and storage of active pineal compounds, it has been shown by electron microscopy that the epiphysial photoreceptors in *Lampetra*, the rudimentary photoreceptor elements in Sauropsida and the pinealocytes in snakes and mammals show signs of secretory activity. Dense-cored vesicles originating in the Golgi zone have been demonstrated. These vesicles migrate to either synaptic or asynaptic end-feet of the basal process of the "sensory" elements. The mode of excretion is discussed. By the fluorescence histochemical technique of Falck and Hillarp and by pharmacological studies it has been shown that serotonin is present in the pineal epithelium of fishes (Owman, personal communication 1970), Sauropsida and mammals. Serotonin (free in the cytoplasm or stored in dense granules of RP cells in *Lacerta*) seems to be present in larger or smaller quantities in all the elements of the sensory line.

From the comparative analysis of the different cell types (including the different types of innervation: Collin 1969d) it is thought that the cells of the sensory line (CSL) are of primary importance in determining the function of any given pineal organ. It is suggested that the epiphysis cerebri is a "photo-neuro(CSL)-endocrine organ".

Acknowledgement

I wish to express my thanks to Mrs S. Verneray for technical assistance, and to Miss Julie Knight for her collaboration in the preparation of the English manuscript.

REFERENCES

ANDERSON, E. (1965) *J. Ultrastruct. Res.* suppl. 8, 1–80.
ARSTILA, A. U. (1967) *Neuroendocrinology* suppl. 1, 1–101.
ARSTILA, A. U. (1971) This volume, pp. 147–164.
BARGMANN, W. (1943) *Handbuch der mikroskopischen Anatomie des Menschen*, VI/4. Berlin: Springer.
BISCHOFF, M. B. (1969) *J. Ultrastruct. Res.* **28**, 16–26.

BREUCKER, H. and HORSTMANN, E. (1965) In *Structure and Function of the Epiphysis Cerebri (Progress in Brain Research* vol. 10), pp. 259–269, ed. Kappers, J. A. and Schadé, J. P. Amsterdam: Elsevier.

COLLIN, J. P. (1966a) *C.r. hebd. Séanc. Acad. Sci., Paris, Sér. D* **262,** 2263–2266.

COLLIN, J. P. (1966b) *C.r. hebd. Séanc. Acad. Sci., Paris, Sér. D* **263,** 660–663.

COLLIN, J. P. (1966c) *C.r. Séanc. Soc. Biol.* **160,** 1876–1880.

COLLIN, J. P. (1967a) *C.r. hebd. Séanc. Acad. Sci., Paris, Sér. D* **264,** 647–650.

COLLIN, J. P. (1967b) *C.r. hebd. Séanc. Acad. Sci., Paris, Sér. D* **265,** 48–51.

COLLIN, J. P. (1967c) *C.r. hebd. Séanc. Acad. Sci., Paris, Sér. D* **265,** 1725–1728.

COLLIN, J. P. (1967d) *C.r. hebd. Séanc. Acad. Sci., Paris, Sér. D* **265,** 1827–1830.

COLLIN, J. P. (1968a) *C.r. hebd. Séanc. Acad. Sci., Paris, Sér. D* **267,** 758–761.

COLLIN, J. P. (1968b) *C.r. hebd. Séanc. Acad. Sci., Paris, Sér. D* **267,** 1047–1050.

COLLIN, J. P. (1968c) *C.r. hebd. Séanc. Soc. Biol.* **162,** 1785–1788.

COLLIN, J. P. (1968d) *C.r. hebd. Séanc. Acad. Sci., Paris, Sér. D* **267,** 1768–1771.

COLLIN, J. P. (1969a) *Archs Anat. microsc. Morph. exp.* **58,** 145–182.

COLLIN, J. P. (1969b) *J. Neuro-visc. Rel.* **31,** 308–333.

COLLIN, J. P. (1969c) *C.r. Séanc. Soc. Biol.* **163,** 1137–1142.

COLLIN, J. P. (1969d) *Annls Stn Biol. Besse-en-Chandesse* suppl. 1, 1–359.

COLLIN, J. P. and KAPPERS, J. A. (1968) *Brain Res.* **11,** 85–106.

COLLIN, J. P. and MEINIEL, A. (1968a) *C.r. hebd. Séanc. Acad. Sci., Paris, Sér. D* **266,** 1293–1295.

COLLIN, J. P. and MEINIEL, A. (1968b) *Archs Anat. microsc. Morph. exp.* **57,** 275–296.

DODT, E. (1963) *Experientia* **19,** 642.

DODT, E. (1964a) In *Lectures on the Diencephalon (Progress in Brain Research* vol. 5), pp. 201–205, ed. Bargmann, W. and Schadé, J. P. Amsterdam: Elsevier.

DODT, E. (1964b) *Mitt. Max-Planck-Ges.* H. 1–2, 64–73.

DODT, E. (1964c) *Vision Res.* **4,** 23–31.

DODT, E. (1966) *Nova Acta Leopoldina* **177,** 219–235.

DODT, E. and HEERD, E. (1962) *J. Neurophysiol.* **25,** 405–429.

DODT, E. and JACOBSON, M. (1963) *J. Neurophysiol.* **26,** 752–758.

DODT, E. and MORITA, Y. (1964) *Vision Res.* **4,** 413–421.

DODT, E. and MORITA, Y. (1967) *Pflügers Arch. ges. Physiol.* **293,** 184–192.

EAKIN, R. M. (1963) In *General Physiology of Cell Specialization,* pp. 398–425, ed. Mazia, D. and Tyler, A. New York: McGraw-Hill.

EAKIN, R. M. (1964) *Vision Res.* **4,** 17–22.

EAKIN, R. M., QUAY, W. B. and WESTFALL, J. A. (1963) *Z. Zellforsch. mikrosk. Anat.* **59,** 663–683.

EAKIN, R. M. and WESTFALL, J. A. (1959) *J. biophys. biochem. Cytol.* **6,** 133–134.

EAKIN, R. M. and WESTFALL, J. A. (1960) *J. biophys. biochem. Cytol.* **8,** 483–499.

FUJIE, E. (1968) *Arch. histol. jap.* **29,** 271–303.

HAFEEZ, M. A. and QUAY, W. B. (1969) *Gen. comp. Endocr.* **13,** 211–217.

HAMASAKI, D. E. and DODT, E. (1969) *Pflügers Arch. ges. Physiol.* **313,** 19–29.

KAPPERS, J. A. (1960) *Z. Zellforsch. mikrosk. Anat.* **52,** 163–215.

KAPPERS, J. A. (1965) In *Structure and Function of the Epiphysis Cerebri (Progress in Brain Research* vol. 10), pp. 87–153, ed. Kappers, J. A. and Schadé, J. P. Amsterdam: Elsevier.

KAPPERS, J. A. (1966) *Bull. Ass. Anat., Paris* **134,** 111–116.

KAPPERS, J. A. (1967) *Z. Zellforsch. mikrosk. Anat.* **81,** 581–618.

KAPPERS, J. A. (1969) *J. Neuro-visc. Rel.* suppl. 9, 140–184.

KELLY, D. E. (1965) In *Structure and Function of the Epiphysis Cerebri (Progress in Brain Research* vol. 10), pp. 270–285, ed. Kappers, J. A. and Schadé, J. P. Amsterdam: Elsevier.

KELLY, D. E. and SMITH, S. W. (1964) *J. Cell Biol.* **22,** 653–674.

LIERSE, W. (1965) *Z. Zellforsch. mikrosk. Anat.* **65**, 397–408.

LUTZ, H. and COLLIN, J. P. (1967) *Bull. Soc. zool. Fr.* **92**, 797–808.

MEINIEL, A. (1970) Thèse (3ème cycle), University of Clermont-Ferrand, **177**, 1–83.

MORITA, Y. (1965a) *Pflügers Arch ges. Physiol.* **283**, R30.

MORITA, Y. (1965b) *Pflügers Arch ges. Physiol.* **286**, 97–108.

MORITA, Y. (1966a) *Experientia* **22**, 402.

MORITA, Y. (1966b) *Pflügers Arch ges. Physiol.* **289**, 155–167.

MORITA, Y. (1969) *Experientia* **25**, 1277.

MORITA, Y. and DODT, E. (1965) *Experientia* **21**, 221–222.

NILSSON, S. E. (1964) *J. Ultrastruct. Res.* **11**, 581–620.

OKSCHE, A. (1968) *Archs Anat. Histol. Embryol.* **51**, 497–507.

OKSCHE, A. and KIRSCHSTEIN, H. (1966a) *Naturwissenschaften* **53**, 46.

OKSCHE, A. and KIRSCHSTEIN, H. (1966b) *Naturwissenschaften* **53**, 591.

OKSCHE, A. and KIRSCHSTEIN, H. (1967) *Z. Zellforsch. mikrosk. Anat.* **78**, 151–166.

OKSCHE, A. and KIRSCHSTEIN, H. (1968) *Z. Zellforsch. mikrosk. Anat.* **87**, 159–192.

OKSCHE, A. and KIRSCHSTEIN, H. (1969) *Z. Zellforsch. mikrosk. Anat.* **102**, 214–241.

OKSCHE, A., MORITA, Y. and VAUPEL-VON HARNACK, M. (1969) *Z. Zellforsch. mikrosk. Anat.* **102**, 1–30.

OKSCHE, A. and VAUPEL-VON HARNACK, M. (1963) *Z. Zellforsch. mikrosk. Anat.* **59**, 582–614.

OKSCHE, A. and VAUPEL-VON HARNACK, M. (1965a) In *Structure and Function of the Epiphysis Cerebri* (*Progress in Brain Research* vol. 10), pp. 237–258, ed. Kappers, J. A. and Schadé, J. P. Amsterdam: Elsevier.

OKSCHE, A. and VAUPEL-VON HARNACK, M. (1965b) *Naturwissenschaften* **24**, 662–663.

OKSCHE, A. and VAUPEL-VON HARNACK, M. (1965c) *Z. Zellforsch. mikrosk. Anat.* **68**, 389–426.

OKSCHE, A. and VAUPEL-VON HARNACK, M. (1966) *Z. Zellforsch. mikrosk. Anat.* **69**, 41–60.

OKSCHE, A. and HARNACK, M. VON (1962) *Naturwissenschaften* **49**, 429–430.

OMURA, Y., KITOH, J. and OGURI, M. (1969) *Bull. Jap. Soc. scient. Fish.* **35**, 1067–1071.

OWMAN, CH. (1964) *Acta physiol. scand.* **63**, suppl. 240, 1–40.

OWMAN, CH. (1965) In *Structure and Function of the Epiphysis Cerebri* (*Progress in Brain Research* vol. 10), pp. 423–453, ed. Kappers, J. A. and Schadé, J. P. Amsterdam: Elsevier.

OWMAN, CH. (1968) *Adv. Pharmac.* **6A**, 167–169.

PETIT, A. (1968) *Z. Zellforsch. mikrosk. Anat.* **92**, 70–93.

PETIT, A. (1969a) *Archs Anat. Histol. Embryol.* **52**, 1–25.

PETIT, A. (1969b) *Z. Zellforsch. mikrosk. Anat.* **96**, 437–465.

QUAY, W. B., KAPPERS, J. A. and JONGKIND, J. F. (1968) *J. Neuro-visc. Rel.* **31**, 11–25.

QUAY, W. B., JONGKIND, J. F. and KAPPERS, J. A. (1967) *Anat. Rec.* **157**, 304–305.

QUAY, W. B. and RENZONI, A. (1963) *Riv. Biol.* **56**, 363–407.

QUAY, W. B., RENZONI, A. and EAKIN, R. M. (1968) *Riv. Biol.* **61**, 371–386.

RALPH, C. I. and DAWSON, D. C. (1968) *Experientia* **24**, 147–148.

RÜDEBERG, C. (1966) *Pubbl. Staz. zool. Napoli* **35**, 47–60.

RÜDEBERG, C. (1968a) *Z. Zellforsch. mikrosk. Anat.* **84**, 219–237.

RÜDEBERG, C. (1968b) *Z. Zellforsch. mikrosk. Anat.* **85**, 521–526.

RÜDEBERG, C. (1969) *Z. Zellforsch. mikrosk. Anat.* **96**, 548–581.

SCHARRER, E. (1964) *Ann. N.Y. Acad. Sci.* **117**, 13–22.

SJÖSTRAND, F. S. (1961) In *The Structure of the Eye*, pp. 1–28, ed. Smelser, G. K. New York and London: Academic Press.

STEYN, W. (1960) *Z. Zellforsch. mikrosk. Anat.* **51**, 735–747.

UECK, M. (1968) *Z. Zellforsch. mikrosk. Anat.* **92**, 452–476.

UECK, M. (1969) *Z. Zellforsch. mikrosk. Anat.* **100**, 560–580.

UECK, M. (1970) *Z. Zellforsch. mikrosk. Anat.* **105**, 276–302.

VIVIEN, J. H. (1964a) *C.r. hebd. Séanc. Acad. Sci., Paris, Sér. D* **258**, 3370–3372.

VIVIEN, J. H. (1964*b*) *J. Microsc.* **3,** 57.
VIVIEN, J. H. (1965) *C.r. hebd. Séanc. Acad. Sci., Paris, Sér. D* **260,** 5370–5372.
VIVIEN, J. H. and ROELS, B. (1967) *C.r. hebd. Séanc. Acad. Sci., Paris, Sér. D* **264,** 1743–1746.
VIVIEN, J. H. and ROELS, B. (1968) *C.r. hebd. Séanc. Acad. Sci., Paris, Sér. D* **266,** 600–603.
VIVIEN-ROELS, B. (1969) *Z. Zellforsch. mikrosk. Anat.* **94,** 352–390.
VIVIEN-ROELS, B. (1970) *Z. Zellforsch. mikrosk. Anat.* **104,** 429–448.
WARTENBERG, H. (1968) *Z. Zellforsch. mikrosk. Anat.* **86,** 74–97.
WARTENBERG, H. and BAUMGARTEN, H. G. (1968) *Z. Anat. EntwGesch.* **127,** 99–120.
WARTENBERG, H. and BAUMGARTEN, H. G. (1969a) *Z. Zellforsch. mikrosk. Anat.* **94,** 252–260.
WARTENBERG, H. and BAUMGARTEN, H. G. (1969b) *Z. Anat. EntwGesch.* **128,** 185–210.
WOLFE, D. E. (1965) In *Structure and Function of the Epiphysis Cerebri* (*Progress in Brain Research* vol. 10), pp. 332–376, ed. Kappers, J. A. and Schadé, J. P. Amsterdam: Elsevier.
WURTMAN, R. J., AXELROD, J. and KELLY, D. E. (1968) *The Pineal.* New York and London: Academic Press.
YOUNG, R. W. and DROZ, B. (1968) *J. Cell Biol.* **39,** 169–184.

DISCUSSION

Kelly: I find the concept that the pinealocyte—the presumed secretory cell of the mammalian pineal organ—is derived evolutionarily from the photoreceptor very attractive; in fact I have often advocated this view. But I think there is still crucial evidence needed here. In the lizard, where you see extensive aggregates of large, dense vesicles, have you also seen synaptic ribbons in the *same cells*?

Collin: In the lizard *Lacerta muralis*, I found two schematic types of cells: secretory rudimentary photoreceptor cells (SRP) and photoreceptor cells (P). I imagine that all intermediate types of cells are present between SRP and P cells. In the SRP cells, which contain large aggregates of large dense vesicles, I was unable to observe typical synaptic connexions or "vesicle-crowned lamellae". Nevertheless, in the P cells which are responsible for the residual photoreceptive potential I found a few scarce synaptic ribbons. Furthermore, in the synaptic pedicles of P cells there are very scarce dense granules, with a mean diameter smaller than that of the numerous dense granules of the SRP cells. In other lizards, *Anguis* and *Chalcides*, "synaptic" components are present.

Kelly: In *Anguis* and *Chalcides*, are the synaptic ribbons or lamellae present in the *same* cell that contains the abundant dense granules?

Collin: I have shown earlier (Collin 1967, 1968, 1969) the differences between the dense granules of the cells of the sensory line in different species of lizards. In *Anguis* and in *Chalcides* the dense granules, originating from the Golgi area, are scarce. In these species the distinction between P and SRP cells is very difficult to make. My own investigations in *Anguis* and *Chalcides* are not so significant as those in *Lacerta* but the presence of rare outer segments with typical disks indicates a residual photoreceptive potential in *Anguis* and *Chalcides* also. I was unable to see the presumed typical synaptic pedicles. Petit (1969) corroborated these observations in *Anguis*. Like me, he found only asynaptic pedicles, probably belonging to the rudimentary photoreceptor cells. These pedicles, in contact with the basal membrane, contain rare dense granules (mean diameter, 100 nm or 1000 Å) and also "vesicle-crowned lamellae" which are not indicative of neurotransmission in the conventional sense (Collin 1969). The presence of typical synaptic ribbons and dense granules in the same pedicle seems to me to be possible in *Anguis* and *Chalcides* (see also *Lampetra;* Collin 1969) but it is very difficult to show them because typical photoreceptors are scarce in these two lizards.

Kelly: The question of course is whether we are talking about *one* cell line, or if it's at all possible that there are *two* cell lines—a secretory cell line and a cell line that is still present in a residual form from the older photoreceptor line.

Kappers: I think that there is one cell line only. At the root of this lineage is the neurosensory epiphysial cell. Principally this element has a direct photosensory function but it also shows a more or less rudimentary capacity to secrete substances. During its phylogenetic evolution, this cell type progressively develops into an exclusively secretory element, its original sensory function becoming gradually lost. That is why, for instance in reptiles, one and the same pineal cell may show ultrastructural features (either well developed or in a residual form) characteristic of a direct photosensory function, next to ultrastructural features characteristic of a secretory function. Even in the mammalian pinealocyte, which is purely secretory, one may observe some rare synaptic ribbons as possible reminders of the original neurosensory function of this cell, next to dense-cored vesicles and other signs of its secretory function.

Kelly: Yes, but there the dense-cored vesicles are often fewer in number. Moreover, they are similar to granule-filled inclusions found in a wide variety of cells. Such profiles are commonly seen scattered among other smaller vesicles in synaptic endings, but they are by no means unique to areas of synaptic contact. Their function is obscure. Because of this, it is difficult to be confident that the cells that produce large amounts of melatonin or serotonin have evolved from photoreceptors unless we know (1) that these products are contained in the vesicles in question, and (2) that the vesicles occupy the same cells as do the ribbons. We should be able to obtain this evidence.

Kappers: As to the chemical nature and the number of the dense-cored vesicles present in mammalian pinealocytes, a recent paper on the pineal of mice by Dr Pellegrino de Iraldi (1969) is relevant. She showed that the number of granule-filled vesicles present in mammalian pinealocytes may vary widely, according to species.

Pellegrino de Iraldi: The granulated vesicles are very abundant in mice (Pellegrino de Iraldi 1969), moderately frequent in the hamster (Pellegrino de Iraldi 1966) and very rare in the rat (Arstila 1967). On morphological grounds the main component characterizing a secretory vesicle is not its contents but the membrane which isolates the product from the cytoplasm of the cell. The cell puts substances which are synthesized to be exported from the cell into a membrane derived from the vacuolar system. The contents of the vesicles may appear electron-dense or not, depending on whether the substance reacts with osmium tetroxide. It is very interesting that the pineals of mammals have in general a similar plan but the concentration of the osmium-reducing material inside these vesicles varies between species. I think that this may be due to some chemical difference in the secretion itself or to different binding of the secretory product in the different kinds of cells.

Wurtman: At the time of the last meeting devoted to the pineal, in Amsterdam in 1963, there was some resistance to the idea that the mammalian pineal functions as a secretory organ, inasmuch as electron micrographs of pineal cells failed to demonstrate characteristic secretory granules. I submit that it is time that we bury this morphological criterion for secretory organs: one should only expect to see secretory granules when one is dealing with a cell that secretes water-soluble hormones like peptides or amines. These subcellular organelles presumably have the special function of protecting the hormones from intracellular enzymes (like monoamine oxidase) that might otherwise destroy them. If the pineal hormones are lipid-soluble substances such as melatonin, there would seem to be little reason why we should expect intracellular pineal granules to be correlated with pineal secretory activity.

Miline: Dr Collin defined the pineal gland of mammals as a photo-neuroendocrine gland. We have observed that the pineal gland is very sensitive to other stimuli besides light. It responds to noise, olfactory stimuli, irradiation, and also emotion, so one should really call it a senso-neuroendocrine organ. Perhaps the sensory capacity, in connexion with the synaptic ribbons, supports this definition.

Wurtman: I wonder if we can list the possible inputs to the pineal, and to the bird pineal in particular? I have been trying to locate the bird pineal on an evolutionary scale. So far in the course of this meeting, seven possible inputs have been mentioned that might influence the bird pineal, or pineals in general. One such influence is environmental lighting. How might one prove that light directly affects avian pineal cells? First one should hope to observe something that looks like a photoreceptor using electron microscopy; secondly, one should be able to measure action potentials or some other physiological response to light within these cells, or in nerves from the pineal to the brain. Thirdly, one might look for photopigments.

A second possible input to the avian pineal could come from post-ganglionic sympathetic neurons. This would perhaps be easiest to examine, since one might hope to find granular vesicles in nerve endings within the pineal, and to show that they disappear after superior cervical ganglionec-tomy. I gather there is some disagreement about whether or not such organelles exist, in avian pineals.

A third possible input would be from postganglionic parasympathetic (cholinergic) neurons. Such neurons might reflect aberrant vagal com-ponents that traversed the superior cervical ganglia without synapsing; their terminals would be expected to contain non-granular synaptic vesicles. A related fourth possible input would consist of postganglionic cholinergic neurons originating from ganglion cells within the substance of the pineal. I gather that such cells have been shown to exist in primate pineals.

A fifth possible input consists of tracts from the habenula and elsewhere in the brain that might ascend via the pineal stalk and release unknown neurotransmitters. Dr Kappers showed some years ago that this is not the case in the rat but I gather from Dr Collin's comments that these tracts might exist in birds.

A sixth input consists of factors that come to the pineal by the blood-stream. For example, in the rat, gonadal hormones have a marked effect on pineal weight and on pineal enzyme activity (Wurtman, Axelrod and Snyder 1965). Dr Miline has considered other factors that come in the bloodstream and affect the size and function of the pineal.

Finally, there is the possible delivery of compounds via the ventricular system. So these are seven possible inputs to the pineal, and it might be useful to consider which of these inputs have been shown to impinge on the bird pineal. In the rat there are only two inputs for which there is experi-mental evidence: a neuronal input from the superior cervical ganglion and a humoral one via the bloodstream. In primates I imagine the con-sensus would be that there are two demonstrated inputs, an input from the superior cervical ganglion and one from intramural ganglion cells.

Axelrod: You can eliminate the sympathetic nervous system for birds, because we find that when the sympathetic innervation to the bird pineal is destroyed, information about lighting still gets through.

Wurtman: That would indicate that the particular network followed by light doesn't involve the sympathetic nervous system but it wouldn't prove that there is no information transfer by the sympathetic nervous system.

Oksche: Sympathetic innervation to the pineal is very abundant in the bird, even if your experiment was negative, Dr Axelrod! (See Ueck 1970.) Furthermore, the stalk of the avian pineal contains a large number of unmyelinated fibres, and also a number of myelinated fibres. Degeneration studies on this pathway are in progress in our laboratory (in a joint project with M. Menaker and associates). We do not know whether these fibres go to the pineal or are coming from the pineal and run to the central nervous system. The number of these fibres is very high compared with the rudiments of sensory cells. This is very puzzling, but we hope to get some more information in our current work.

Martini: Dr Wurtman said just now that melatonin is a typical pineal hormone. Dr Axelrod indicated in his paper that, in the pineal gland, serotonin may be the victim of monoamine oxidase and that because of this a lot of methoxytryptophol can be formed. Is it known whether the preferential way of disposing of serotonin is through the formation of methoxytryptophol or through the formation of melatonin?

Axelrod: Monoamine oxidase is by far the greatest destroyer of serotonin in the pineal, but you have to think of serotonin in the context of its sub-cellular dynamics. All kinds of forces are acting on serotonin. Part of the pineal serotonin is taken up by sympathetic nerves and part is metabolized by other enzymes, such as N-acetyltransferase and hydroxyindole-O-methyltransferase.

Wurtman: If one cultures a pineal with radioactive tryptophan and then examines the fate of the resulting radioactive serotonin, one observes several very surprising things. For example, it is seen that very much more tryptophan is transferred to other indoles than is incorporated into proteins. It is generally held that the neurotransmitter amines are a minor by-product of tryptophan and tyrosine, in terms of total body metabolism. This is true in terms of general body metabolism, but not for the small number of individual cells that synthesize these amines. A second point, more germane to Professor Martini's question, is that *in vitro*, much more serotonin is converted to melatonin than to 5-hydroxyindole acetic acid. This suggests that melatonin synthesis is more important as a pathway for pineal serotonin metabolism than is oxidative deamination by monoamine oxidase.

Owman: With regard to the statement that the pineal contains serotonin, one must be very careful before one identifies a yellow formaldehyde-induced fluorescence as serotonin. Firstly, it's possible that there is storage of 5-hydroxytryptophan (see Wilhoft and Quay 1965), and the 5-hydroxy-tryptophan fluorophore is indistinguishable from the serotonin fluorophore. Secondly, we have found that some of the yellow fluorophores which previously have been identified as serotonin are actually 5-methoxy-tryptamine. Thirdly, we have made a microspectrophotometric analysis of the fluorescence characteristics of the yellow fluorophore in the pineal of fishes and amphibians, and this curve is not typical for serotonin (Owman and Rüdeberg 1970). There are thus several pieces of evidence indicating that a yellow fluorescence in some pineals may represent another indole than serotonin.

REFERENCES

ARSTILA, A. U. (1967) *Neuroendocrinology* suppl. 1, 1–101.
COLLIN, J. P. (1967) *C.r. hebd. Séanc. Acad. Sci., Paris, Sér. D* **265**, 1725–1728 and 1827–1830.
COLLIN, J. P. (1968) *C.r. Séanc. Soc. Biol.* **162**, 1785–1788.
COLLIN, J. P. (1969) *Annls Stn Biol. Besse-en-Chandesse* suppl. 1, 1–359.
OWMAN, CH. and RÜDEBERG, C. (1970) *Z. Zellforsch. mikrosk. Anat.* **107**, 522–550.
PELLEGRINO DE IRALDI, A. (1966) *Anat. Rec.* **154**, 481.
PELLEGRINO DE IRALDI, A. (1969) *Z. Zellforsch. mikrosk. Anat.* **101**, 408–418.
PETIT, A. (1969) *Z. Zellforsch. mikrosk. Anat.* **96**, 437–465.
UECK, M. (1970) *Z. Zellforsch. mikrosk. Anat.* **105**, 276–302.
WILHOFT, D. C. and QUAY, W. B. (1965) *Comp. Biochem. Physiol.* **15**, 325–338.
WURTMAN, R. J., AXELROD, J. and SNYDER, S. H. (1965) *Endocrinology* **76**, 798–800.

SENSORY AND GLANDULAR ELEMENTS OF THE PINEAL ORGAN*

A. OKSCHE

Department of Anatomy, University of Giessen, Germany

RECENT investigations in our laboratory have been concerned with: (1) pineal sense organs of fishes, anurans and lizards; (2) intermediate forms of pineal organs containing both sensory and secretory ultrastructural elements (in lizards); and (3) intermediate forms of pineal organs which are predominantly secretory and fail to show an electrical response to direct illumination (in birds) (Fig. 1). These investigations have been conducted with Professor E. Dodt and his co-workers. The electrophysiological aspects of the problem will be discussed by Professor Dodt (see p. 164). In our laboratory we have been concerned mainly with structural analysis in species used in physiological experiments, such as the shark, *Scyliorhinus canicula*; the rainbow trout, *Salmo gairdneri*; frogs, *Rana esculenta* and *Rana catesbeiana*; the lizard, *Lacerta sicula*, and the house sparrow, *Passer domesticus*.

The conclusions presented by Dr Collin in his paper (pp. 79–120; see also Collin 1969) are in good agreement with our phylogenetic and cytological concepts of pineal evolution. We believe that the secretory pinealocyte is derived from the pineal photoreceptor cells of lower vertebrates.

The experiments of Professor Dodt and co-workers (see Dodt, Ueck and Oksche 1970) have shown that the pineal systems in fishes, anurans and lizards respond to light with nervous impulses which are conducted to other parts of the brain. Two different types of impulse patterns have been observed (cf. Dodt, Ueck and Oksche 1970): (1) achromatic responses consisting of a depression of impulse activity in response to light stimuli of all wavelengths, and (2) chromatic responses consisting of an increase of impulse frequency upon stimulation with medium and long wavelengths (excitatory component) and a decrease of impulse frequency upon stimulation with short wavelengths, including ultraviolet radiation (inhibitory component). Chromatic responses have been observed in the frontal

* With contributions by H. G. Hartwig, H. Kirschstein, E. Paul, G. Möller and M. Langbein, C. Rüdeberg, and M. Ueck, Giessen.

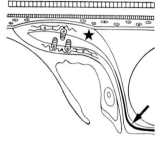

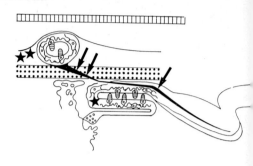

A Teleostei   B Anura

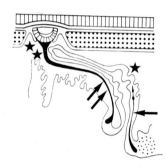

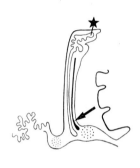

C Lacertilia   D Aves

FIG. 1. Diagram showing different types of pineal organs in submammalian vertebrates. The pineal organs (or complexes) of fishes, amphibians and lizards are functional photoreceptors (Dodt, Ueck and Oksche 1970).

A. *Teleostei:* Sac-like pineal organ (★) as observed in *Salmo gairdneri*. Pineal tract (arrow).

B. *Anura:* Frontal organ (★★) and epiphysis (★). Continuous pineal pathway formed by frontal (two arrows) and pineal (arrow) tracts.

C. *Lacertilia:* Parietal eye (★★) and pineal organ (★). Parietal (two arrows) and pineal (arrow) tracts.

D. *Aves:* Pineal organ (★) with bundles of intraparenchymal axons (arrow). The avian pineal organ failed to show electrical responses to illumination.

organ of frogs, in the parietal eye of lizards and in the pineal body (epiphysis) of a few anuran species (*Rana catesbeiana*, *Rana esculenta*; see Morita 1969). There is physiological evidence for one or two different photopigments in one particular pineal organ.

The following neurohistological and electron microscopic evidence, related to the above physiological findings, will be presented here:

(1) a survey of different modifications of the receptor outer segment;

(2) observations on different synaptic and synaptoid structures;

(3) a structural analysis of different types of pineal neurons and their connexions; and

(4) further neuroanatomical identification of afferent (epiphysio-fugal) pathways of pineal sense organs, including counts of myelinated and unmyelinated nerve fibres.

For a detailed analysis of pineal sense organs, see Dodt and Oksche (1971). A considerable number of our recent investigations on this project are still in progress.

(1) OUTER SEGMENTS OF PINEAL RECEPTORS (Figs. 2–4)

The outer segments of pineal sensory cells are formed by multiple invaginations of the outer plasma membrane. According to the criteria used for the identification of retinal cones and rods, the outer segments resemble the cones. However, the structural type of a photoreceptor cell does not determine the mode of retinal action (Dodt 1962). In the pineal complex, the length of the pineal outer segment varies between 15 μm (in the lizard parietal eye) and 1–2 μm (in the fish pineal organ). Outer segments of the anuran frontal organ have a length of approximately 3–6 μm (cf. Eakin 1961; Oksche and von Harnack 1963). In the frontal organ of *Rana temporaria*, 2·5–3·5 μm long outer segments consist of 60–110 lamellar discs. Compared with the 55 μm long (1000 discs) outer segment of a rod in the frog, the outer segments of pineal receptor cells appear to be rudimentary. However, Nilsson and Crescitelli (1970) have recently shown that in the lateral eye of developing frog tadpoles (*Rana pipiens*), the first electroretinographic response to light corresponds to the first appearance of the outer segment discs. At this stage, the number of newly formed discs is comparable with the number of the discs in the shortest outer segments of pineal sensory cells.

Much diversity has been encountered among the pineal outer segment structures although they belong basically to the cone type. Mushroom-like and overlapping outer segments have been observed in pineal organs of several teleost fishes (Rüdeberg 1968), the lungfish, *Protopterus dolloi* (Ueck 1969), and some primitive anuran species (Ueck 1968). Luxuriant basal development of the lamellae seems to initiate degeneration, possibly followed by a process of renewal. Furthermore, many outer segments of the light-sensitive pineal system of frogs show the formation of tubules and vesicles, followed by disintegration and phagocytosis (see also Kelly 1965). It has been suspected that in a pineal outer segment a certain degree of

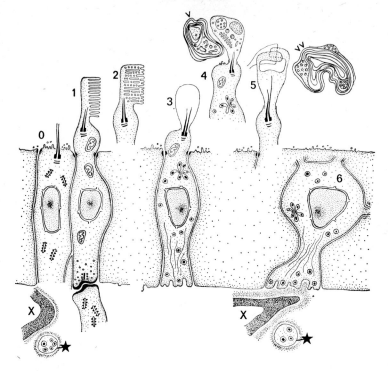

FIG. 2. Different types of pinealocytes.

Sensory pinealocytes: (1) regular cone-like outer segment (discovered by Eakin 1961); (2) outer segment showing tubular and vesicular structures. O, supportive cell.

Rudimentary sensory pinealocytes: (3) bulbous cilium (9+0 type); (4) degenerated outer segment showing fragments of lamellae, vesicles and segregated membrane whorls (V); (5) bulbous cilium (9+0 type) with ectopic lamellar complexes (VV). Note the secretory activity (dense-cored vesicles) of the vestigial receptors.

Secretory mammalian pinealocyte (6). X, blood vessels; ★, autonomic nerve fibres.

Outer segments of types 1 and 2 have been observed in the pineal organs of fishes and anurans. Type 1 shows variations in length and form (also cup-like). Long outer segments of type 1 are predominant in the parietal eye of lizards; the lacertilian pineal organ shows the outer segment types 1, 2, 3 and 4. Type 5 is the characteristic vestigial outer segment structure of the avian pineal organ.

ultrastructural differentiation is needed to produce a primary photoreceptor response. In the retina, vesicular alterations of rod outer segments are familiar signs of degeneration leading to night blindness (Dowling and Gibbons 1961).

The pineal organ of *Lacerta sicula* shows a distinct electrical response to light stimulation (Hamasaki and Dodt 1969). Regular outer segments of

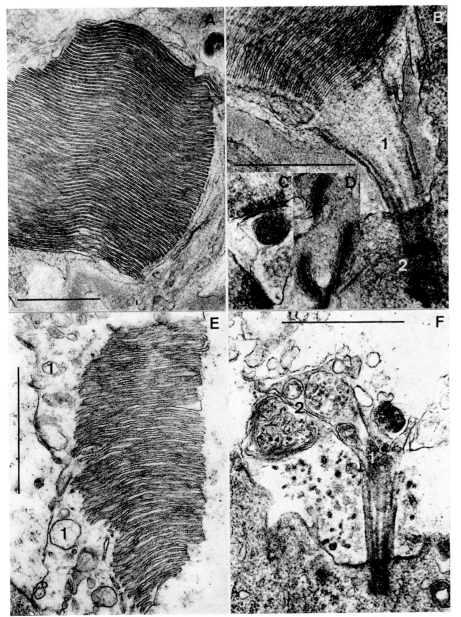

Fig. 3. A, B. Regular cone-like outer segments in the pineal organ of the European minnow (*Phoxinus laevis*). *P. laevis* shows a very spectacular light sensitivity of the diencephalic roof. A × 22 500, B × 33 000. Bar 1 μm. In B, (1) connecting piece, (2) centrioles.

C, D. Synaptic structures in the pineal organ of *Phoxinus laevis*. C, conventional contacts, × 36 250. D, synaptic ribbons, × 26 500.

E, F. Different types of outer segments in the pineal organ of *Lacerta sicula*. The pineal organ of *Lacerta sicula* shows an achromatic response to direct illumination (Hamasaki and Dodt 1969). E, regular discs associated with some vesicular structures, × 33 600. F, degenerated outer segment showing an axial cilium (1) and numerous vesicles (2). Bar 1 μm. × 33 000.

(A. Oksche and H. Kirschstein, unpublished.)

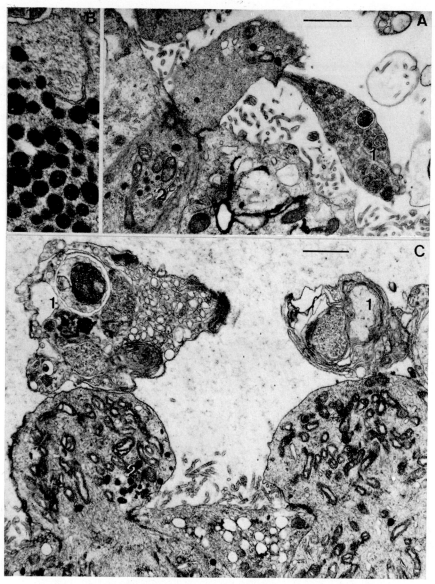

FIG. 4. Pineal organ of *Lacerta sicula*. Rudimentary sensory pinealocytes show secretory activity.

A. Degenerated outer segment (1), dense-cored vesicles (2). × 13 000.

B. Fine structure of dense-cored vesicles; nucleus (1). × 33 600.

C. Segregated outer segment structures (1), secretory granules (2). × 12 500. Bar 1 μm.

(A. Oksche and H. Kirschstein, unpublished.)

pineal receptor cells are still conspicuous in this lizard species (Fig. 3E). However, in lacertilian species a considerable number of pinealocytes show a vestigial or degenerating outer segment (Figs. 3, 4 and 10).

In spite of the presence of rudimentary receptor-type pinealocytes with bulbous cilia, the avian pineal organ fails to show electrical responses to illumination (see details in section 6). However, the lamellar complexes connected with these 9 + 0 type of cilia are completely irregular, resembling the final stage of degeneration in vitamin A-deficient retinas—vesiculation of lamellar "sacs" of the pineal outer segments has also been described as a fixation artifact (cf. Rüdeberg 1969).

The ultrastructural pattern of the outer segments in different pineal organs does not provide a basis for understanding the achromatic and chromatic reactions.

A kind of ultrastructural dimorphism of the outer segments has been observed recently by Ueck (1970) in the epiphysis of *Rana esculenta*. After prolonged treatment with osmium tetroxide, as introduced by Eakin and Brandenburger (1970), the membrane complexes of some outer segments show a characteristic darkening while other outer segments remain completely negative. If the theory of Eakin and Brandenburger is correct, the blackened spots should indicate the site of a photopigment or at least of a vitamin A-containing compound. Under the same conditions, osmiophilic granular material appears in adjacent supportive cells.

Radioautographic investigations with labelled vitamin A are in progress (Ueck and Rüdeberg).

(2) DIFFERENT PINEAL SYNAPTIC STRUCTURES (Fig. 5)

According to the duplicity theory, photopigment of the outer segment as well as upstream and horizontal neuronal connexions determine the reactions of cones and rods (cf. Dodt, Ueck and Oksche 1970). In contrast to the detailed information available for the retina, the synaptic relationships in the pineal sense organs are not yet well known. The following synaptic structures have been observed in the pineal complex: "club-foot" endings of receptor cells containing clear vesicles of mean diameter 30–50 nm (300–500 Å) and "synaptic ribbons"; conventional synapses; synapses containing some dense-cored vesicles of diameter 80–120 nm (800–1200 Å) (for details see Fig. 5). Synaptic ribbons have been observed in the pineal systems of amphibia (Kelly 1965; Oksche and von Harnack 1963), cyclostomes (Collin 1969) and teleost fishes (Takahashi 1969; Oksche and Kirschstein 1970). In the frog (*Rana temporaria, Rana esculenta*), synaptic endings similar to those in the frontal organ (response of the chromatic type) also occur in the epiphysis (response of the achromatic type). All of our histochemical attempts to demonstrate acetylcholinesterase activity in the terminals of the frog pineal receptors have so far been negative. The same sections show a considerable number of acetylcholinesterase-positive nerve cells (Ueck, in press; see Owman, Rüdeberg and Ueck 1970). Reconstructions from electron microscopic serial sections of pineal synapses are very much needed for accurate interpretation.

In the frog retina, synaptic ribbons are characteristic of rod-bipolar cell contacts; synapses of conventional type are formed by horizontal cells and

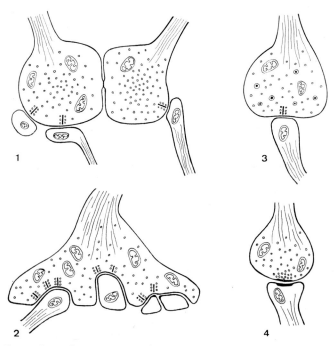

Fig. 5. Synaptic structures in the pineal organs of lower vertebrates (C. Rüdeberg, unpublished diagram).

(1) Synaptic ribbons are probably responsible for the transmission from pineal receptor terminals to dendrites of nerve cells in most, if not all, lower vertebrates. In many teleosts the vesicle-filled, bulbous terminal contains only a few synaptic ribbons. In *Esox*, tight junctions between receptor terminals may represent points of electrotonic transmission.

(2) The receptor terminals in the pineal organs of certain forms, especially amphibians, have an enlarged contact surface provided with a relatively large number of synaptic ribbons. Postsynaptically, the membrane may or may not show a thickening.

(3) Some receptor terminals in the amphibian pineal contain granulated vesicles as well as normal synaptic vesicles. The significance of the former is yet unknown.

(4) Synapses of the conventional type have been found in the pineal complex of certain amphibians.

amacrine cells (Dowling 1968). In *Necturus* ribbons are associated with different types of synaptic terminals on rods and cones (Dowling and Werblin 1969). In pineal sense systems, synaptic ribbons occur in receptor cells bearing a cone-like outer segment. The exact position of pineal receptors in this classification remains to be determined.

In our electron microscopic material, the most complex synaptic junctions have been demonstrated in the frontal organ of the frog (Oksche and von Harnack 1963). The chromatic response of the frontal organ requires sensory cells with different photopigments which converge upon one nerve cell in a complicated way (Dodt, Ueck and Oksche 1970). This important problem of the exact convergence ratio of sensory cells to nerve cells must be re-examined by modern morphometric methods.

(3) DIFFERENT TYPES OF PINEAL NEURONS AND THEIR GROUPINGS (Fig. 6)*

The structure and organization of the neuronal chain in pineal sense organs is important in all functional interpretations. Our previous findings and the results of Collin (1969) seemed to be in favour of a bineuronal chain. Since knowledge of the existence of bipolar, amacrine and horizontal cells is extremely important for the functional interpretation of the chromatic and achromatic responses, some of our recent studies may be mentioned. For these investigations modifications of classical neurohistological methods (Golgi; methylene blue) have been valuable. Our new Golgi-Colonnier material has produced precise images of pineal receptors, neurons and their synaptic connexions (E. Paul, unpublished). The results obtained with intravital methylene blue staining procedures (H. G. Hartwig, unpublished), based on the classical work of Holmgren (1917/ 1918), are also promising. There is no doubt that the epiphysis of *Rana esculenta* contains large stellate neurons contributing to the formation of the pineal tract. Furthermore, there are smaller bipolar or scarcely ramified neurons in juxtaposition or in a chain-like arrangement with the stellate cells (for details see Fig. 6). So far there is no evidence for typical horizontal cells. Some of the pineal neurons resemble amphibian amacrine cells. The arrangement of the bipolar neurons observed in the frog pineal is quite different from that in the retina. A number of pineal bipolar cells seem to contribute to the formation of the pineal tract (unmyelinated fibres?). There is a good correlation between the number of the large stellate neurons, or the large neurons rich in Nissl substance, and the myelinated fibres of the pineal tract (60–80).

* For further details of sections 3 and 5 see Paul, Hartwig and Oksche (1970).

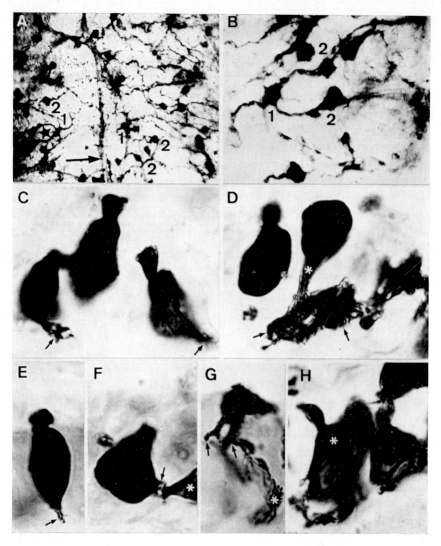

FIG. 6. Cells in the epiphysis of *Rana esculenta* stained by methylene blue (A, × 150; B, × 400) and Golgi–Colonnier methods (C–H, × 1340).

A. Cleared total preparation. Low-power micrograph showing multipolar (1) and bipolar (2) nerve cells. Axonal processes extend from both nerve cell types into the pineal tract (arrow). ★ indicates the area illustrated at higher magnification in B.

B. Convergence in the arrangement of two smaller neurons, probably interneurons (2), and one large multipolar (1) nerve cell. (H. G Hartwig, unpublished.)

C. Three receptor cells. Distinct terminals (arrow).

D. Nerve or receptor (?) cell with a single process (★) showing an extensive plexiform terminal formation (arrows).

E. Receptor cell with a typical terminal (arrow).

F. Receptor cell terminal (arrow) forming a synaptic contact with a nerve cell (★).

G. Receptor cell terminals (arrow) and a reticular formation (★).

H. Overlapping receptor cells (★). Processes with terminal convolutions and twigs. (E. Paul, unpublished; preparations by G. Möller and M. Langbein; see also Paul, Hartwig and Oksche 1970.)

We conclude that a limited number of interneurons appear to exist in the pineal sense organs of Anura. These interneurons differ in type from those seen in the amphibian retina.

(4) NERVOUS TRACTS OF PINEAL SENSE ORGANS (Fig. 7, Table I)

The nervous pathways of pineal organs have been reviewed by Kappers (1965, p. 89). The term "afferent" has been applied to epiphysio-fugal axons, while "efferent" nerve fibres run to the pineal body. The achromatic response observed in different pineal systems is mediated by nerve fibres of fast conduction velocity, whereas the chromatic response of the anuran frontal organ is transmitted by axons of fast and slow conduction velocity (Dodt, Ueck and Oksche 1970).

The frontal and epiphysial component of the afferent pineal tract of *Rana esculenta* has been explored systematically in electron micrographs. We counted 1–22 myelinated and 35–146 unmyelinated nerve fibres in the extracranial portion of the frontal tract ("pineal nerve") (Oksche and Vaupel-von Harnack 1965). Some of these frontal organs have shown a chromatic, and others an achromatic or even a chromatic and achromatic response (Morita, in Oksche and Vaupel-von Harnack 1965). However, the number of myelinated and unmyelinated fibres or the ratio of myelinated to unmyelinated elements do not provide an anatomical basis for understanding the chromatic or achromatic response mechanism. The diameter of the nerve fibres varies considerably. Exact histograms of axon calibres should provide valuable new anatomical information for functional interpretations. In the pineal tract of *Rana esculenta* conducting achromatic impulses, 60–80 myelinated fibres (1–6 μm in diameter) have been observed (Oksche and Vaupel-von Harnack 1965). In one *Rana esculenta*, 54 myelinated and 605 unmyelinated fibres of the pineal tract have been counted (Ueck, see Dodt, Ueck and Oksche 1970).

The parietal eyes of *Lacerta sicula* and *Iguana iguana* display reactions of the chromatic type. The parietal nerve of *Lacerta sicula* contains 10–40 myelinated and about 300 unmyelinated fibres, whereas the parietal nerve of *Iguana iguana* has only 200–300 unmyelinated fibres. The origin of the unmyelinated axons is still debatable. They may originate from smaller, less conspicuous nerve cells. A contribution to the pineal tracts by the axonal processes of the primary receptor cells cannot be ruled out completely. However, surgical interruption of the frontal organ nerve is not followed by a degeneration of receptor cells (Morita, Ueck and Vaupel-von Harnack, unpublished).

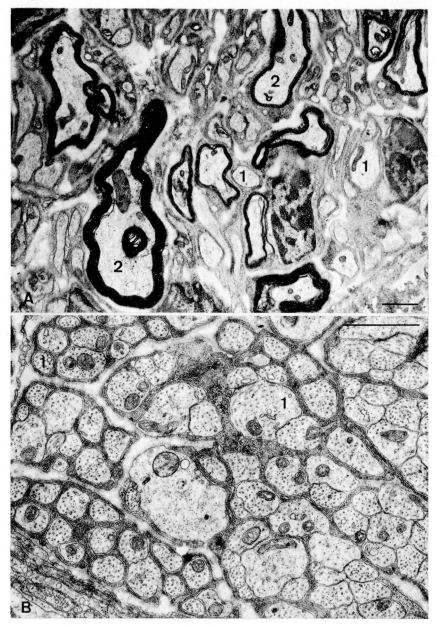

FIG. 7. Different fibre types in the parietal tract (parietal eye nerve) of
lizards.
    A. *Lacerta sicula.* Unmyelinated(1) and myelinated(2) axons. × 10 000.
    B. *Iguana iguana.* Unmyelinated axons (1).   × 21 600. See details in
section 4. Bar 1 μm.
    (A. Oksche and H. Kirschstein, unpublished.)

TABLE I

NUMBERS OF NERVE FIBRES IN DIFFERENT NERVE TRACTS OF THE PINEAL COMPLEX

Species	Tract	Nerve fibres Myelinated	Unmyelinated	Type of response* (impulse pattern)	
		1–22	35–146		
Rana esculenta	Tr. frontalis	1	35	Chromatic and achromatic	Oksche and Vaupel-von Harnack (1965)
		3	71	Chromatic	
		6	39	Achromatic	
		3	130	Achromatic	
		2	67	Chromatic and achromatic	
	Tr. pinealis	60–80	~200	Achromatic	Oksche and Vaupel-von Harnack (1965)
	Tr. pinealis	54 (5**)	605 (20**)		Ueck, see Dodt, Ueck and Oksche (1970)
Rana catesbeiana	Tr. frontalis, proximal div.	20	95	Chromatic	Ueck, see Dodt, Ueck and Oksche (1970)
	distal div.	9	30		Ueck, see Dodt, Ueck and Oksche (1970)
Lacerta sicula	Tr. parietalis	12–39	279–308	Chromatic	Oksche and Kirschstein (1968)
Iguana iguana	Tr. parietalis		~300	Chromatic	Oksche and Kirschstein (1968)
Lacerta vivipara	Tr. parietalis		~300		
Anguis fragilis	Tr. parietalis		~200		Oksche and Kirschstein (1968)
Anguis fragilis	Tr. parietalis		371		Petit (1968)
Sceloporus occidentalis	Tr. parietalis		~250		
Lacerta viridis	Tr. pinealis	34	241	(Achromatic)	Eakin and Westfall (1960)
Lacerta viridis	Tr. pinealis	1–16	73–93		Wartenberg and Baumgarten (1968)
Lacerta muralis	Tr. pinealis		124–148		Collin (1969)
					Collin (1969)

* Dodt and co-workers (for references see Dodt, Ueck and Oksche 1970)
** Number of frontal tract fibres joining the pineal tract.

New functional evidence (Morita, unpublished results) speaks in favour of efferent (fronto-petal) fibres within the anuran frontal nerve. Neuro-histological investigations with degenerating frontal nerves (due to surgical interruption) are in progress, using Nauta preparations.

(5) CENTRAL PROJECTION OF THE AFFERENT PINEAL TRACTS (Figs. 8–9)

The central projection of the pineal tracts is of great functional interest. The axons of the pineal tract can be traced easily to the diencephalic-mesencephalic border area where they are seen in juxtaposition with the subcommissural organ. In *Lacerta viridis*, subependymal terminals of the pineal tract have been described by Kappers (1967). In *Rana temporaria* and *Rana esculenta*, Paul and Hartwig (unpublished results) have interrupted the pineal tract surgically and studied fibre degeneration in Nauta prepara-tions. Degenerating fibre elements have been observed in the upper and lower divisions of the posterior commissure, *in the nuclear areas of the "periventricular gray"*, in the vicinity of nucleus Darkschewitsch, and some-times also in the pretectal region. The basal tegmentum of the mesence-phalon is always free of degenerating fibre elements.

The basal tegmentum in the frog contains reticular (extrapyramidal motor) and also aminergic centres (cf. Braak 1970). Degenerated pineal fibres have not been demonstrated within the aminergic areas described by Braak (1970). In regard to reticular centres, it should be remembered that in the sockeye salmon the negative phototactic response strongly depends on an intact pineal organ (Hoar 1955).

A considerable part of our work concerned with the problem of central projections of the pineal tract is still in progress.

(6) ASPECTS OF THE AVIAN PINEAL ORGAN

Some comment should be made on the avian pineal organ. This discussion will be limited to problems of general functional interest.

Our recent investigations of the avian pineal organ have been largely limited to the house sparrow, *Passer domesticus*. The structural findings reported here have been obtained from our joint project with Professor M. Menaker and Professor E. Dodt and their groups.

The pineal organ of birds has a remarkable secretory capacity (for references see Oksche and Kirschstein 1969) with light-dependent rhythmic changes in 5-hydroxytryptamine (5-HT) content. Our ultrastructural findings on avian secretory pinealocytes are in good agreement with the

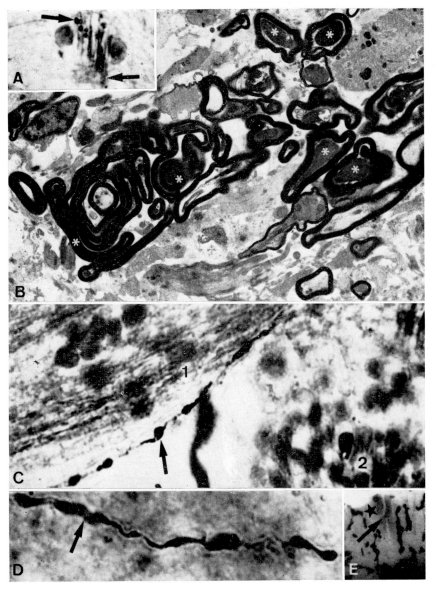

FIG. 8. Degeneration of pineal axons after microsurgical transection of the pineal tract.

A. *Rana temporaria*. Swollen fibres of the pineal tract (arrow) 8 days after injury. × 875.

B. *Rana esculenta*. Electron microscopic picture of degenerating pineal tract fibres (*) 8 days after injury. × 3750.

C. *Rana temporaria*. Degenerating pineal tract fibre (arrow) running with the posterior commissure (1); (2), subcommissural organ; 20 days after injury. × 1400.

D. *Rana temporaria*. Higher magnification of a swollen and distorted pineal tract fibre 19 days after injury (arrow). × 2170.

E. *Rana temporaria*. Dorsal view of the brain roof showing the transected (arrow) pineal tract. Dislocated proximal stump (★).

(A, C, D, E, E. Paul, unpublished, preparations by G. Möller and M. Langbein; B, A. Oksche and H. Kirschstein, unpublished.)

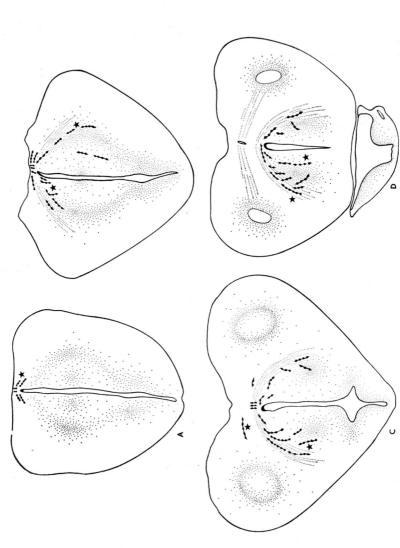

FIG. 9. *Rana esculenta*. Outline drawings of cross-sections through representative levels of the diencephalic–mesencephalic border area showing the distribution of degenerated pineal tract fibres (★swollen and bead-like structures). Nauta-Fink-Heimer method. Levels: A, pineal tract; B, subcommissural organ; C, posterior commissure; D, nuclei of the "central gray".

findings of Collin (1969). When compared with a characteristic outer segment of a pineal receptor cell, the bulbous cilium of avian pinealocytes appears vestigial. The lamellar complexes connected with these bulbous cilia are very irregular. Under conditions of vitamin A deficiency, causing severe damage of retinal outer segment structures, the further disintegration of pineal lamellar whorls is only gradual.

The following functional facts are related to these anatomical features. The pineal organ of *Passer domesticus* fails to show an electrical response to direct illumination (Ralph and Dawson 1968; Hamasaki, in Oksche and Kirschstein 1969). Similar tests with other avian species are also negative (for references see Oksche and Kirschstein 1969). On the other hand, surgical removal of the pineal organ in the house sparrow results in the loss of the circadian locomotor rhythms in constant darkness (Gaston and Menaker 1968). However, in the chicken, complete blinding does not interfere with the rate of enzymic synthesis of melatonin in the pineal organ. Furthermore, the pineal organ of *Passer domesticus* contains, in spite of its rudimentary receptor-type pinealocytes, puzzling synaptoid structures and intraparenchymal nerve bundles.

(7) SECRETORY ACTIVITY (BIOGENIC AMINES) OF SOME PINEAL SENSE ORGANS

The significant secretory activity of lacertilian and avian pineal organs has been investigated to some extent in our laboratory (Oksche, Ueck and Rüdeberg 1971). Hamasaki and Dodt (1969) have clearly proved that the pineal organ of a lizard, *Lacerta sicula*, is a functional photoreceptor showing an electrical response of the achromatic type. In *Lacerta sicula* a considerable number of pinealocytes bearing a vestigial or degenerating outer segment form secretory granules within the Golgi complex (Fig. 10).

A puzzling problem is the secretory activity of the teleost and anuran pineal sense organs (see Oksche, Ueck and Rüdeberg 1971). Owman, Rüdeberg and Ueck have investigated the pineal organ of the pike (Owman and Rüdeberg 1970) and the frog (Owman, Rüdeberg and Ueck 1970) with the fluorescence and electron microscopes. Both pineal organs contain large amounts of 5-HT in their sensory and supportive cells. A part of this fluorescent material may represent an agranular fraction of 5-HT. It may be suggested that in such sensory cells, rich in biogenic amines, photic impulses may be converted into a neuroendocrine reaction. In addition, in the pike and in the frog, noradrenergic nerve fibres appear in the connective tissue capsule of the pineal organ—these are new aspects of pineal biology. They deviate from the standard hypothesis based on the

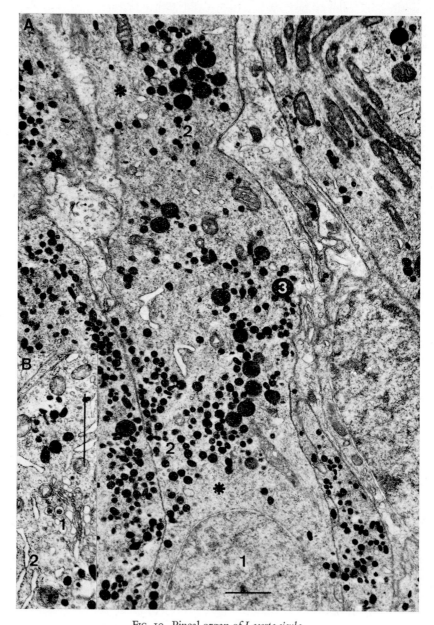

FIG. 10. Pineal organ of *Lacerta sicula*.

A. Secretory pinealocyte (★). Nucleus (1), 100 nm (1000 Å)-range dense-core vesicles (2), cytosomes (3). × 12 500.

B. Formation of secretory material within the Golgi complex (1); 2, endoplasmic reticulum. × 19 500. Bars 1 μm.

(A. Oksche and H. Kirschstein, unpublished.)

idea that secretory activity and sympathetic innervation of the pineal organ are products of a phylogenetic transformation characterized by a gradual or complete loss of receptor structures.

CONCLUSION

The ultrastructure of pineal sense organs has been studied quite thoroughly in terms of descriptive comparative morphology. In the future, more emphasis should be put on a direct correlation between neurophysiological and structural findings. Consequently, our recent studies have been extended to models providing further support for concepts of pineal regulatory systems.

SUMMARY

Pineal systems of fishes, anurans, lizards and birds (*Passer domesticus*) have been examined in the present studies. These studies have been correlated with the physiological investigations of Dodt and Menaker and their co-workers. The uniform structure of the cone-like pineal sensory cells does not explain the mechanism of the achromatic and chromatic responses to direct illumination. It is suggested that a certain degree of ultrastructural differentiation is needed in the pinealocyte outer segment to produce a primary photoreceptor response. Attempts have been made to demonstrate pineal photopigment and to analyse the nervous connexions of pineal neurons. A comparison of the structural composition of different epiphysio-fugal (afferent) pineal tracts has seemed to be helpful in judging the conduction velocities of achromatic and chromatic responses. Some pineal sense organs of lower vertebrates contain 5-HT and receive adrenergic nerve fibres. Thus in some pineal photoreceptors, the photic information may initiate a neuroendocrine reaction. This observation deviates to some extent from the prevalent concept of a gradual phylogenetic transformation of the pineal sense organ into a glandular organ. Degenerating epiphysio-fugal (afferent) fibres have been traced within the posterior commissure and the "central gray" after transection of the pineal tract in *Rana esculenta* and *Rana temporaria*.

Acknowledgements

The investigations reported in this paper were supported by research grants from the Deutsche Forschungsgemeinschaft and the Alexander von Humboldt Foundation.

The author is greatly indebted to Dr J. Priedkalns, Cambridge, and Miss I. Lyncker, Giessen, for their generous help in preparing this manuscript, to Miss D. Vaihinger for her drawings (Figs. 1, 2, 5, and 9) and to Mr W. Kramer for his excellent technical assistance.

REFERENCES

BRAAK, H. (1970) *Z. Zellforsch. mikrosk. Anat.* **106,** 269–308.

COLLIN, J. P. (1969) *Annls Stn Biol. Besse-en-Chandesse* suppl. 1, 1–359.

DODT, E. (1962) *Naturwissenschaften* **49,** 530–533.

DODT, E. and OKSCHE, A. (1971) In *Zoophysiology and Ecology*, ed. Burkhardt, D., Farner, D. S., Hoar, W. S., Jacobs, J. and Lindauer, M. Berlin, Heidelberg and New York: Springer. In press.

DODT, E., UECK, M. and OKSCHE, A. (1970) In *Proc. J. E. Purkyně Centenary Symposium, Prague*, ed. Kruta, V. In press.

DOWLING, J. E. (1968) *Proc. R. Soc. B.* **170,** 205–228.

DOWLING, J. E. and GIBBONS, I. R. (1961) In *The Structure of the Eye*, pp. 85–89, ed. Smelser, G. K. New York and London: Academic Press.

DOWLING, J. E. and WERBLIN, F. S. (1969) *J. Neurophysiol.* **32,** 315–338.

EAKIN, R. M. (1961) *Proc. natn. Acad. Sci. U.S.A.* **47,** 1084–1088.

EAKIN, R. M. and BRANDENBURGER, J. L. (1970) *J. Ultrastruct. Res.* **30,** 619–641.

EAKIN, R. M. and WESTFALL, J. A. (1960) *J. biophys. biochem. Cytol.* **8,** 483–499.

GASTON, S. and MENAKER, M. (1968) *Science* **160,** 1125–1127.

HAMASAKI, D. I. and DODT, E. (1969) *Pflügers Arch. ges. Physiol.* **313,** 19–29.

HOAR, W. S. (1955) *J. Fish. Res. Bd. Can.* **12,** 178–185.

HOLMGREN, N. (1917/1918) *Ark. Zool.* **11,** No. 24, 1–13.

KAPPERS, J. A. (1965) In *Structure and Function of the Epiphysis Cerebri (Progress in Brain Research* vol. 10), pp. 87–153, ed. Kappers, J. A. and Schadé, J. P. Amsterdam: Elsevier.

KAPPERS, J. A. (1967) *Z. Zellforsch. mikrosk. Anat.* **81,** 581–618.

KELLY, D. E. (1965) In *Structure and Function of the Epiphysis Cerebri (Progress in Brain Research* vol. 10), pp. 270–287, ed. Kappers, J. A. and Schadé, J. P. Amsterdam: Elsevier.

MORITA, Y. (1969) *Experientia* **25,** 1277.

NILSSON, S. E. G. and CRESCITELLI, F. (1970) *J. Ultrastruct. Res.* **30,** 87–102.

OKSCHE, A. and HARNACK, M. VON (1963) *Z. Zellforsch. mikrosk. Anat.* **59,** 239–288.

OKSCHE, A. and KIRSCHSTEIN, H. (1968) *Z. Zellforsch. mikrosk. Anat.* **87,** 159–192.

OKSCHE, A. and KIRSCHSTEIN, H. (1969) *Z. Zellforsch. mikrosk. Anat.* **102,** 214–241.

OKSCHE, A. and KIRSCHSTEIN, H. (1970) *Z. Zellforsch. mikrosk. Anat.* In press.

OKSCHE, A. and VAUPEL-VON HARNACK, M. (1965) *Z. Zellforsch. mikrosk. Anat.* **68,** 389–426.

OKSCHE, A., UECK, M. and RÜDEBERG, C. (1971) In *Symposium on Subcellular Organization and Function in Endocrine Tissues. Mem. Soc. Endocrinology* no. 19, ed. Heller, H. and Lederis, K. London: Cambridge University Press. In press.

OWMAN, CH. and RÜDEBERG, C. (1970) *Z. Zellforsch. mikrosk. Anat.* In press.

OWMAN, CH., RÜDEBERG, C. and UECK, M. (1970) *Z. Zellforsch. mikrosk. Anat.* **111,** 550–558.

PAUL, E., HARTWIG, H. G. and OKSCHE, A. (1970) *Z. Zellforsch. mikrosk. Anat.* In press.

PETIT, A. (1968) *Z. Zellforsch. mikrosk. Anat.* **92,** 70–93.

RALPH, C. L. and DAWSON, D. C. (1968) *Experientia* **24,** 147–148.

RÜDEBERG, C. (1968) *Z. Zellforsch. mikrosk. Anat.* **84,** 219–237.

RÜDEBERG, C. (1969) *Z. Zellforsch. mikrosk. Anat.* **96,** 548–581.

TAKAHASHI, H. (1969) *Bull. Fac. Fish. Hokkaido Univ.* **20,** 143–157.

UECK, M. (1968) *Z. Zellforsch. mikrosk. Anat.* **92,** 452–476.

UECK, M. (1969) *Z. Zellforsch. mikrosk. Anat.* **100,** 560–580.

UECK, M. (1970) 64. Jahresvers. Zool. Ges., Köln 1970. *Verh. Zool. Ges.* in press.

WARTENBERG, H. and BAUMGARTEN, H. G. (1968) *Z. Anat. EntwGesch.* **127,** 99–120.

[For discussion of this paper see pp. 164–175.]

SECRETORY ORGANELLES OF THE RAT PINEAL GLAND: ELECTRON MICROSCOPIC AND HISTOCHEMICAL STUDIES *IN VIVO* AND *IN VITRO*

Antti U. Arstila, Hannu O. Kalimo and Markku Hyyppä

Laboratory of Electron Microscopy and Department of Anatomy,
University of Turku, Finland

Although the fine structure of the rat pineal gland has been rather extensively studied (De Robertis and Pellegrino de Iraldi 1961; Arstila and Hopsu-Havu 1967; Wolfe 1965; Arstila 1967; Kappers 1969), many important problems still await elucidation. From biochemical studies it is well known that the rat pineal gland contains large amounts of mono-amines: noradrenaline, serotonin, melatonin and dopamine (for references see Wurtman, Axelrod and Kelly 1968; Kappers 1969). In previous reports of electron microscopic studies a variety of organelles have been observed in the pinealocytes and in the nerve endings which could be the morphological equivalents of the storage and release of these secretory products. However, the exact identification of the secretory organelles has so far failed in the pinealocytes, whereas in sympathetic nerve endings it has been possible to localize both serotonin and noradrenaline by electron microscopic, histochemical and radioautographic means (Wolfe *et al.* 1962; Taxi and Droz 1966; Jaim-Etcheverry and Zieher 1968*a*, *b*; Bak, Kim and Hassler 1970; Louis 1970). Furthermore, it has been difficult to clarify the relationship between the nerve endings and the pinealocytes, mainly because of the close structural similarity between the nerve endings and the terminations of the pinealocyte processes (the so-called terminal clubs). For instance, even though the morphology of the pinealocytes has been studied extensively, it was not until 1969 that Ariëns Kappers described the presence of synapses between at least some of the nerve endings and the pinealocyte perikarya.

We shall describe here some new electron microscopic findings on the rat pineal gland *in vivo* which are relevant to this point. However, the main emphasis in this paper will be placed on our electron microscopic, histochemical and radioautographic observations on the pineal gland cultured *in vitro*. It is our belief that many of the problems concerning the secretory organelles of the pinealocytes may be more easily elucidated *in vitro*, since nervous and humoral factors are excluded from this model.

THE RELATIONSHIP OF THE TERMINAL CLUBS TO THE NERVE ENDINGS

The majority of pinealocyte processes terminate at the periphery of the pericapillary spaces. The nerve fibres, which closely follow the capillaries, are, on the other hand, mostly adjacent to the capillary endothelial cells. From previous studies on the rat pineal gland it is well established that this difference in the localization of these two types of cell processes is by no means absolute and that the nerve endings can often be seen at the periphery of the pericapillary spaces or even within the pineal parenchyma (Wolfe 1965; Pellegrino de Iraldi, Zieher and De Robertis 1965; Arstila 1967; Kappers 1969). In these areas especially, the distinction between nerve endings and pinealocyte processes is often difficult. This problem is, of course, overcome if one is able to follow the pinealocyte process in a thin section from its origin, the cell perikaryon, to its termination, but in our material this has been possible only in a few instances. Therefore adequate distinction between the terminations of the pinealocyte processes (terminal clubs) and nerve endings has to rely on differences in their organelle contents. However, the nerve endings and especially the pinealocyte terminal clubs vary in their structure, which makes reliable distinction even more difficult. Because of this we shall briefly summarize the major variations in the structure of the pinealocyte terminal clubs as observed in our material.

(1) The majority of the clubs are filled with small agranular vesicles (about 40 nm in diameter), among which tubular structures, mitochondria and lipid inclusions are present. A few granular vesicles (about 100 nm) are also frequently seen in these clubs. (2) Another variant, although less frequently observed, is typified by the presence of vesicle-crowned lamellae. (3) A number of terminal clubs are characterized by the presence of numerous, quite electron-dense, membrane-limited bodies varying from 100 to 300 nm in diameter. In some of these bodies, especially the smaller ones, a distinct electron-lucent halo can be seen underneath the limiting membrane, and these bodies therefore resemble the larger granular vesicles in the nerve endings.

The nerve endings and/or the varicosities of the nerve fibres are usually distinguished by their smaller size and by the presence of numerous even-sized agranular vesicles (about 40 nm) within them. A few larger granular vesicles are also present within these endings. Another variant of the nerve

endings and/or varicosities closely resembles the Herring body: it is characterized by its larger size (up to 2 μm) and by the presence of numerous
mitochondria and dark membrane-limited bodies, while the number of
both granular and agranular vesicles is small (Fig. 1). Thus these structures
closely resemble those pinealocyte terminal clubs which are filled with
electron-dense, membrane-limited bodies, which makes their erroneous
identification possible.

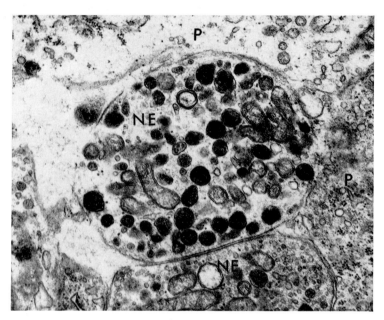

FIG. 1. Electron micrograph of the rat pineal *in vivo*, showing a Herring
body-like nerve ending, which contains numerous mitochondria and
dark membrane-limited bodies, but only a few agranular and granular
vesicles. P, pinealocyte; NE, nerve ending. × 15 200.

As mentioned, the nerve endings are by no means limited to the areas
around the capillary, but are also observed either within the pineal parenchyma or adjacent to the terminal clubs. In the case of the latter localization
we have recently found that the nerve endings and the terminal clubs at the
periphery of the pericapillary spaces sometimes appear to form "mixed"
clusters, in which both types of cell processes are intermingled. In these
instances it is difficult to identify reliably the individual structures as
terminal clubs or as nerve endings.

What then is the relationship of the nerve endings to the pinealocytes in
those instances where they are closely apposed to each other? In previous

studies Wolfe (1965) observed close apposition of the nerve endings with the pinealocytes and packing of vesicles in the nerve endings along the apposed membrane. He suggested that these sites may function as specific synapses. Arstila (1967) also observed close appositions of these structures with each other but considered it unlikely that they represented synapses, since they lacked membrane thickenings and since the packing of the vesicles also occurred towards intercellular spaces and interstitial cells. Additional interest to this question has been given by the recent observations of Kappers (1969), who found in some instances typical synapses

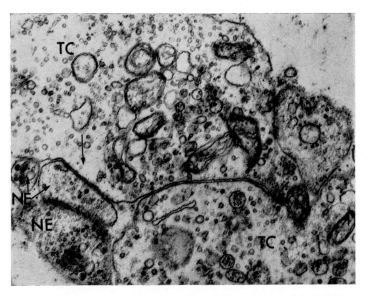

FIG. 2. A mixed cluster of nerve endings (NE) and terminal clubs (TC) in the pericapillary space of the rat pineal *in vivo*. The nerve ending is separated from the terminal club by a narrow intercelluar space (arrow), in which quite electron-dense material is present. × 10 400.

between nerve endings and pinealocyte perikarya. These were characterized by the accumulation of vesicles on the presynaptic side and by the accumulation of dense material under the postsynaptic membrane. He also suggested that the innervation of the gland might be quite similar to the innervation of smooth muscle by sympathetic fibres and could therefore have several different modes of transmission. Nerve fibres in the pericapillary spaces could exert their effect by releasing transmitter substances into the pericapillary spaces, whereas the nerve endings terminating against the pinealocyte perikaryon could exert their effect directly. In addition, the vesicle-crowned lamellae and fasciae adhaerentes between the pinealocytes could participate in the propagation of impulses between the pinealocytes.

Although we have not observed synapse-like structures between nerve endings and pinealocytes it is evident that a close spatial relationship often exists between them. This relationship is especially distinct in the "mixed" clusters of nerve endings and terminal clubs (Fig. 2). It is typified by the narrowing of the intercellular space to about 10 nm and by the presence of electron-dense material in the intercellular space between the apposed plasma membranes.

From the morphological point of view these contacts do indeed resemble the apposition of autonomic nerve endings and smooth muscle cells (Burnstock 1968). The innervated terminal club is, in turn, associated with neighbouring terminal clubs by modified tight junctions. Thus it can be assumed that the nerve impulse could spread from the innervated terminal club to adjacent terminal clubs by means of these low-resistance pathways.

Serotonin has been demonstrated in pinealocytes by fluorescence microscopy (Owman 1964; Bertler, Falck and Owman 1964; Falck, Owman and Rosengren 1966). However, the ultrastructural localization of serotonin and melatonin in the pinealocytes has remained unclarified, even though Taxi and Droz (1966), Jaim-Etcheverry and Zieher (1968b) and Bak, Kim and Hassler (1970) have succeeded in localizing serotonin to small granular vesicles in the nerve endings using both electron micro-scopic–histochemical and radioautographic techniques. For some reason both these techniques have failed to demonstrate serotonin in the pinealo-cytes, possibly because of the smaller concentration of serotonin per unit area in the pinealocytes than in the nerve endings. By analogy to nerve endings one could assume that serotonin is also stored in or secreted from the pinealocytes in the form of granular vesicles. However, even the presence of granular vesicles in rat pinealocytes has been controversial (De Robertis and Pellegrino de Iraldi 1961; Wolfe 1965; Rodin and Turner 1965; Arstila 1967; Halaris, Ruther and Matussek 1967), partly at least be-cause of the difficulties in distinguishing nerve endings from terminal clubs. From our previous and present observations it is evident that granular vesicles do occur in the pinealocytes *in vivo* and *in vitro*, although in many cells their number is relatively small. However, the question of whether these vesicles are storage or secretory organelles for indoleamines remains unsolved. It is well known that in the Golgi apparatus many other sub-stances are also packed into similar vesicles. For instance, many of the similar looking small bodies in the pinealocytes display acid phosphatase activity and therefore are most probably primary lysosomes (Arstila 1967).

FINE STRUCTURAL CHARACTERISTICS OF THE PINEAL GLAND *IN VITRO*

In our efforts to elucidate the morphological characteristics of secretion in the rat pineal gland we have recently turned our attention to organo-typic pineal gland cultures. This model not only eliminates the effects of nervous and humoral factors on the pinealocytes, but also serves as an easier experimental system for such techniques as radioautography, which is relatively difficult to do *in vivo*. In these experiments male albino rats weighing from 150 to 250 g were used and the animals were killed between 12.00 noon and 1.00 p.m. The pineal glands were cultivated by a modification of Trowell's method (1959). The cultivation time varied from four to eight days.

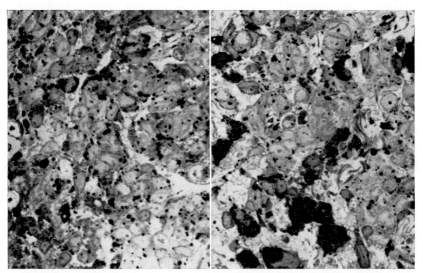

Fig. 3. (*left*). A light micrograph of the rat pineal gland *in vitro*. The pinealocytes contain numerous darkly stained lipid droplets. Epon-Araldite-embedded 1 μm section stained with toluidine blue. × 450.
Fig. 4 (*right*). A light micrograph of the pineal gland cultured in the presence of exogenous 5-hydroxytryptophan and nialamide. A number of pinealocytes contain abundant lipid inclusions, which fill the whole cell perikaryon. Epon-Araldite-embedded section stained with toluidine blue. × 450.

Since the fine structure of the pineal gland maintained *in vitro* has not been previously described the major relevant characteristics will be briefly summarized:

The fine structural features of the cultured pineal cells resemble those seen *in vivo*. The architecture of the gland is also rather similar, and the cells are arranged in irregular lobules surrounded by the former pericapillary spaces (Figs. 3 and 4). At the centre of the culture the cells are often necrotic or display alterations typical of hypoxic injury. The pinealocytes and interstitial cells are readily distinguishable from each other. In addition, there are small spindle-shaped cells at the periphery of the culture which resemble fibrocytes and are most probably derived from the capsule of the gland. After seven days of culture all nerve fibres and endings have completely disappeared.

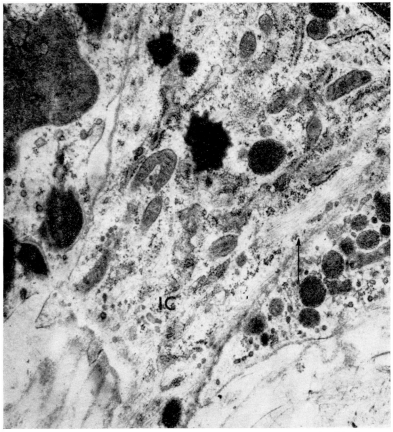

FIG. 5. Rat pineal cultured *in vitro*, showing a typical interstitial cell (IC) which displays granular endoplasmic reticulum, lipid inclusions and microfilaments (arrow). × 11 250.

The interstitial cells have elongated nuclei with a few indentations. Compared to the pinealocyte nuclei they have more heterochromatin at the periphery, and this gives them a rather dark appearance. Typical features of the cytoplasm are the microfilaments and the abundance of rough-surfaced endoplasmic reticulum (Fig. 5). Numerous single-membrane-limited bodies are observed, whereas the number of lipid inclusions is much smaller than in the pinealocytes.

The structure of the pinealocytes varies to some extent depending upon the culture medium. Typically the cells closely resemble those seen *in vivo* (Figs. 6 and 7). The nucleus is large with numerous deep indentations and contains only a little heterochromatin. In the cytoplasm the most conspicuous features are the abundant lipid inclusions, membrane-limited bodies and agranular vesicles. The lipid inclusions are about 0·3 μm in diameter and they are often arranged in tightly packed clusters of ten to

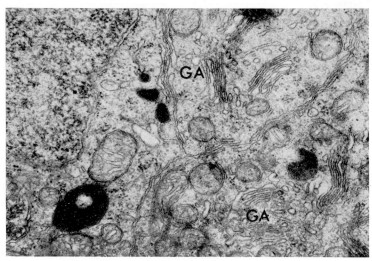

FIG. 6. Rat pineal cultured *in vitro*, showing three adjacent pinealocytes which display a conspicuous Golgi apparatus (GA) and dense lysosome-like bodies in the cytoplasm. The nucleus on the left is closely similar to that seen in pinealocytes *in vivo*. × 19 200.

thirty inclusions. The single-membrane-limited bodies display wide variations in their structure. Most of them are from 0·1 to 0·3 μm in diameter and composed of homogeneous material of intermediate electron density. Some of them are larger, up to 2 μm in diameter, and contain heterogeneous material typical of auto- and heterolysosomes. There is a continuous spectrum of bodies from the small granular vesicles measuring about 100 nm in diameter to large lysosome-like bodies. The membrane-limited bodies are often closely associated with the lipid inclusions and concentrated in the cell processes. The agranular vesicles are about 40 nm in diameter and are especially numerous in the Golgi area. Sometimes terminations of the cell processes are observed which are filled with the agranular vesicles. The Golgi apparatus is extensive and usually made up of five to ten dictyosomes. The endoplasmic reticulum is mostly of the smooth type, and the number of ribosomes is small.

A feature of the pinealocytes *in vitro* as opposed to those *in vivo* is the absence of vesicle-crowned lamellae. The junctional complexes are similar to those seen *in vivo*, and could be regarded as modified tight junctions (gap junctions), with an intercellular gap of about 10 nm.

When L-tryptophan (TP) or DL-5-hydroxytryptophan (5-HTP) is added to the culture medium at approximate concentrations of 10^{-3} mol/l

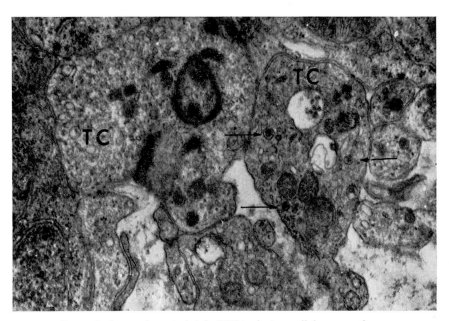

FIG. 7. A cluster of terminal clubs (TC) in the intercellular space of a rat pineal cultured *in vitro*. The terminal clubs are filled with agranular vesicles among which dense membrane-limited bodies are present. The smaller membrane-limited bodies (arrows) have a distinct halo underneath the membrane and therefore resemble granular vesicles containing monoamines. × 14 400.

and 10^4 mol/l the number of the lipid inclusions increases markedly, and often most of the cytoplasm is filled with them (Fig. 4). The appearance of the nucleus is also changed from a lobulated to a more regularly oval shape, and the rough-surfaced endoplasmic reticulum is more abundant.

The fine structure of the pinealocytes *in vitro* is quite similar to that of the pinealocytes *in vivo*, as described above. Both are composed of those organelles which have been thought to participate in the storage and secretion of the indoleamines, with the exception that pinealocytes *in vitro* do not have vesicle-crowned lamellae. Since the pineal gland is able to synthesize both serotonin and melatonin *in vitro* and secrete them into the culture medium (Shein, Wurtman and Axelrod 1967; Klein *et al.* 1970), it is unlikely that these organelles would be alone responsible for the secretion of the amines. It is interesting that vesicle-crowned lamellae are present *in vivo* if only the sympathetic nerve fibres are cut (Arstila 1967), but absent if the pinealocytes completely lack nervous and humoral contacts.

SECRETORY ORGANELLES OF THE PINEALOCYTES *IN VITRO*

Previous reports have shown that serotonin and melatonin can be synthesized by the pineal gland *in vitro* (Shein, Wurtman and Axelrod 1967;

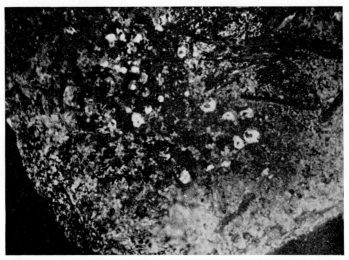

FIG. 8. A fluorescence histochemical preparation of the pineal gland cultured in the presence of 5-hydroxytryptophan and nialamide. A granular (yellow) fluorescence is seen in the majority of the cells. × 320.

Klein *et al.* 1970). We have done a series of experiments to characterize the localization of indoleamines histochemically by the fluorescence technique of Falck and Hillarp according to Eränkö (1967). In the preparations cultured without any added precursors of serotonin a yellowish fluorescence which disappears rapidly under ultraviolet light is seen throughout the tissue in the paraffin and Araldite-embedded sections (Hökfelt 1965). When tryptophan (TP) is added to the medium a more pronounced yellow fluorescence is noticed, which also disappears rapidly under ultraviolet light. This fluorescence is distinctly localized in the pinealocyte cytoplasm. When the tryptophan hydroxylase inhibitor, α-propyl-dopacetamide (H 22/54 Hässle; Carlsson, Corrodi and Waldeck 1963) is added to the medium at a concentration of o·3 mg/ml together with tryptophan, the fluorescence is weaker and is localized in the cells but is distributed diffusely throughout the culture. When 5-hydroxytryptophan (5-HTP) is added, with or without the inhibitor, a yellow fluorescence is again seen in the pinealocytes. In this case an exceptionally strong yellow granular fluorescence is localized in some of the pinealocyte perikarya, whereas the rest of the cells display less intense fluorescence (Fig. 8).

Under light microscopy of 1 μm sections stained with toluidine blue, distinct morphological alterations are also seen when TP or 5-HTP is added to the medium. These are typified by an increase in the number of lipid inclusions and/or membrane-limited bodies, especially in the perikarya of the pinealocytes (Fig. 4). It is likely that these cells are the same as those seen in fluorescent preparations, which display intense granular yellow fluorescence.

In the previous chemical studies it has been suggested that serotonin, melatonin and dopamine are present in pinealocytes (for references see Wurtman, Axelrod and Kelly 1968). The direct demonstration of serotonin and dopamine in pinealocytes has also been possible by a fluorescence histochemical technique (Bertler, Falck and Owman 1964; Owman 1964; Falck, Owman and Rosengren 1966). Since serotonin is also seen in the nerve fibres it has been more difficult to pinpoint the actual site of its synthesis. On the basis of experimental studies Owman (1964) and Wragg and co-workers (1967) reported that serotonin is synthesized in the pinealocytes and transported from them into the nerve endings. As mentioned above it has also been demonstrated by chemical means that serotonin is synthesized *in vitro* when TP or 5-HTP is added to the culture medium. Our findings, showing intensive yellow fluorescence in pinealocytes *in vitro* after the addition of TP or 5-HTP, also favour the idea that serotonin is synthesized in the pinealocytes and that this synthesis is not dependent upon nervous or humoral factors if TP or 5-HTP is present in the medium. On the other hand, we do not know if the bright yellow fluorescence is exclusively serotonin, since both TP and 5-HTP can induce a weak fluorescence themselves (Jonsson 1967).

In order to identify the organelles responsible for the granular yellow fluorescence we have done a series of electron microscopic histochemical studies. In these studies an intense acid phosphatase activity is seen in large single-membrane-bound bodies in the interstitial cells, whereas less activity is seen in the pinealocytes (Fig. 9). These large bodies are also morphologically typical lysosomes. Only about half of the smaller membrane-limited bodies can be identified as lysosomes on the basis of the lead phosphate reaction product. From these and previous results it is

6*

apparent that many, if not all, of the membrane-limited bodies seen both *in vivo* and *in vitro* are lysosomes. The larger number of them in both interstitial cells and pinealocytes *in vitro* is probably only a non-specific response to the conditions *in vitro*, typical of tissue cultures in general.

Since histochemical methods have been developed for demonstrating monoamines at a fine structural level it was of interest to do a series of experiments to demonstrate serotonin. In preparations fixed in sodium

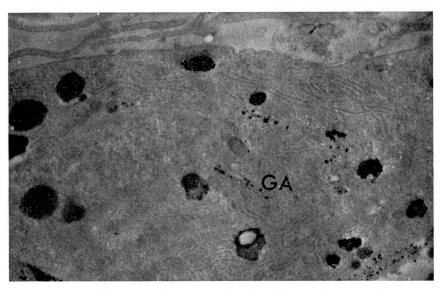

Fig. 9. A pinealocyte from a rat pineal cultured *in vitro*, showing acid phosphatase activity within the membrane-limited bodies and in the Golgi apparatus (GA). The lipid inclusions, on the other hand, are negative. × 14 000.

permanganate (Hökfelt and Jonsson 1968) the lipid inclusions and membrane-limited bodies are darkly stained, as are also all the membranous components in the interstitial cells and the pinealocytes. No staining is, on the other hand, observed using the technique of Jaim-Etcheverry and Zieher (1968*a*, *b*) to demonstrate serotonin. It should be pointed out that the sodium permanganate method is by no means specific to indole-amines but most probably stains all lipoprotein components of the cell.

The *in vitro* model of the pineal gland offers still another possibility for localizing indoleamines more precisely, by using light and electron micro-scopic radioautographic techniques. Although our results are still prelim-inary, some comments can already be made. These studies were done by adding tritiated 5-hydroxytryptophan to the culture medium at a concentration of 100 μCi/ml (specific activity 3·5 Ci/mM). To half of the specimens the monoamine oxidase inhibitor nialamide was added at a concentration of 0·25 mg/ml. The cells were fixed after four hours of incubation. For control studies some glands were incubated in a medium to which only nialamide was added. The radioautographic procedures were done according to the methods of Caro and Van Tubergen (1962) and Maunsbach (1966).

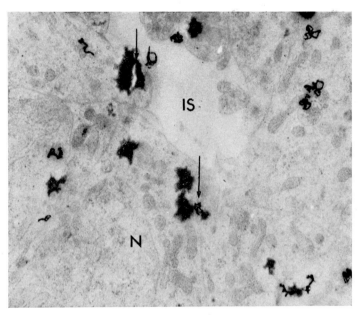

FIG. 10. An electron microscopic radioautograph of a rat pineal cultured *in vitro*, showing the distribution of grains over the cytoplasm of pinealocytes. Most of the grains are seen at a short distance from the lipid inclusions. The arrows point to grains over the lipid inclusions. IS, intercellular space; N, nucleus. × 10 800.

The light and electron microscopic radioautographs reveal that very little radioactivity is present in areas other than the pinealocyte cytoplasm (Figs. 10 and 11). When the distribution of grains is studied qualitatively by serial-section autoradiography, counting only those areas in which grains are seen over or adjacent to the same organelle in at least two serial sections, the following grain distribution is observed. Grains are seen over or close to lipid inclusions, membrane-limited bodies, agranular and granular vesicles and the Golgi apparatus. The quantitative analysis of the distribution of grain density in relation to lipid inclusions is shown in

Fig. 12 (Salpeter, Bachmann and Salpeter 1969). The grain density is maximal at a distance of 150 nm (1 HD) from the edge of the lipid inclusion, fairly high over the inclusions, but rapidly decreases when the distance from the lipid inclusion increases. These results suggest that radioactive 5-HTP is localized either in the lipid inclusions or in the cell sap in their immediate

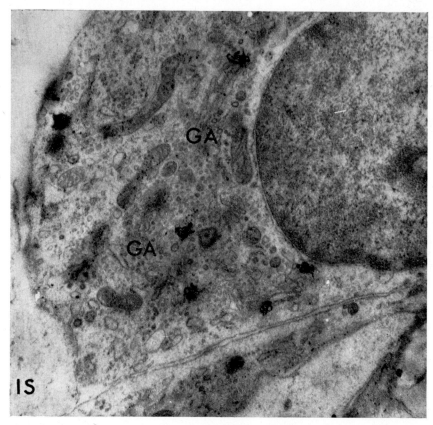

FIG. 11. An electron microscopic radioautograph of a pinealocyte of a rat pineal cultured *in vitro*. Grains are seen over the Golgi area (GA) and over the areas containing numerous small vesicles. IS, intercellular space. × 20 800.

vicinity. Although it is too early to speculate whether this localization represents uptake, storage or a secretory phase in serotonin synthesis, it is in accordance with the fluorescence histochemical studies demonstrating intense granular yellow fluorescence in the pinealocytes when 5-HTP is added to the culture medium. On the other hand the grains are not confined to lipid inclusions only; the areas around the Golgi apparatus especially, and those areas rich in agranular or granular vesicles and the larger membrane-limited bodies, display distinct radioactivity. Since the Golgi apparatus is known to participate in the formation of secretory vacuoles in many cell types this result seems to indicate that some stage in the secretory cycle of serotonin and/or melatonin occurs in the Golgi apparatus. Furthermore it is of interest that the grain density is especially high over the pinealocyte process whereas very little radioactivity is seen at four hours over the intercellular spaces. Bak, Kim and Hassler (1970) have recently described

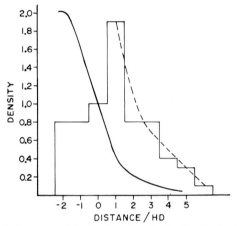

FIG. 12. A histogram of the developed grain-density distribution relative to lipid inclusions. The solid curve corresponds to the distribution expected if the lipid inclusions were homogeneously labelled with [³H]5-hydroxytryptophan. In the histogram the maximum grain density is seen at one HD (= 150 nm) from the edge of the lipid inclusions. The dotted curve shows that the grain density rapidly decreases when the distance from the lipid inclusions increases. The grain density was analysed according to Salpeter, Bachmann and Salpeter (1969) and Budd and Salpeter (1969). HD = 150 nm. The lipid inclusions were regarded as round bodies with a mean diameter of 0·3 μm. The histograms were obtained from 50 electron micrographs taken at × 7500 magnification.

the localization of tritiated 5-HTP in the nerve endings in the pineal gland *in vivo*, whereas only a few grains were seen over the pinealocyte cytoplasm and nuclei. Our preliminary studies on the localization of tritiated 5-HTP have demonstrated that in an *in vitro* model intense radioactivity is seen over the pinealocytes and that this model should be especially advantageous in future studies aimed at elucidating the secretory mechanisms of pinealocytes.

CONCLUSIONS AND SUMMARY

Our electron microscopic data on the rat pineal gland *in vivo* support the hypothesis of Kappers (1969) that the sympathetic nerve fibres may exert their effect on the pinealocytes in two different ways: (1) By a "slow" action through the release of neurotransmitters into the pericapillary space, from where they reach the pinealocytes by diffusion. (2) By a "fast" action through the gap junction-like contacts between the nerve endings and pinealocytes. In regard to the latter mechanism, the direct contacts of the nerve endings with the secretory processes of the pinealocytes may have a special functional significance, if one assumes that the sympathetic nerves either inhibit or facilitate the secretion of stored indoleamines from the pinealocytes into the circulation.

Klein and co-workers (1970) have shown that the pineal gland retains *in vitro* its ability to synthesize and secrete serotonin and melatonin. Since the cultured gland is totally denervated, this indicates that most probably it is the pinealocytes that synthesize these indoleamines and the action of nerves is not essential for this synthesis. The relationship between the serotonin pools in the pinealocytes and nerve endings as well as the exchange of serotonin between these two compartments remain, however, unknown. From our present results one can infer that serotonin is synthesized by the pinealocytes and thereafter secreted into the pericapillary space. So far no substantial evidence has been presented to identify the organelles in the pinealocytes responsible for the storage and/or release of serotonin and melatonin, since the cytochemical method for demonstrating serotonin introduced by Jaim-Etcheverry and Zieher (1968*a*, *b*) has failed to localize serotonin in the pinealocytes. Our present studies demonstrate that the pinealocytes also retain *in vitro* their fine structural characteristics with the exception of the disappearance of vesicle-crowned lamellae and the anticipated absence of nerves. The vesicle-crowned lamellae have been suggested as possible organelles taking part in the secretion of indoleamines in the rat pineal gland, but on the basis of our results *in vitro* we consider this unlikely.

The distinct yellow fluorescence, which is most probably induced by serotonin, is seen in the pinealocytes *in vitro*, and this finding is in agreement with the chemical studies of Shein, Wurtman and Axelrod (1967) and Klein and co-workers (1970). The distinct granularity of this fluorescence, together with the increase in the number of lipid inclusions in the presence of exogenous 5-HTP in the culture medium, suggests that the lipid inclusions are associated with the synthesis, storage or release of serotonin. This is also supported by our electron microscopic radioautographic results using exogenous tritiated 5-HTP as a precursor for serotonin. Part of the radioactivity is localized in and/or close to the lipid inclusions, and this localization is confirmed by the quantitative analysis of the autoradiographs according to Salpeter, Bachmann and Salpeter (1969). Another part of the radioactivity is localized in the pinealocyte cytoplasm over the areas which contain the Golgi apparatus, small agranular and granular vesicles and large membrane-limited bodies. These results would imply that the Golgi apparatus may participate in the synthesis and "packaging" of serotonin. As far as the small agranular and granular vesicles are concerned, it is too early to make any definite comments on their role in serotonin metabolism from our studies. Many of the large membrane-limited bodies might not be directly associated in the secretory processes, since they were identified as lysosomes on the basis of the positive reaction for phosphatase. It should, however, be borne in mind that the lysosomes also originate in the Golgi apparatus. The abundance of lysosomes in the interstitial cells and in the pinealocytes *in vitro* probably reflects only a sublethal injury due to the conditions *in vitro*.

The previous chemical and the present fluorescence microscopic, histochemical, radioautographic and electron microscopic findings show that the rat pineal gland in organotypic culture offers a suitable model for further characterization of the indoleamine secretory mechanisms. Furthermore the specificity with which the serotonin can be labelled by radioactive precursors may make this *in vitro* model useful in future studies of these mechanisms.

Acknowledgements

The work reported from the authors' laboratories was supported by grants from the Finnish National Research Council for Medical Sciences, from the Sigrid Juselius Foundation and from the Yrjo-Jahnsson Foundation.

REFERENCES

ARSTILA, A. U. (1967) *Neuroendocrinology*, suppl. 1, 1–101.
ARSTILA, A. U. and HOPSU-HAVU, V. K. (1967) *Z. Zellforsch. mikrosk. Anat.* **80,** 22.
BAK, I. J., KIM, J. H. and HASSLER, R. (1970) *Z. Zellforsch. mikrosk. Anat.* **105,** 167.
BERTLER, Å., FALCK, B. and OWMAN, CH. (1964) *Acta physiol. scand.* **63,** suppl. 239.
BUDD, G. C. and SALPETER, M. M. (1969) *J. Cell Biol.* **41,** 21.
BURNSTOCK, G. (1968) *Proc. XXIV Int. Congr. Physiol. Sci.* **6,** 7.
CARLSSON, A., CORRODI, H. and WALDECK, B. (1963) *Helv. chim. Acta* **46,** 2271.
CARO, L. G. and VAN TUBERGEN, R. P. (1962) *J. Cell Biol.* **15,** 173.
DE ROBERTIS, E. and PELLEGRINO DE IRALDI, A. (1961) *J. biophys. biochem. Cytol.* **10,** 361.
ERÄNKÖ, O. (1967) *Jl R. microsc. Soc.* **87,** 259.
FALCK, B., OWMAN. CH. and ROSENGREN, E. (1966) *Acta physiol. scand.* **67,** 300.
HALARIS, A., RUTHER, E. and MATUSSEK, N. (1967) *Z. Zellforsch. mikrosk. Anat.* **76,** 100.
HÖKFELT, T. (1965) *J. Histochem. Cytochem.* **13,** 518.
HÖKFELT, T. and JONSSON, G. (1968) *Histochemie* **16,** 45.
JAIM-ETCHEVERRY, G. and ZIEHER, L. M. (1968a) *Z. Zellforsch. mikrosk. Anat.* **86,** 393.
JAIM-ETCHEVERRY, G. and ZIEHER, L. M. (1968b) *J. Histochem. Cytochem.* **16,** 162.
JONSSON, G. (1967) *Histochemie* **8,** 288.

KAPPERS, J. A. (1969) *J. Neuro-visc. Rel.* suppl. 9, 140.

KLEIN, D. C., BERG, G. R., WELLER, J. and GLINSMANN, W. (1970) *Science* **167**, 1738.

LOUIS, C. J. (1970) *Histochem. J.* **2**, 29.

MAUNSBACH, A. B. (1966) *J. Ultrastruct. Res.* **15**, 197.

OWMAN, CH. (1964) *Acta physiol. scand.* **63**, suppl. 240.

PELLEGRINO DE IRALDI, A., ZIEHER, L. M. and DE ROBERTIS, E. (1965) In *Structure and Function of the Epiphysis Cerebri (Progress in Brain Research* vol. 10), pp. 389–422, ed. Kappers, J. A. and Schadé, J. P. Amsterdam: Elsevier.

RODIN, A. E. and TURNER, R. A. (1965) *Lab. Invest.* **14**, 1644.

SALPETER, M. M., BACHMANN, L. and SALPETER, E. E. (1969) *J. Cell Biol.* **41**, 1.

SHEIN, H. M., WURTMAN, R. J. and AXELROD, J. (1967) *Nature, Lond.* **213**, 730.

TAXI, J. and DROZ, B. (1966) *C.r. hebd. Séanc. Acad. Sci., Paris, Sér. D* **263**, 1326.

TROWELL, O. A. (1959) *Expl Cell Res.* **16**, 118.

WOLFE, D. E. (1965) In *Structure and Function of the Epiphysis Cerebri (Progress in Brain Research* vol. 10), pp. 332–369, ed. Kappers, J. A. and Schadé, J. P. Amsterdam: Elsevier.

WOLFE, D. E., POTTER, L. T., RICHARDSON, K. C. and AXELROD, J. (1962) *Science* **138**, 440.

WRAGG, L. E., MACHADO, C. R. S., SNYDER, S. H. and AXELROD, J. (1967) *Life Sci.* **6**, 31.

WURTMAN, R. J., AXELROD, J. and KELLY, D. E. (1968) *The Pineal.* New York and London: Academic Press.

DISCUSSION

Dodt: In the frontal organ of the pineal of most species of frogs anatomists describe typical signs of structural regression of the outer segments. The functional performance, however, is surprisingly good in most cases. As far as the absolute threshold is concerned, the values obtained compare favourably to the absolute threshold in man. This implies a highly developed nervous organization including a convergence mechanism of several sense cells on to one ganglion cell. In respect of the functional state of the photoreceptor outer segments of the pineal end vesicle of the frog and the epiphysis cerebri in lizards, we note that the individual outer segment has only about 5 per cent of the number of lamellated discs and only about 3 per cent of the volume of the individual outer segments of rods in the frog's lateral eye. Consequently, only a small amount of photopigment will be present. Yet the light threshold in the dark-adapted state is about the same in the pineal organ and in the lateral eye. In the epiphysis cerebri of *Lacerta* the light threshold in the dark-adapted state is about a thousand times higher. This, however, does not necessarily mean that the outer segments are less functional. It indicates that the converging mechanism of sensory cells towards ganglion cells is less pronounced in the epiphysis cerebri of lizards than in the pineal system of the frog.

By comparison it is interesting to note that the first electroretinographic response to light in developing tadpoles of frogs is a cornea-negative potential corresponding in time with the first appearance of outer segments of retinal receptors, as revealed by electron microscopy (Nilsson and Crescitelli 1970). No signs were noted of receptor synaptic structures or of the outer plexiform layer. The potential recorded may therefore be an isolated receptor potential, since the appearance of the cornea-positive potential somewhat later corresponded in time with the maturation of the receptor synaptic apparatus. Within the pineal system of some species of fishes synaptic structures are scarcely developed or even absent. Nevertheless, besides the slow potential, propagated impulses from ganglion cells as well as from tract fibres can be recorded at light intensities close to the absolute threshold of the human eye. In order to avoid the conclusion that we are dealing with neurons of primary receptor cells, we are forced to believe that propagation of impulses within the pineal system somehow differs from that in the lateral eye.

Structurally the outer segments of pineal and parietal photoreceptors are clearly of the cone type. According to current concepts of retinal function, it is not the type of sensory cell (rod or cone) which determines the type of response, but rather the photopigment in the outer segments and the upstream and horizontal nervous connexions of neural elements. Physiologically, both the chromatic and achromatic responses are different from what recording from the third optic neuron of the vertebrate retina has shown. The achromatic response may be understood as the result of inhibitory action of sensory cells on the second-order neurons from which recordings are made. The sensory cells governing this type of response may contain one (fishes) or two (frogs) photopigments absorbing light at or near 500 nm (fishes, frogs) and at 570 nm (frogs). In the so-called chromatic response of the pineal system, the situation is different since two types of sensory cells may be present, one absorbing in the ultraviolet (fishes, frogs) or in the blue (lizards), the other in the green (fishes, frogs and lizards). As far as the nervous organization of the pineal organ is concerned, the structural findings available provide only a narrow basis for understanding the physiological findings. It is mainly the apparent lack of cells comparable to the bipolar, amacrine and horizontal cells which suggests a two-neuron pathway in the pineal organs.

In order to achieve the chromatic response, sensory cells absorbing short wavelengths may exert their effect either by inhibiting presynaptically the excitatory effect of the green-absorbing sensory cell or by using a different transmitter substance. A third possibility would be the presence of inhibitory interneurons. For the two-neuron pathway of the frog's pineal eye, Hamasaki proposed a model demonstrating the possible relationship of two photoreceptors synapsing on the same ganglion cell (Fig. 1). His hypothesis is based on the recording of the slow potentials from the *Stirnorgan* which he regards as the summated inhibitory and excitatory postsynaptic potentials of the ganglion cells transmitted electrotonically along the nerve to the recording electrode (Baumann 1962; Hamasaki 1970). Like the excitatory postsynaptic potentials of the central nervous system of vertebrates, Hamasaki believes the positive slow potential to be the generator potential of the spike of the ganglion cells. In regard to the significantly shorter latencies of the inhibitory (ultraviolet) system, Hamasaki suggests that these photoreceptors synapse on the soma of the

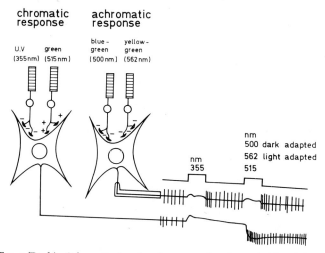

FIG. 1 (Dodt). Schematic drawing demonstrating the probable relationship between the photoreceptor and ganglion cells for the chromatic and achromatic system of the frog's pineal organ (modified after Hamasaki 1970).

ganglion cells while the longer latency and summation period of the excitatory system would indicate that the excitatory photoreceptors synapse on the dendrites.

From Oksche and Vaupel-von Harnack (1965) we know the number and diameter of medullated and unmedullated nerve fibres as well as the number and diameter of ganglion cells within the pineal system of the frog. Physiologically, there is good agreement between these observations on the presence of medullated and unmedullated nerve fibres and the conduction velocities measured in the pineal nerve and tract (Dodt and Morita 1967).

A possible approach to the identification of structures involved in the achromatic and chromatic responses may be the observation that achromatic responses were never obtained when recordings were made from unmedullated nerve fibres. Furthermore, in the frog's pineal end vesicle the chromatic photic response is found more regularly than the achromatic response, which is a prominent response of the frog's epiphysial stalk. Similarly to the frog and still more clearly separated are the two types of response in the lizard's pineal system. Only chromatic responses are recorded from the parietal eye of *Lacerta*, whereas only achromatic responses are obtained from its epiphysis cerebri.

According to Morita (1963, quoted by Dodt 1964), repetitive electrical stimuli applied to the frog's pineal nerve cause long-lasting (2–5 minutes) changes in afferent impulse activity in the pineal nerve both for the spontaneous discharge in the absence of light and for the sustained excitation following stimulation of the *Stirnorgan* by red light (chromatic response). The question arises whether or not the effects may be due to antidromic hyperpolarization of pineal ganglion cells or by the activation of efferent nerve fibres making synaptic contact with the pineal ganglion cells. Since post-tetanic facilitation frequently occurs in Morita's experiments there is evidence that part of the pineal nerve fibres somehow transmit efferent signals into the neural network of the *Stirnorgan*. Furthermore, there is some evidence that unmedullated nerve fibres are involved. According to a model proposed by Collin (1969), efferent autonomic nerve fibres in lizards approach the inner segment of the photoreceptors close to their synaptic junctions with the ganglion cells in the epiphysis cerebri. It is highly desirable for degeneration experiments to be made on pineal nerves in order to see where the efferent fibres end.

Oksche: Degeneration experiments of this type are in progress in our laboratory. With regard to Dr Hamasaki's model, we have never seen axo-somatic contacts between the pineal receptor endings and the perikaryon (soma) of the nerve cells in our electron micrographs; all synaptic contacts are located in a plexiform neuropile area and they seem to be axo-dendritic. The axo-somatic contacts observed in light microscopic preparations are not conclusive with respect to the synaptic character of the contact zone.

Miline: Professor Oksche, what happens in the proximal segment of neurons after transection of the pineal tract? Is there regeneration? Secondly, do the afferent fibres come from the habenula?

Oksche: The examinations of the proximal segment of the transected anuran pineal tract are still in progress. We were able to examine only 51 distal segments, 2 to 28 days after transection of the pineal tract in the frog, and we never saw any degenerating structures in the habenula.

Mess: There has been terrible confusion in the last ten years about the histology of the pineal body, and anything from one cell type to five different cells types has been described. Is there any agreement now that the pineal body of mammals, at least, consists of two different cell types: the pinealocyte and the remnants of the original photosensitive cells? Secondly, if both cell types really exist, do both equally secrete all members of the series of indoleamines, that is to say melatonin and serotonin, or do the phylogenetically older remnants of photosensitive cells perhaps secrete only up to the step of serotonin and a more developed cell type takes the synthesis further to melatonin? Can we agree now on what is the structure and the related function, from the histological point of view, of the mammalian pineal?

Oksche: I think you forgot the astrocytes in the mammalian pineal organ. I would say that this organ consists of secretory pinealocytes and astrocytes. On the basis of our own findings, in the lizard *Lacerta sicula*, I am ready to accept Dr Collin's hypothesis of a progression from a fully differentiated receptor, through a form with a vestigial outer segment, to the classical secretory pinealocyte. In the mammalian pineal there are no vestigial sensory cells, at least in adult animals.

Kappers: In the mammalian pineal gland there is, indeed, only one characteristic cell type, the pinealocyte, which is exclusively secretory. Another cell type of ectodermal origin is also present in varying numbers. This is the so-called "interstitial cell", which, however, can better be termed "fibrous astrocyte" to avoid confusion with the interstitial cells of Cajal, which are utterly different in structure and function and are not present in the pineal.

Arstila: I also think that there is only one major cell type in the rat pineal gland, the so-called pinealocyte. On the other hand, I would hesitate to call the other cell type an astrocyte, because for the present we do not know enough about the metabolism and function of these cells. The astrocytes of the central nervous system have a very characteristic metabolism as compared for instance to oligodendrocytes. However, morphologically, the second cell type resembles astrocytes somewhat.

Collin: In all pineals one type of cell is always numerically important and invariably accompanies the cells of the sensory line (photoreceptors, rudimentary photoreceptors, pinealocytes and the presumed intermediate forms) and sensory nerve cells. All the terms proposed for this type are inadequate ("supportive cells", "ependymal cells" of the lower vertebrates). Their functional significance is uncertain (Collin 1969). In pineal organs of higher vertebrates, lacking a lumen, such cells are generally termed "glial cells" or "interstitial cells" or "astrocytes". In terms of the phylogeny of the pineal, it seems possible that "glial" or "interstitial cells" are the equivalent of the "supportive cells" or "ependymal cells" of lower vertebrates. All these cells generally contain numerous microfilaments.

In terms of an evolutionary series of such cells, we must suppose that the polarity (lumen—basement membrane) found in the Anamniota and Sauropsida disappears in snakes and mammals, where the lumen is lost from the pineal. In all vertebrates I provisionally term these elements "interstitial cells" (Wolfe 1965, in the laboratory rat). The functional aspects are not involved here, but there can be confusion with the "interstitial cells" of Cajal. The term "satellite cell" cannot be used because lemmocytes are present in the pineals of lower vertebrates such as *Lampetra*. So the problem of the terminology and the function of such cells remains open.

Pellegrino de Iraldi: There are certain species differences in the morphology of the pineal secretory cells in mammals. These differences are most evident in the perivascular space. Light and electron microscopic studies have demonstrated that the mammalian pineal gland is made up of two cell types: the pinealocytes and a small proportion of glial and/or interstitial cells. The organ is mainly, if not exclusively, innervated by the superior cervical ganglia (Kappers 1965). The pinealocyte was described by del Rio Hortega (1922) as a polymorphic cell with processes ending in club-shaped enlargements which are situated in the perivascular and intercellular spaces. This pattern has been confirmed in all studies of the structure of the mammalian pineal.

Electron microscopic studies have demonstrated that there are at least two kinds of processes in the perivascular and intercellular spaces. One of them shows the structure now considered to be characteristic of adrenergic nerves (De Robertis and Pellegrino de Iraldi 1961; Bondareff 1965), and the other is more polymorphic, resembling the structure of the pinealocyte. They will be called polar processes, following the nomenclature proposed by Wolfe (1965). The former processes disappear and the latter remain after bilateral superior cervical ganglionectomy (Pellegrino de Iraldi, Zieher and De Robertis 1965).

The polar processes of the rat pineal are characterized (Fig. 1) by clear vesicles of different sizes. Exceptionally, some electron-dense vesicles may be observed. In the cytoplasm clear vesicles are also predominant. Our observations (Pellegrino de Iraldi, Zieher and De Robertis 1965) agree with those of Dr Arstila (1967). A similar pattern has been observed in cow and lamb (Anderson 1965), cat (Duncan and Micheletti 1966), monkey (Wartenberg 1968) and rabbit (Wartenberg and Gusek 1965).

In the pineal of the hamster (Fig. 2) the polar processes are characterized by abundant granulated vesicles intermingled with clear vesicles. Similar kinds of vesicles may be found in the cytoplasm although in a smaller concentration (Pellegrino de Iraldi 1966).

In the mouse pineal the polar processes (Fig. 3) are filled with granulated

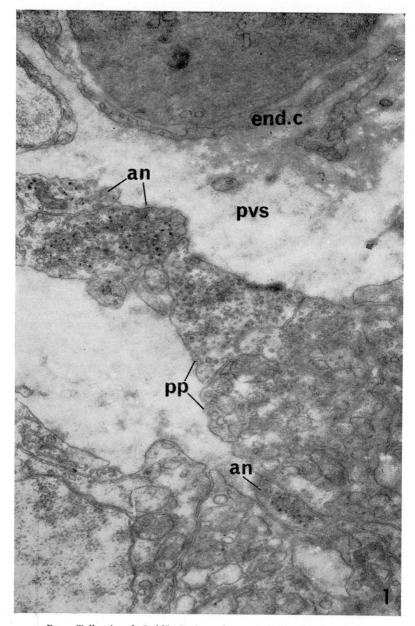

FIG. 1 (Pellegrino de Iraldi). Perivascular space (pvs) of the rat pineal, fixed in osmium tetroxide. Adrenergic nerve endings (an) with small granulated vesicles and polar processes (pp) with stippled vesicles and clear vesicles of different size may be observed. End. c, endothelial cell.

×25 000.

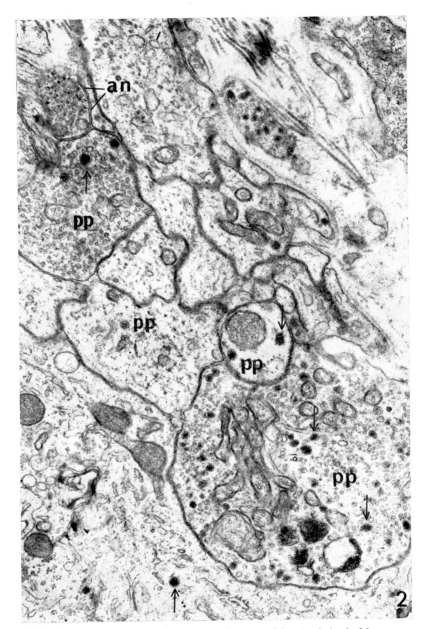

Fig. 2 (Pellegrino de Iraldi). Perivascular space of the pineal gland of the hamster, fixed in osmium tetroxide. Adrenergic nerve endings (an) with small granulated vesicles and different kinds of polar processes (pp) are observed. Large granulated vesicles (arrows) are seen in some polar processes and in the perikaryon. × 25 000.

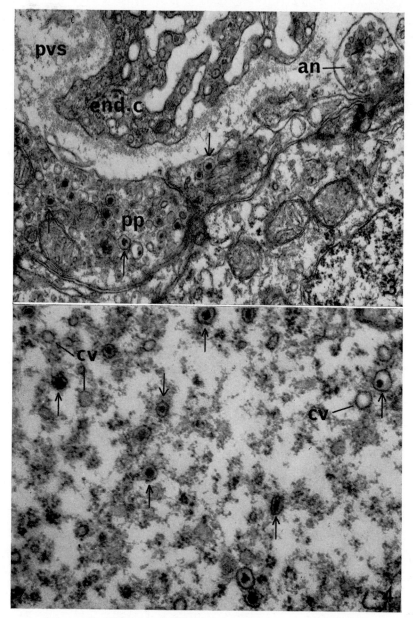

FIGS. 3 and 4 (Pellegrino de Iraldi). Pineal gland of the mouse, fixed in
osmium tetroxide.
Fig. 3 (*upper*). Perivascular space (pvs) with an adrenergic nerve
ending (an) and polar processes (pp) with large granulated vesicles
(arrows). × 45 000.
Fig. 4 (*lower*). Perikaryon of a pinealocyte showing clear (cv) and
granulated vesicles of similar size (arrows). × 45 000.

and clear vesicles of similar size. They are also abundant in the cytoplasm (Fig. 4) (Pellegrino de Iraldi 1969).

Comparing these different patterns we conclude that the granulated vesicles observed in the pineals of the mouse and hamster are the homologue of clear vesicles found in many mammals and that both kinds of vesicles may correspond to morphological signs of the secretory activity of the pinealocytes. At present we have no explanation for these species differences.

Wurtman: I should like to return to the question raised earlier by Dr Owman (p. 124) of whether all that glitters is really serotonin. This issue came up at the previous pineal meeting (Kappers and Schadé 1965) when the fact that the pineal contained so much serotonin as indicated by histochemical fluorescence assays caused its relatively high concentration of noradrenaline to be missed entirely. What I am questioning now is whether we can extrapolate from the localization of noradrenaline in sympathetic nerve endings to granular vesicles, to the assumption that serotonin will also be stored in granular vesicles within pinealocytes. I'm afraid the evidence is more against this assumption than for it. Dahlström, making fluorescence studies of noradrenergic and serotoninergic neurons in the central nervous system, has shown (1970) that while in the noradrenergic neurons most of the neurotransmitter is located at the region of the nerve ending among the granules, in the serotoninergic cells the yellow fluorescence is distributed throughout the cell. There is not the same intense concentration of colour in the region of the nerve ending. With this sort of evidence it seems dangerous to conclude from the fact that sympathetic-neuronal noradrenaline is concentrated within granules that serotonin will have a similar distribution in pinealocytes. One important experiment that should be done before one can make this assumption is to homogenize pineals previously incubated with radioactive tryptophan and demonstrate on sucrose-density gradients that the resulting radioactive serotonin is present in the granular fraction. From the studies to be described by Dr Shein (pp. 197–207) it appears that most of the serotonin and melatonin formed by the pineal is not retained inside the pinealocytes; about a thousand times as much is released into the medium. So the notion that there is a specific secretory mechanism for pineal serotonin should not be accepted uncritically. The indole may be released upon being made.

Arstila: I agree that this is a possibility. I would also emphasize that there is no conclusive radioautographic evidence yet that noradrenaline is present inside the small granular vesicles in sympathetic nerve terminals, because of the poor resolution of electron microscopic radioautography and the small size of the granular vesicles. From our own radioautographic studies on the localization of serotonin it appears that radioactive 5-hydroxy-tryptophan is localized in the pinealocyte cytoplasm, whereas there is little radioactivity in the nuclei of the pinealocytes, in the interstitial cells or in the intercellular spaces. Of course, the radioactive material would be washed out from the intercellular spaces during the processing of the tissue for electron microscopy.

Owman: We should remember that serotonin has a very rapid turnover in the pineal (see Falck, Owman and Rosengren 1966) and that the diurnal fluctuations are very marked. When trying to find the submicroscopic storage site for serotonin we should consider as one possibility—and I only say *possibility*—that serotonin might not even be stored in the pineal in the classical sense but synthesized according to the needs. It is thus not necessary that it is stored in a type of organelle of the same kind as in neurons or in enterochromaffin cells.

Kordon: Professor Dodt, has anyone tried to block the light-induced responses that you have recorded using drugs that interfere with mono-amine metabolism? Such experiments could help to determine whether serotonin or other monoamines are involved in these evoked responses.

Dodt: Nobody has done this yet, but it's a very good suggestion.

Miline: Dr Arstila, have you observed lamellar bodies in pinealocytes? In rats Wolfe has described pineal lamellar concentric formations which come from mitochondria (Wolfe 1965). We have shown that they occur in the wild rabbit in response to emotion (Miline, Devečerski and Krstić 1966). Secondly, do you think that synaptic ribbons are evidence of secretion, or are they specialized synaptic formations? We have observed great numbers of this formation after stress conditions (such as immobili-zation and cold). Can we speak of physiological degeneration of ribbon synapses or regeneration of ribbon synapses?

Arstila: One sees in rat pinealocytes *in vivo* so-called lamellar bodies, which somewhat resemble stacks of myelin lamellae. This is interesting, since the photoreceptor organelles are made of similar looking lamellae. These lamellar bodies may have some special functional significance.

The mitochondria are quite peculiar in many pinealocytes since they look like the vesicular mitochondria in steroid-secreting cells. As to the synaptic ribbons, we have mostly looked at normal pineal glands and therefore have not observed alterations in their structure or in their number. The only thing we know in this regard, is that when we culture the pineal gland *in vitro* in the dark the synaptic ribbons disappear. Whether they are secretory or whether they have electrophysiological activity, we do not know.

REFERENCES

ANDERSON, E. (1965) *J. Ultrastruct. Res.* suppl. 8, 1–80.

ARSTILA, A. U. (1967) *Neuroendocrinology*, suppl. 1, 1–101.

BAUMANN, CH. (1962) *Pflügers Arch. ges. Physiol.* **276**, 56–65.

BONDAREFF, V. (1965) *Z. Zellforsch. mikrosk. Anat.* **67**, 211–218.

COLLIN, J. P. (1969) *Annls Stn Biol. Besse-en-Chandesse* suppl. 1, 1–359.

DAHLSTRÖM, A. (1970) *Neurosci. Res. Prog. Bull. Brain Monoamines and Endocrine Function*, ed. Wurtman, R. J. In press.

DE ROBERTIS, E. and PELLEGRINO DE IRALDI, A. (1961) *Anat. Rec.* **139**, 299.

DODT, E. (1964) *Vision Res.* **4**, 23–31.

DODT, E. and MORITA, Y. (1967) *Pflügers Arch. ges. Physiol.* **293**, 184–192.

DUNCAN, D. and MICHELETTI, G. (1966) *Texas Rep. Biol. Med.* **24**, 576–587.

FALCK, B., OWMAN, CH. and ROSENGREN, E. (1966) *Acta physiol. scand.* **67**, 300–305.

HAMASAKI, D. I. (1970) *Vision Res.* **10**, 307–316.

HORTEGA, P. DEL RIO (1922) *Archs Neurol.* **3**, 359–389.

KAPPERS, J. A. (1965) In *Structure and Function of the Epiphysis Cerebri (Progress in Brain Research* vol. 10), pp. 87–153, ed. Kappers, J. A. and Schadé, J. P. Amsterdam: Elsevier.

KAPPERS, J. A. and SCHADÉ, J. P. (ed.) (1965) *Structure and Function of the Epiphysis Cerebri (Progress in Brain Research* vol. 10). Amsterdam: Elsevier.

MILINE, R., DEVEČERSKI, V. and KRSTIĆ, R. (1966) In *Symposium Internationale sur la Neuroendocrinologie*, pp. 229–256. Paris: Expansion Scientifique Française.

NILSSON, S. E. G. and CRESCITELLI, F. (1970) *J. Ultrastruct. Res.* **30**, 87–102.

OKSCHE, A. and VAUPEL-VON HARNACK, M. (1965) *Z. Zellforsch. mikrosk. Anat.* **68**, 389–426.

PELLEGRINO DE IRALDI, A. (1966) *Anat. Rec.* **154**, 481.

PELLEGRINO DE IRALDI, A. (1969) *Z. Zellforsch. mikrosk. Anat.* **101**, 408–418.

PELLEGRINO DE IRALDI, A., ZIEHER, L. M. and DE ROBERTIS, E. (1965) In *Structure and Function of the Epiphysis Cerebri (Progress in Brain Research* vol. 10), pp. 389–422, ed. Kappers, J. A. and Schadé, J. P. Amsterdam: Elsevier.

WARTENBERG, H. (1968) *Z. Zellforsch. mikrosk. Anat.* **86**, 74–97.

WARTENBERG, H. and GUSEK, W. (1965) In *Structure and Function of the Epiphysis Cerebri (Progress in Brain Research* vol. 10), pp. 296–315, ed. Kappers, J. A. and Schadé, J. P. Amsterdam: Elsevier.

WOLFE, D. E. (1965) In *Structure and Function of the Epiphysis Cerebri (Progress in Brain Research* vol. 10), pp. 332–376, ed. Kappers, J. A. and Schadé, J. P. Amsterdam: Elsevier.

TWO COMPARTMENTS IN THE GRANULATED VESICLES OF THE PINEAL NERVES

Amanda Pellegrino de Iraldi and Angela María Suburo

Instituto de Anatomía General y Embriología, Facultad de Medicina,
Buenos Aires, Argentina

Axons and nerve endings of the pineal gland of the rat contain a pluri-vesicular component which is characteristic of adrenergic nerves (De Robertis and Pellegrino de Iraldi 1961). This component is made up of clear and granulated vesicles of about 40–60 nm (400–600 Å) and a few granulated vesicles of about 80–90 nm (800–900 Å) (Bondareff 1965). Both types of granulated vesicles are characterized by an electron-dense core and a clear space between the core and the surrounding membrane. Until now the dense core has attracted the attention of most investigators, since it can be visualized with the usual fixation techniques. Moreover, the hypothesis was made (De Robertis and Pellegrino de Iraldi 1961) that the dense cores were the sites of storage of biogenic amines in autonomic nerves, and this assumption was confirmed using different experimental approaches (Pellegrino de Iraldi and De Robertis 1963; Pellegrino de Iraldi, Zieher and De Robertis 1965; Bloom and Giarman 1967; Jaim-Etcheverry and Zieher 1968; Pellegrino de Iraldi and Gueudet 1969a). However, the clear space is an important component of the granulated vesicle. Taking into account that the diameter of the core is less than half the total diameter of the vesicle, it can be calculated that the volume of the clear space is about three times larger than that of the core. From now on the clear space will be called the *matrix* of the vesicle.

The core can be visualized with osmium tetroxide alone (Fig. 1) or glutaraldehyde followed by osmium tetroxide, although these two fixations are not equivalent (Pellegrino de Iraldi and Gueudet 1969a). The core is the only site of the vesicle which gives a positive reaction with the histochemical technique of Wood (1967) for catechol and indoleamines (Fig. 2). The matrix and the core may be stained differently with the Champy-Maillet mixtures (Pellegrino de Iraldi and Suburo 1970), depending on the composition of the mixture employed. Those con-taining zinc iodide (ZIO) give a full reaction with the matrix leaving a

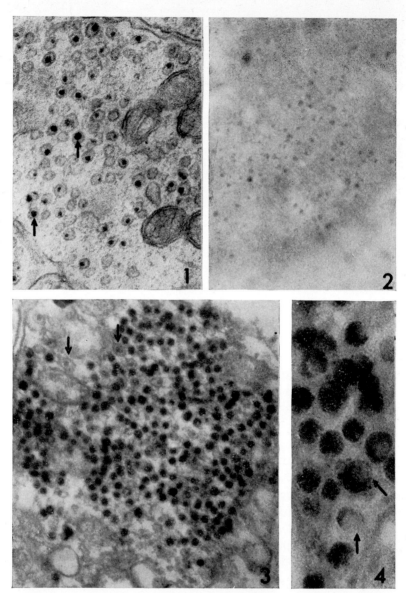

FIG. 1. Electron micrograph of a control nerve ending from the pineal gland of the rat as revealed by osmium tetroxide. In a certain proportion of the synaptic vesicles a core of 28 nm (280 Å) (arrows) may be observed. A clear space or matrix is evident between the core and the surrounding membrane. × 60 000.

FIG. 2. The same as Fig. 1, fixed in glutaraldehyde and treated with potassium dichromate (histochemical technique of Wood for catechol and indoleamines). Numerous reactive granules of 20–30 nm (200–300 Å) and one of 60 nm (600 Å) can be observed. Compare these granules with the dense cores of Fig. 1. × 55 000.

FIG. 3. The same as Fig. 1, fixed with the osmium tetroxide–zinc iodide (ZIO) mixture. Most of the synaptic vesicles are completely stained. Only a few are unstained or show a pale core (arrows). × 60 000.

FIG. 4. A higher power view of ZIO-fixed vesicles. In many of them a pale core of diameter 28 nm (280 Å) (arrows) may be distinguished. The space surrounding the core shows a very intense reaction. × 220 000.

paler core (Figs. 3 and 4). Although the matrix reaction is considerably denser, the core reacts more quickly and may be visualized after half an hour of impregnation, while the matrix takes two hours or more to give a full reaction.

These considerations led us to think that on morphological and on histochemical grounds two main compartments can be considered in the granulated vesicles, namely the core and the matrix.

As shown in Figs. 3 and 4, the matrix of practically all the synaptic vesicles reacts intensely with ZIO. Generally, only a few of the large vesicles remain unstained or show a pale core. Thus, the vesicular morphology revealed by ZIO in the pineal nerves of the rat may be considered as a negative image of that shown with osmium tetroxide or glutaraldehyde-osmium tetroxide. The ZIO reaction is not the same in all adrenergic vesicles. In the vas deferens (see Fig. 6) only the core reacts, while even after two hours the matrix remains unstained.

The nature of the substance or substances revealed by ZIO in synaptic vesicles remains uncertain and at first sight it seems to be quite unspecific. A positive reaction has been observed in the matrix of cholinergic (Akert and Sandri 1968) and non-cholinergic vesicles (Pellegrino de Iraldi and Gueudet 1968, 1969b), while in others of proved adrenergic nature, such as those of the vas deferens, the matrix remains unreactive. However, it is interesting that the core of adrenergic vesicles is more constantly stained by the different Champy-Maillet mixtures assayed (Pellegrino de Iraldi and Suburo 1970).

Test-tube experiments done in our laboratory show that ZIO reacts with noradrenaline, dopamine and serotonin and with its precursors DOPA, 5-hydroxytryptophan and tryptophan. Catechols reduce ZIO immediately and a fine precipitate appears within 30 minutes. A small black precipitate can be observed with phenylalanine after two hours. The reduction of ZIO by indoles takes a few minutes but a heavy precipitate appears with serotonin and 5-hydroxytryptophan in 15 minutes, with tryptophan in 20 minutes and with melatonin in 30 minutes. Among the substances tested the most reactive were 5-hydroxydopamine, 6-hydroxydopamine and pyrogallol. These tri-hydroxylated substances reduce and precipitate ZIO in a few seconds. The amino acids cysteine, methionine and glutamic acid also react with ZIO in less than 30 minutes. Certain inorganic ions, such as phosphates, also give a precipitate in a few seconds. Heparin reduces ZIO in 10 minutes, but after 2 hours only a microscopic precipitate can be observed. Some other substances give a microscopic precipitate without reduction of the ZIO mixture. This group includes tyramine, ATP and serum albumin. After 24 hours ATP and

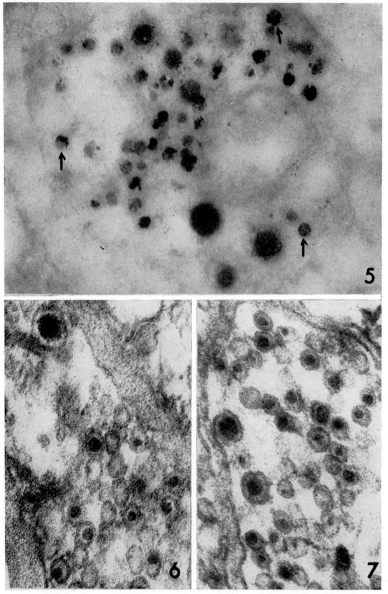

FIGS. 5, 6 and 7. Nerve endings of the vas deferens of the rat, fixed with ZIO. In Figs. 6 and 7 the grids were stained with uranyl acetate.

FIG. 5. After treatment with 5-hydroxydopamine small and large granulated vesicles have a very electron-dense material in their matrix. In some of them a paler core (arrows) can be observed. × 100 000.

Fig. 6. In the control vas deferens, no ZIO-reactive material can be observed in the vesicular matrix. × 100 000.

Fig. 7. After treatment with nialamide-DOPA the matrix of granulated vesicles remains unreactive, like those from the controls. × 100 000.

acetylcholine give a yellow-black macroscopic precipitate and the precipitate of tyramine is still microscopic after the same time. No reaction was observed with mescaline, histamine, GABA and cholesterol.

These assays indicate that a reaction of ZIO with the biogenic amines and their precursors cannot be excluded. In this respect it is significant that 5-hydroxydopamine changes the reaction of ZIO with the matrix of the granulated vesicles in the adrenergic nerves of the vas deferens. Tranzer and Thoenen (1967) have offered strong evidence that 5-hydroxydopamine accumulates in the vesicles of sympathetic nerve terminals, filling them completely. Since the matrix of granulated vesicles from the vas deferens is unreactive to ZIO, we thought that it would be an appropriate structure in which to study the ability of ZIO to reveal storage of 5-hydroxydopamine in tissues. Rats injected with 5-hydroxydopamine (4×20 mg/kg intraperitoneally over a period of 48 hours) were killed 4 hours after the last injection. The vas deferens was fixed in ZIO and the pineal gland in ZIO and 1 per cent osmium tetroxide in Periston (Bayer). The vas deferens of animals treated with nialamide (400 mg/kg intraperitoneally for 6 hours) and DOPA (100 mg/kg intraperitoneally for 30 minutes) was also fixed in ZIO. As shown in Fig. 5, the matrix of granulated vesicles of the vas deferens nerves, which remained unstained in controls (Fig. 6), became intensely reactive in the 5-hydroxydopamine-treated animals. No reaction could be detected in the vesicular matrix of animals treated with nialamide and DOPA (Fig. 7). In the pineal glands fixed with ZIO the normal reaction was so enhanced that it was difficult to distinguish the central cores from the matrix. When fixed with osmium tetroxide the central cores of small and large granulated vesicles appeared denser than usual and although the matrix remained pale, it was slightly denser than in the controls.

Summarizing, it can be said that our findings and those of other authors suggest that more than one substance may be responsible for the ZIO reactions observed in the synaptic vesicles. Furthermore, biogenic amines, their precursors or structurally related substances, as well as other components of the vesicle may participate in this reaction. In any case the vesicle morphology revealed by ZIO, together with other staining and histochemical techniques, is useful to distinguish two compartments in adrenergic vesicles.

PHARMACOLOGICAL STUDY

In order to obtain more information about these compartments the effect of different drugs which act on biogenic amine stores was studied.

Reserpine

The action of reserpine on both compartments of granulated vesicles of the pineal nerves has already been described. This drug depletes the central core revealed with osmium tetroxide (Pellegrino de Iraldi and De Robertis 1961), with glutaraldehyde-osmium tetroxide (Pellegrino de Iraldi 1969) or with the histochemical technique of Wood (1967) for catechol and indole-amines (Jaim-Etcheverry and Zieher 1969). This treatment also depletes the ZIO-reactive material (Pellegrino de Iraldi and Gueudet 1968). After reserpine (5 mg/kg intraperitoneally for two hours) the vesicles appear empty (Fig. 8) and many of them have an elliptical or tubular shape. However, an improved resolution technique has allowed us to observe a small and faint core of 15 nm (150 Å) in many vesicles (around 45 per cent) in glands fixed with ZIO (Fig. 8).

DL-p-Chlorophenylalanine (p-CPA)

This drug depletes serotonin by inhibiting tryptophan hydroxylase (Koe and Weissman 1966). In a previous study (Pellegrino de Iraldi and Gueudet 1969a) we confirmed the observation of Bloom and Giarman (1967) that this drug depletes serotonin in the pineal gland of the rat, whereas noradrenaline and dopamine levels do not decrease (Table I). We also found that the dense cores of granulated vesicles disappeared in glands fixed in glutaraldehyde–osmium tetroxide but remained in those fixed with osmium tetroxide alone (Table II), which thus explained the apparent contradiction between the findings of Bloom and Giarman and previous data from our laboratory about the nature of dense cores. The correlation between the morphological and biochemical data suggested that both catechol and indoleamines are stored in the granulated vesicles in the pineal nerves. It also showed that the two fixation methods, done as described in Pellegrino de Iraldi and Gueudet (1969a), preserve different

TABLE I

EFFECT OF DL-p-CHLOROPHENYLALANINE ON SEROTONIN AND CATECHOLAMINE CONTENT OF THE PINEAL GLAND

	Control	DL-p-Chlorophenylalanine	Percentage of control	t*	P
Serotonin	(8) $30 \cdot 66 \pm 2 \cdot 6$	(7) $3 \cdot 9 \pm 2 \cdot 7$	-87	$7 \cdot 101$	$< 0 \cdot 001$
Noradrenaline	(11) $5 \cdot 8 \pm 1 \cdot 1$	(3) $9 \cdot 4 \pm 2 \cdot 2$	$+62$	$1 \cdot 468$	$> 0 \cdot 1$**
Dopamine	(9) $20 \cdot 3 \pm 2 \cdot 5$	(3) $18 \cdot 3 \pm 4 \cdot 3$	-10	$0 \cdot 390$	$> 0 \cdot 7$**

Data are expressed as μg/g wet weight (mean standard error) of serotonin, noradrenaline and dopamine. Number of determinations in parentheses. Animals injected with saline were used as controls.

* t, Student's "t" value.
** Non-significant value.

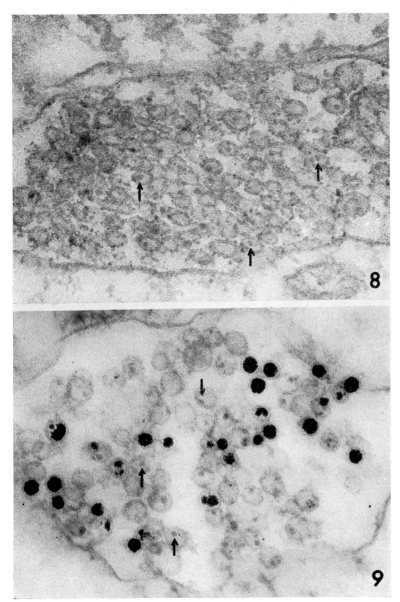

FIG. 8. Nerve ending from the pineal of a reserpinized rat, fixed with ZIO. The reactive material of the matrix has completely disappeared and a very small and faint core (arrows) is present in many vesicles. × 110 000.

FIG. 9. Nerve ending from the pineal of a rat treated with *p*-chlorophenylalanine; fixed with ZIO. The matrix is unreactive in about 60 per cent of the vesicles. A central core (arrows) is observed in many vesicles but it is smaller and less electron-dense than those from the controls. × 110 000.

TABLE II

EFFECT OF DL-*p*-CHLOROPHENYLALANINE ON GRANULATED VESICLES IN NERVE ENDINGS OF THE PINEAL GLAND

	Percentage of total vesicles		Percentage of control	$t\star$	P
	Control	DL-p-*Chlorophenylalanine*			
Osmium tetroxide					
1% Periston Bayer	(7) 37 ± 3	(7) 47 ± 3	$+25$	$1\cdot893$	$>0\cdot05\star\star$
Glutaraldehyde 3%					
phosphate buffer	(7) 33 ± 1	(7) 5 ± 1	-85	$14\cdot860$	$<0\cdot001$

Data are expressed as mean percentage of total number of vesicles ± S.E.
Number of pineals studied in parentheses; 1000 vesicles were counted in each gland. Animals injected with saline were used as controls.
★ t, Student's "t" value.
★★ Non-significant value.

components of the pineal nerves. The storage of noradrenaline and serotonin in the dense cores and the action of *p*-CPA was also confirmed by us with Wood's histochemical technique (1967). The results obtained indicated that both amines are stored in the same morphological entity. However, this does not exclude a different biochemical storage site at a molecular level.

In this study we have used ZIO after the same treatment with *p*-CPA (i.e. 300 mg/kg intraperitoneally. The injection was repeated 2 days later and the animals killed 24 hours after the second injection). It was observed that the ZIO-reactive material of the matrix disappears in about 60 per cent of the vesicles (Fig. 9). Central cores can still be observed but they are smaller and less electron-dense than those in the controls. When the staining of the cores with ZIO after *p*-CPA is correlated with the histochemical reactivity of the cores after the same treatment (Pellegrino de Iraldi and Gueudet 1969*a*), the ZIO reaction seems to be related to catechol and indoleamines. The fact that *p*-CPA depletes the ZIO-reactive material from the matrix where the Wood technique does not detect indole or catecholamines deserves further discussion. This fact suggests either that there is a serotonin store in the matrix not revealed by the Wood technique, or that ZIO reacts with a different substance which is also depleted by *p*-CPA. Koe and Weissman (1966) observed that *p*-CPA reduces the normal increase of brain serotonin and 5-hydroxyindole acetic acid resulting from 5-hydroxytryptophan administration and they postulated an inhibition by *p*-CPA of 5-hydroxytryptophan uptake. It may be hypothesized that the matrix-reactive material represents a binding site for 5-hydroxytryptophan.

Oxypertine

According to Spector, Melmon and Sjoerdsma (1962), oxypertine or

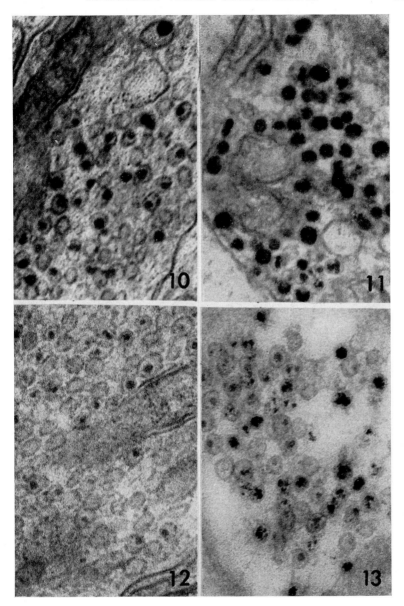

FIG. 10. Nerve terminal from the pineal of a control rat, fixed with osmium tetroxide. × 120 000.

FIG. 11. The same as Fig. 10, fixed with ZIO. × 120 000.

FIGS. 12 and 13. Pineal nerve endings of oxypertine-treated rats.
Fig. 12. After osmium tetroxide fixation the cores are fewer in number and smaller than those of the control. × 120 000.
Fig. 13. After ZIO fixation the matrix appears negative, decreased in density or irregularly stained. × 120 000.

WIN 18501–2 specifically depletes noradrenaline in brain and heart, although some authors accept that serotonin is also partially depleted. Rats were injected intraperitoneally with one dose of 140 mg/kg and killed 2 hours later. It was observed that dense cores stained with osmium tetroxide decreased in size and density (compare Figs. 10 and 12). The relative proportion of clear and granulated vesicles showed a decrease in granulated vesicles of only 15 per cent but because the total number of vesicles per surface area of the nerve endings was also decreased, it could be calculated that the granulated vesicles had diminished by 50 per cent. A larger decrease has been reported by Bak and Hassler (1968). After ZIO fixation the matrix appears negative, decreased in density or irregularly stained in oxypertine-treated rats (compare Figs. 13 and 11).

Tyramine

In recent years considerable evidence has accumulated which strongly suggests that noradrenaline stores in sympathetic nerve terminals are not homogeneous and that there are at least two metabolic pools, which can be characterized as tyramine-releasable and tyramine-resistant (Trendelenburg 1961; Axelrod *et al.* 1962; Chidsey and Harrison 1963). We decided to study the pineal glands of rats treated with tyramine under the electron microscope. Two dosage schedules were assayed: in one the animals were killed 15 minutes after one dose of 50 mg/kg intraperitoneally and in the other the animals received 10 doses of 50 mg/kg intraperitoneally at 15-minute intervals and were killed 15 minutes after the last dose. As shown in Fig. 14, the acute treatment produces a great decrease in the ZIO-reactive material of the matrix, while many of the central cores (around 52 per cent of all the vesicles) are preserved. However, their mean diameter seems to be slightly decreased, being around one-third of the total diameter of the vesicles instead of half. After the 10 injections of tyramine, ZIO-reactive material has practically disappeared. A well-preserved matrix can occasionally be seen. The central cores are drastically reduced in number (they remain in only 25 per cent of all vesicles) and in size (they reach a mean diameter of about 15 nm, 150 Å). However, a few relatively well preserved cores can be observed (Fig. 15).

The action of tyramine has also been observed in material fixed in osmium tetroxide. After a single dose of tyramine the proportion of granulated vesicles is about 42 per cent, which can be considered to be the normal one with this fixative, but the cores appear smaller than in the control. After 10 doses there is also a considerable reduction in the proportion of granulated vesicles. With the Wood technique the catechol

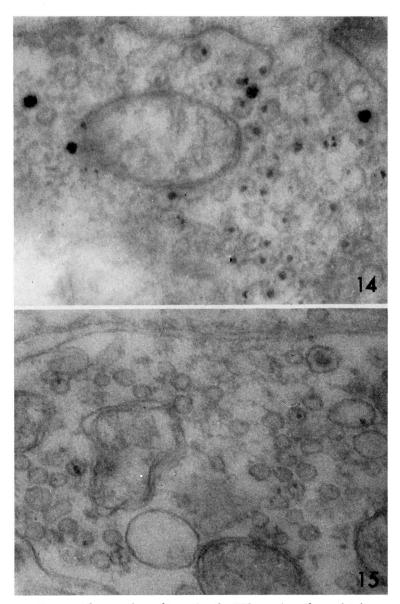

FIG. 14. After one dose of tyramine the ZIO reaction of granulated vesicles of pineal nerves is considerably diminished. The matrix reaction has disappeared in most of the vesicles, whereas the cores are only slightly modified. × 100 000.

FIG. 15. Pineal nerves after 10 doses of tyramine; fixed with ZIO. The cores are drastically reduced in number and size. No matrix reaction is observed. × 100 000.

and indoleamine-reactive sites can still be seen after one dose, although they are of lower electron density, but after the 10 doses of tyramine they have almost disappeared, being confined to the large granulated vesicles. The release of serotonin by tyramine in the pineal nerves, shown by this failure of the Wood technique to demonstrate reactive sites after the long treatment with this drug, is in line with the serotonin-releasing activity of tyramine in blood platelets (Da Prada, Bartholini and Pletscher 1965) and in the small intestine of the dog (Burks and Long 1966).

Summarizing, the effect of tyramine on the compartments of the granulated vesicles of the pineal nerves seems to be more intense at first on the matrix than on the central core. However, an initial action of the drug may also be considered to occur on the core, from the results observed after fixation with osmium tetroxide. But with a more protracted treatment the central compartment is obviously affected.

DISCUSSION AND CONCLUDING REMARKS

From the staining properties, histochemical reactions and responses to pharmacological treatment we conclude that the granulated vesicles of the pineal nerves of the rat are made up of two concentric compartments of different volume: the central core and the surrounding matrix. Although there are individual differences, this may be considered as a general pattern of organization for the granulated vesicles of adrenergic nerves. The fact that the core can be revealed by a variety of techniques made it possible to establish some ultrastructural, pharmacological, histochemical and bio-chemical correlations. Such correlations have confirmed the earlier hypothesis (Pellegrino de Iraldi, Zieher and De Robertis 1965) that the pineal nerves of the rat were of a tryptaminergic and adrenergic nature. This hypothesis was based on biochemical and pharmacological deter-minations of serotonin (Bertler, Falck and Owman 1963; Pellegrino de Iraldi, Zieher and De Robertis 1963), histochemical fluorescence (Bertler, Falck and Owman 1963), radioautography at the level of the electron microscope (Wolfe *et al.* 1962), and pharmacological findings obtained by electron microscopy (Pellegrino de Iraldi and De Robertis 1963; Pellegrino de Iraldi, Zieher and De Robertis 1965). The storage of noradrenaline in the pineal nerves of the rat has also been demonstrated biochemically in normal and denervated pineal glands (Pellegrino de Iraldi and Zieher 1966). The use of *p*-CPA and Wood's histochemical technique to reveal catechol and indoleamines at the electron microscopic level demonstrated that both amines are localized in the central cores (Bloom and Giarman 1967; Jaim-

Etcheverry and Zieher 1968; Pellegrino de Iraldi and Gueudet 1969*a*) and suggested that noradrenaline and serotonin are stored in the same granule (Pellegrino de Iraldi and Gueudet 1969*a*).

The reaction of the matrix with the ZIO mixture enabled us to show that certain drugs interfering with the storage of catechol and indoleamines have a marked action on this compartment. Thus, the matrix may be partially or totally depleted by *p*-CPA, oxypertine, reserpine and tyramine. These findings, together with the experiments *in vitro* and the ZIO reaction in 5-hydroxydopamine-treated rats, indicate that catechol and indole-amines, their precursors or other related substances might be responsible, at least partially, for the ZIO reaction in adrenergic vesicles.

However, the fact that the ZIO reaction is positive in non-monoamin-ergic vesicles (Akert and Sandri 1968; Pellegrino de Iraldi and Gueudet 1969*b*) and other structures, and the greater reaction in the matrix than in the core (where catechol and indoleamines can be histochemically localized) suggest the possibility that substances other than catechol and indole-amines or related substances may be implicated. Alternatively it may be postulated that a common substance is present in both adrenergic and non-adrenergic vesicles. The possibility must be considered that the amine depletors assayed are not strictly specific and perhaps are depleting some non-monoaminic component of the vesicle, such as chromogranins, to which a role in the storage of noradrenaline has been assigned.

Taking into account that much of the current thinking on noradrenaline pools is based on evidence that the amine is stored in tyramine-releasable and tyramine-resistant pools, it may be of interest to discuss the action of tyramine on ZIO-reactive material in the matrix and the core. From the slight reduction in the diameter of the cores and the smaller reaction with the Wood technique after treatment with one dose of tyramine, the possi-bility that the releasable pool is in the core must be considered. However, if we speculate that the action of tyramine on ZIO-reactive material reflects in some way the action of the drug on noradrenaline pools, it may be suggested that the tyramine-releasable pool is in intimate connexion with the matrix or outer compartment, while the tyramine-resistant pool is mainly related to the core or central compartment. Tyramine acts at first more intensely on the matrix but also has an effect on the core. Later the matrix disappears almost completely and the cores are drastically reduced. Both compartments of the vesicle are affected—although to different degrees—during the action of the drug, as if they were in dynamic equilibrium in an open two-compartment system, as in the theoretical model proposed by Neff and co-workers (1965) to integrate the formation, storage, release and metabolism of noradrenaline.

7*

SUMMARY

The granulated vesicles of the pineal nerves of the rat have two components, a central core and a space between the core and the surrounding membrane, or matrix, which have different staining properties. Histochemical, biochemical and pharmacological correlations demonstrate that catechol and indoleamines are localized in the central core. This localization has been confirmed by treatment with p-chlorophenylalanine. The matrix can be visualized with the osmium tetroxide–zinc iodide mixture of Champy-Maillet. The nature of the material reacting with this mixture is uncertain. Treatment with 5-hydroxydopamine and assays done *in vitro* suggest that biogenic amines, their precursors or structurally related substances and/or other components of the vesicle may participate in this reaction.

The fact that this Champy-Maillet mixture is reactive with the matrix allowed us to demonstrate that drugs interfering with the metabolism or storage of biogenic amines act not only on the core but also on the matrix. Thus, it is shown that p-chlorophenylalanine, oxypertine, reserpine and tyramine can partially or totally remove the osmium tetroxide–zinc iodide reactive material from the matrix. Tyramine acts at first more intensely on the matrix but with a more prolonged treatment the central core is obviously affected. From the staining properties, histochemical reactions and results of the pharmacological treatment we conclude that the granulated vesicles of the pineal nerves of the rat are formed by two concentric compartments, the central core and the surrounding matrix. Although individual differences exist, this may be considered as a general pattern of organization of the granulated vesicles of adrenergic nerves.

Acknowledgements

The original research contained in this report has been supported by grants of the Consejo Nacional de Investigaciones Científicas y Técnicas, Argentina and the National Institutes of Health, U.S.A. (2 Ro1 NS 06953-04 NEVA).

We are grateful to Professor E. De Robertis for his critical reading of the manuscript; and to Miss Margarita López and Mr Alberto Saenz for their skilful technical assistance. We also thank CIBA Argentina for a generous supply of reserpine, and Pfizer Argentina for nialamide.

REFERENCES

AKERT, K. and SANDRI, C. (1968) *Brain Res.* **7**, 286–295.

AXELROD, J., GORDON, E., HERTTING, G., KOPIN, I. J. and POTTER, L. T. (1962) *Br. J. Pharmac. Chemother.* **19**, 56–63.

BAK, I. J. and HASSLER, R. (1968) *Agressologie* **9**, 3–12.

BERTLER, A., FALCK, B. and OWMAN, CH. (1963) *Kl. fysiogr. Sällsk. Lund Förh.* **33**, 13–16.

BLOOM, F. and GIARMAN, N. J. (1967) *Anat. Rec.* **157,** 351.

BONDAREFF, W. (1965) *Z. Zellforsch. mikrosk. Anat.* **67,** 211–218.

BURKS, T. F. and LONG, J. P. (1966) *J. Pharmac. Sci.* **55,** 1383–1386.

CHIDSEY, C. A. and HARRISON, D. C. (1963) *J. Pharmac. exp. Ther.* **140,** 217–223.

DA PRADA, M., BARTHOLINI, G. and PLETSCHER, A. (1965) *Biochem. Pharmac.* **14,** 1721–1726.

DE ROBERTIS, E. and PELLEGRINO DE IRALDI, A. (1961) *Anat. Rec.* **139,** 299.

JAIM-ETCHEVERRY, G. and ZIEHER, L. M. (1968) *Z. Zellforsch. mikrosk. Anat.* **86,** 393–400.

JAIM-ETCHEVERRY, G. and ZIEHER, L. M. (1969) *J. Cell Biol.* **42,** 855–860.

KOE, B. K. and WEISSMAN, A. (1966) *J. Pharmac. exp. Ther.* **154,** 499–516.

NEFF, H. H., TOZER, N. T., HAMMER, W. and BRODIE, B. B. (1965) *Life Sci.* **4,** 1869–1875.

PELLEGRINO DE IRALDI, A. (1969) *Z. Zellforsch. mikrosk. Anat.* **101,** 408–418.

PELLEGRINO DE IRALDI, A. and DE ROBERTIS, E. (1961) *Experientia* **17,** 122–123.

PELLEGRINO DE IRALDI, A. and DE ROBERTIS, E. (1963) *Int. J. Neuropharmac.* **2,** 231–239.

PELLEGRINO DE IRALDI, A. and GUEUDET, R. (1968) *Z. Zellforsch. mikrosk. Anat.* **91,** 178–185.

PELLEGRINO DE IRALDI, A. and GUEUDET, R. (1969a) *Int. J. Neuropharmac.* **8,** 9–14.

PELLEGRINO DE IRALDI, A. and GUEUDET, R. (1969b) *Z. Zellforsch. mikrosk. Anat.* **101,** 203–211.

PELLEGRINO DE IRALDI, A. and SUBURO, A. M. (1970) *J. Microscopy* **91,** part 2, 99–103.

PELLEGRINO DE IRALDI, A. and ZIEHER, L. M. (1966) *Life Sci.* **5,** 149–154.

PELLEGRINO DE IRALDI, A., ZIEHER, L. M. and DE ROBERTIS, E. (1963) *Life Sci.* **9,** 691–696.

PELLEGRINO DE IRALDI, A., ZIEHER, L. M. and DE ROBERTIS, E. (1965) In *Structure and Function of the Epiphysis Cerebri (Progress in Brain Research* vol. 10), pp. 389–422, ed. Kappers, J. A. and Schadé, J. P. Amsterdam: Elsevier.

SPECTOR, S., MELMON, K. and SJOERDSMA, A. (1962) *Proc. Soc. exp. Biol. Med.* **3,** 79–81.

TRANZER, J. P. and THOENEN, H. (1967) *Experientia* **23,** 743–745.

TRENDELENBURG, U. (1961) *J. Pharmac. exp. Ther.* **134,** 8–17.

WOLFE, D. E., POTTER, L. T., RICHARDSON, K. C. and AXELROD, J. (1962) *Science* **138,** 440–441.

WOOD, J. G. (1967) *Anat. Rec.* **157,** 343–344.

DISCUSSION

Axelrod: Have you considered whether the larger (80 nm) vesicles contain any biogenic amines?

Pellegrino de Iraldi: Yes. From our results with Wood's histochemical technique, they contain catechol and indoleamines in the pineal nerves of the rat. Two different types of granules are seen with this technique. They correspond in diameter with the dense cores of the two types of granulated vesicles described in the pineal nerves. Both types disappear after treatment with drugs interfering with the synthesis or storage of indole and/or catecholamines (Pellegrino de Iraldi and Gueudet 1969; Jaim-Etcheverry and Zieher 1969). However, the larger vesicles show a dense core after treatment with reserpine if they are fixed with glutaraldehyde–osmium tetroxide (Hökfelt 1966) or glutaraldehyde–phosphotungstic acid (Jaim-Etcheverry and Zieher 1969), suggesting that these fixatives preserve a non-amine component of the larger vesicles.

Axelrod: I asked about the larger vesicles because I don't know whether there are many smaller vesicles in the cell bodies of the nerves and there is some speculation whether the larger vesicles will form the smaller ones in some way, perhaps by splitting off.

Pellegrino de Iraldi: There are no intermediate types; there are two populations of distinct sizes in the pineal nerves. There are other differences as well as size. The ZIO reaction does not occur in the matrix of the larger vesicles. To make things more complicated, these larger vesicles in the vas deferens can be filled with 5-hydroxydopamine, but in the pineal gland, after the same treatment, whereas the small vesicles are loaded with the dense material (the core is difficult to see), we see some larger vesicles with a clear matrix.

Herbert: It seems that large (80–100 nm) dense-cored vesicles may also be found in endings which by other criteria are cholinergic, not adrenergic, which makes it unlikely that they are part of the same system as the small vesicles.

Wurtman: Dr Pellegrino de Iraldi has, I believe, made some very important observations. For a decade investigations have sought a relationship between the "easily releasable" and "storage" pools of noradrenaline and specific organelles within the terminals of sympathetic nerve endings. Most authors have placed the "easily releasable" material within the cytoplasm and the "less releasable" material in the granular synaptic vesicles; the notion that *both* pools might be present within one and the same vesicle is original and exciting. It has been suggested by S. S. Kety (unpublished) and others that some of the synaptic vesicles might be located within the plasma membrane of the presynaptic neuron, and that the material released after nerve stimulation derives selectively from these vesicles. When you deplete with tyramine, do you find any selective change in the vesicles that are closer to the membrane as opposed to vesicles that are deeper in the cytoplasm?

Pellegrino de Iraldi: No. In the peripheral nerve endings it is difficult to see the so-called active points commonly observed in the central nervous system, because the connexions between the nerves and the subsynaptic areas are different. Usually the vesicles are distributed uniformly in the nerve endings or varicosities in the control animals. I have not tried stimulation, which would be a more physiological stimulus, but drugs act in the same way on all the vesicles distributed in the nerve endings.

Wurtman: There is confusion about whether pineal granular vesicles in which serotonin has replaced noradrenaline retain their granular appearance; your data suggest that this depends on what stain one uses. I wonder, in view of the facts that there are enormous daily rhythms in the contents of serotonin and noradrenaline in the pineal and that these rhythms are out of phase with each other, if it would be possible, using the right stain (and I imagine the right stain here would be glutaraldehyde) to see striking differences in the percentages of vesicles with dense granular cores?

Pellegrino de Iraldi: I think so, but I have not done it.

Wurtman: Finally, you showed that repeated doses of tyramine cause a loss of granularity. We know that a large amount of the tyramine injected is taken up within the granular vesicles and converted to octopamine (β-hydroxytryptamine). This would suggest that octopamine, unlike many other amines, does not react with glutaraldehyde or osmium tetroxide to yield a stainable product. This is surprising, since you showed that many similar compounds react to give a stainable product. Have you checked on octopamine directly, *in vitro*?

Pellegrino de Iraldi: We have not assayed octopamine *in vitro* with osmium tetroxide–zinc iodide (ZIO) nor with glutaraldehyde–osmium tetroxide or osmium tetroxide alone. We have assayed ZIO *in vitro* with different substances. It is interesting that tyramine behaves in a different way from catechol and indoleamines. While these latter reduce and precipitate ZIO in a few seconds, tyramine does not reduce ZIO and it forms a very small precipitate only after 24 hours. This may be important, because if a substance reacts immediately and precipitates, it can be revealed later in the electron microscope, but if substances react slowly they may be washed out.

Wurtman: Dr Axelrod has shown that octopamine is normally present in nerve endings, and one would imagine that very large amounts would be present after repeated treatment with tyramine.

Herbert: Dr Pellegrino de Iraldi, it is my impression that *p*-chlorophenylalanine does deplete noradrenaline and dopamine, but over a much shorter time than serotonin. The result might depend on when the animals were killed after the injection.

Pellegrino de Iraldi: According to studies by Koe and Weissman (1966), Bloom and Giarman (1967) and by us (Pellegrino de Iraldi and Gueudet 1969), *p*-chlorophenylalanine depletes serotonin specifically. Catecholamines are not depleted in the peripheral nervous system although a smaller release of noradrenaline has been shown in the central nervous system.

Herbert: You observed a difference between the dense cores in glutaraldehyde-fixed and osmium-fixed material after treating with *p*-chlorophenylalanine. Have you tried using a mixture of paraformaldehyde and glutaraldehyde (the Palay mixture), and do you get the same results?

Pellegrino de Iraldi: No. I have tried only glutaraldehyde–osmium tetroxide and osmium tetroxide alone. Our fixation schedules seem to preserve different amines in the granulated vesicles of the pineal nerves. We also tried Wood's technique; with this, when the tissue is fixed in glutaraldehyde and then treated with dichromate, noradrenaline and serotonin react; if formaldehyde is used before glutaraldehyde, dichromate does not react with noradrenaline but only with serotonin. After *p*-chlorophenylalanine, reactive granules were present in the nerves treated with glutaraldehyde–dichromate but they do not appear in those treated with formaldehyde–glutaraldehyde–dichromate. In the controls, reactive granules were seen after both histochemical procedures.

One important difference between this histochemical technique and our observations with glutaraldehyde–osmium tetroxide is that Wood treats the tissues for 4 hours with glutaraldehyde, whereas we do the fixation overnight.

Owman: In the pineal preparations where you have evidence for a storage site for serotonin in the nerve terminals, what do you find in the pinealocytes? Do you find anything similar?

Pellegrino de Iraldi: I couldn't identify a storage site for serotonin in the pinealocytes with Wood's technique, and I must add that with this technique I couldn't identify a storage site for serotonin in the central nervous system. But the vesicles in the pinealocytes and also in the central nervous system are morphologically different from those in the pineal nerve endings, and perhaps serotonin is stored in different ways, and is more easily releasable by histological processing in some places. Alternatively, its concentration could be too weak for the sensitivity of this technique. Another possibility is that serotonin is not in the granules. However, if serotonin and/or melatonin are secreted by the pinealocytes, what we know about the morphology of secretory processes at present suggests that they should be stored in vesicles.

Miline: In the same experimental conditions, have you observed any changes in the ribbon synapses of the pinealocytes?

Pellegrino de Iraldi: No, I haven't, but synaptic ribbons are not common enough in the pineal gland to make a quantitative study.

Shein: You have depleted either serotonin or noradrenaline and then observed the effect of this depletion on the granule morphology. Perhaps it would be useful to deplete both serotonin and noradrenaline with reserpine and then selectively return serotonin, say, by giving 5-hydroxytryptophan?

Pellegrino de Iraldi: We haven't done that in the pineal gland.

Arstila: It is very interesting that you get differential release of substances from the outer matrix and from the inner core of the vesicles. This situation may be somewhat similar to the storage of substances within lysosomes, some of which, according to Koenig (1969), may be electrostatically bound to the matrix of the lysosomes, whereas others may be retained within the lysosomes by the lysosomal membrane. In this regard it would be interesting to see whether you get differential release of catecholamines from the granular vesicles using various types of membrane labilizers and stabilizers such as vitamin A, chloroquine or cortisone.

Pellegrino de Iraldi: I think it would be possible, but we have not used these substances.

REFERENCES

BLOOM, F. and GIARMAN, N. J. (1967) *Anat. Rec.* **157,** 351.
HÖKFELT, T. (1966) *Experientia* **22,** 56.
JAIM-ETCHEVERRY, G. and ZIEHER, L. (1969) *J. Cell Biol.* **42,** 855–860.
KOE, B. K. and WEISSMAN, A. (1966) *J. Pharmac. exp. Ther.* **154,** 499–516.
KOENIG, H. (1969) In *Lysosomes in Biology and Pathology,* pp. 111–162, ed. Dingle, J. T. and Fell, H. B. Amsterdam: North Holland Publishing Company.
PELLEGRINO DE IRALDI, A. and GUEUDET, R. (1969) *Int. J. Neuropharmac.* **8,** 9–14.

CONTROL OF MELATONIN SYNTHESIS BY NORADRENALINE IN RAT PINEAL ORGAN CULTURES

HARVEY M. SHEIN

McLean Hospital Research Laboratory, Belmont, Massachusetts; and Department of Psychiatry, Harvard Medical School, Boston, Massachusetts

DURING the past ten years, comparative investigations of the melatonin and serotonin content of pineals of intact, blinded and ganglionectomized rats housed under continuous light or darkness have established that the sympathetic innervation to the rat pineal gland controls the daily rhythmic fluctuations in the pineal melatonin and serotonin content which occur in response to environmental lighting (Wurtman, Axelrod and Kelly 1968). Although these *in vivo* investigations have demonstrated that intact sympathetic innervation is essential for maintenance of the diurnal rhythms in pineal indole content, many unanswered questions have remained concerning the mechanisms by which the innervation brings about these effects. Since the sympathetic nerves to the pineal contain large amounts of both noradrenaline and serotonin in the nerve endings (Pellegrino de Iraldi and Zieher 1966; Quay 1963), it is not immediately obvious whether the nerves exert their effects on the pineal parenchymal cells by release of the usual sympathetic neurotransmitter, noradrenaline, or by release of the serotonin also contained in the nerve endings. Moreover, if noradrenaline is the responsible agent, it may be asked whether it acts upon a classical alpha or beta adrenergic receptor located in the pineal cell membrane, and whether some or all of its actions are mediated by a "second messenger", cyclic adenosine monophosphate (cyclic AMP), produced in response to noradrenaline-induced stimulation of an adenyl cyclase system. If cyclic AMP does in fact mediate some of the effects of noradrenaline on the pineal gland, one may inquire further which enzymic step in the pineal indole pathway is affected by cyclic AMP.

Organ culture of the rat pineal gland provides a useful experimental system in which to study these questions. The effects of noradrenaline, cyclic AMP and adrenergic blocking agents on pineal indole synthesis can be studied in organ cultures free from hormonal, neuronal and other complicating influences of the *in vivo* milieu.

Studies of the effects of noradrenaline and cyclic AMP on adult rat pineal glands in organ cultures have been pursued independently by Wurtman, Axelrod and the present author, and by Klein and co-workers, using different techniques of organ culture. Shein, Wurtman and Axelrod (1967) culture individual pineal glands by clotting each gland to the walls of a Wasserman tube, adding 0·5 ml of nutrient medium, sealing the culture with a rubber stopper, and incubating on a roller wheel at 37 °C. Klein and co-workers (Klein *et al.* 1970) culture individual rat pineal glands in a Petri dish according to a modification by Raisz (1965) of the method of Trowell (1959). Each pineal is incubated in 0·5 ml of culture medium in a stationary position at 37 °C and continually gassed with a mixture of 95 per cent oxygen and 5 per cent carbon dioxide.

With both techniques of culture, radioactively labelled precursors of the various pineal indoles included in the culture media are incorporated into these indoles *in vitro* and the melatonin, serotonin and 5-hydroxy-indole acetic acid thus synthesized are rapidly released into the culture media. Each of the labelled indoles can be assayed quantitatively by liquid scintillation spectrophotometry after its extraction from the media by organic solvents. The content of the labelled tryptophan and other pre-cursors remaining in the pineal gland and the content of labelled pineal gland protein can then be measured separately (Wurtman *et al.* 1969). Klein and co-workers have also measured the activity in the cultured pineal gland of the melatonin-forming enzyme, hydroxyindole-O-methyl-transferase (HIOMT), and of the enzyme, *N*-acetyltransferase, which con-verts serotonin to *N*-acetylserotonin (Klein 1969; Klein, Berg and Weller 1970; Klein *et al.* 1970; Klein and Weller 1970).

In the rat pineal grown in organ culture the synthesis of melatonin from tryptophan proceeds by the same steps as in the innervated pineal gland (Wurtman *et al.* 1968): tryptophan→5-hydroxytryptophan→serotonin→ *N*-acetylserotonin→melatonin. Serotonin can also be metabolized in the pineal cultures, as *in vivo*, by deamination and oxidation to form 5-hydroxy-indole acetic acid (5-HIAA). Also as *in vivo*, the rate-limiting step for serotonin synthesis from tryptophan in the pineal cultures is the formation of 5-hydroxytryptophan (Shein, Wurtman and Axelrod 1967). All of the enzymes of the pineal indole pathway remain active at a stable level in the pineal cultures for more than two days after explantation (Wurtman *et al.* 1968). The pineal organ cultures also incorporate [^{14}C]tryptophan into proteins at a nearly constant rate for at least two days after explantation (Wurtman *et al.* 1969).

In order to determine whether the addition of exogenous noradrenaline or serotonin could reproduce *in vitro* the stimulating effect of the sym-pathetic innervation on melatonin synthesis, Axelrod, Shein and Wurtman

TABLE I

STIMULATION OF MELATONIN FORMATION FROM [^{14}C]TRYPTOPHAN BY
L-NORADRENALINE IN RAT PINEAL ORGAN CULTURES

Concentration of noradrenaline	Percentage formation from [^{14}C]tryptophan		
	[^{14}C]melatonin	[^{14}C]serotonin	[^{14}C]5-HIAA
o*	0·45±0·05	2·1±0·18	1·1±0·10
3 × 10^{-5} M	0·65±0·10	2·1±0·35	0·9±0·18
1 × 10^{-4} M	0·79±0·16	2·6±0·5	0·9±0·18
3 × 10^{-4} M	1·20±0·15**	2·7±0·32	0·6±0·09†

* Each experimental group included eight pineal cultures.
** $p < 0.001$, † $p < 0.05$, differs from cultures without noradrenaline.

(Modified from Axelrod, Shein and Wurtman 1969.)

(1969) added *l*-noradrenaline or serotonin to the nutrient medium of rat pineal organ cultures and compared the effects of these compounds on the synthesis of [^{14}C]melatonin from [^{14}C]tryptophan. Exogenous serotonin had no effect on [^{14}C]melatonin synthesis in concentrations as high as 3×10^{-4} M; addition of similar concentrations of exogenous melatonin and 5-HIAA was also without effect. In marked contrast to the ineffectiveness of these indoles, the addition of noradrenaline to the pineal culture medium in a concentration of 3×10^{-4} M caused a threefold increase in the formation of [^{14}C]melatonin from [^{14}C]tryptophan (1×10^{-4} M) during a two-day incubation period (Table I). At lower concentrations, 1×10^{-4} M and 3×10^{-5} M, noradrenaline also stimulated melatonin synthesis but to a lesser extent. In pineals cultured in an atmosphere of 95 per cent O_2, the addition of noradrenaline in a concentration as low as 1×10^{-5} M caused a six to seven-fold increase in the synthesis of [^{3}H]melatonin from [^{3}H]tryptophan during a one-day incubation period (Klein 1969).

In contrast to the marked enhancement of melatonin synthesis, addition of noradrenaline produced no change in the net amount of [^{14}C]serotonin present and produced only a slight decrease in the amount of [^{14}C]5-HIAA during a two-day incubation period (Table I). When the effects of noradrenaline were studied after 4, 16 and 48 hours of incubation, the stimulating effect on melatonin synthesis was apparent at as early as four hours. The finding that physiological concentrations of *l*-noradrenaline markedly stimulated the synthesis of [^{14}C]melatonin in cultured pineals within so short a period strongly suggests that *l*-noradrenaline is the substance released by the sympathetic innervation to the pineal which controls melatonin synthesis *in situ*.

In order to determine the degree of specificity of the melatonin stimulation induced by *l*-noradrenaline, Axelrod, Shein and Wurtman (1969) compared compounds structurally related to *l*-noradrenaline for their capacity to stimulate melatonin synthesis from [^{14}C]tryptophan (1×10^{-4} M)

TABLE II

EFFECT OF VARIOUS PHENYLETHYLAMINE DERIVATIVES ON THE FORMATION OF
MELATONIN IN RAT PINEAL ORGAN CULTURES

	Percentage formation from [^{14}C]tryptophan		
Amine	[^{14}C]melatonin	[^{14}C]serotonin	[^{14}C]5-HIAA
None*	0·45±0·05	1·3 ±0·2	0·80±1·6
l-Noradrenaline	1·31±0·20†	1·4 ±1·8	0·61±1·2
d-Noradrenaline	1·68±0·15**	2·85±0·2†	0
l-Adrenaline	0·84±0·16	2·21±0·3‡	0·76±0·2
Dopamine	0·87±0·18†	2·4 ±0·3‡	0
Tyramine	0·72±0·06†	6·4 ±0·05**	0
dl-Octopamine	2·7 ±0·30**	7·4 ±0·71**	1·0 ±0·11
Tryptamine	1·4 ±0·16**	3·4 ±0·6‡	0·25±0·05**
Catron	1·1 ±0·20†	3·5 ±0·8‡	0·22±0·07**

* Each experimental group included six pineal cultures.
** $P < 0·001$, † $P < 0·01$, ‡ $P < 0·05$, differs from cultures without amines.

(Modified from Axelrod, Shein and Wurtman 1969.)

in the pineal cultures during a two-day incubation period. The compounds studied were l- and d-noradrenaline, l-adrenaline, dopamine, dl-octopamine and tyramine. At a concentration of 3×10^{-4} M, all of the phenylethyl-amine derivatives, as well as tryptamine, significantly stimulated the synthesis of melatonin from [^{14}C]tryptophan (Table II). However, the β-hydroxylated primary amines, l- and d-noradrenaline and octopamine, produced the greatest stimulation. A high degree of specificity in the action of l-noradrenaline on [^{14}C]melatonin synthesis was indicated by the finding that only l-noradrenaline, among the compounds tested, had little or no effect on the formation of [^{14}C]serotonin and [^{14}C]5-hydroxy-indole acetic acid. In contrast to l-noradrenaline, all the other phenylethyl-amine derivatives and tryptamine elevated the [^{14}C]serotonin content and markedly inhibited the formation of [^{14}C]5-HIAA. This suggests that only l-noradrenaline directly stimulates [^{14}C]melatonin synthesis by acting on one of the two steps in the indole pathway to melatonin subsequent to serotonin formation, and that, in contrast, the other phenylethylamine derivatives and tryptamine primarily act to inhibit the activity of mono-amine oxidase in deaminating [^{14}C]serotonin to [^{14}C]5-HIAA and thereby divert serotonin metabolism to the alternative pathway of N-acetylation, O-methylation and melatonin formation. This hypothesis is supported by finding that addition of Catron (α-methylphenethylhydrazine), a potent monoamine oxidase inhibitor, also almost completely inhibits the form-ation of [^{14}C]5-HIAA and increases both [^{14}C]melatonin and [^{14}C]sero-tonin levels (Table II).

One possible mechanism by which l-noradrenaline could stimulate pineal glands to incorporate more [^{14}C]tryptophan into melatonin would be by stimulating the uptake of [^{14}C]tryptophan by the pineal parenchymal cells. To examine this possibility, Wurtman and co-workers (Wurtman *et al.* 1969) undertook studies of the effects of *l*-noradrenaline and related catecholamines on the uptake of [^{14}C]tryptophan into pineal cells and on the content of labelled protein in the cells.

In pineals incubated for two days in the presence of *l*-noradrenaline (3×10^{-4} M) the tryptophan content was increased by 70 per cent over controls. Addition of *l*-noradrenaline also stimulated the uptake of the non-utilizable amino acid α-aminoisobutyric acid within 20 minutes after the start of incubation, but *l*-noradrenaline failed to stimulate the uptake of [^{14}C]leucine, [^{14}C]methionine or [^{14}C]tyrosine. Pineals incubated for two days with *l*-noradrenaline (3×10^{-4} M) also contained 50–125 per cent more [^{14}C]protein than organs incubated without the catecholamine (Table III). Various other catecholamines—*d*-noradrenaline, *l*-adrenaline and dopamine—when added in the same concentration (3×10^{-4} M), were also found to stimulate the incorporation of [^{14}C]tryptophan into protein (Table III). In contrast, the addition of serotonin, melatonin or 5-HIAA to the medium had no effect on [^{14}C]protein synthesis. The enhanced accumulation of [^{14}C]protein in pineals incubated with *l*-noradrenaline was found not to represent primarily an increase in pineal [^{14}C]protein synthesis but rather to represent an increase in the intracellular specific activity of the precursor amino acid, [^{14}C]tryptophan, secondary to the increased uptake of the amino acid. Evidence against a primary effect on [^{14}C]protein synthesis was provided by the observation that *l*-noradrenaline failed to stimulate [^{14}C]protein synthesis from labelled utilizable amino acids other than [^{14}C]tryptophan, such as [^{14}C]methionine or [^{14}C]leucine.

These findings indicate that *l*-noradrenaline and related catecholamines stimulate the uptake of [^{14}C]tryptophan by pineal cells and thereby enhance

TABLE III

EFFECT OF VARIOUS CATECHOLAMINES ON THE INCORPORATION
OF [^{14}C]TRYPTOPHAN INTO PROTEIN BY RAT PINEAL ORGAN CULTURES

Amine	[^{14}C]protein content (c.p.m.)
None*	134 ± 3
l-Noradrenaline	299 ± 24**
d-Noradrenaline	298 ± 24**
l-Adrenaline	233 ± 28†
Dopamine	412 ± 24**

* Each experimental group included six pineal cultures.
** $P < 0.001$, † $P < 0.05$, differs from cultures without amine.

(Modified from Wurtman *et al.* 1969.)

its incorporation into pineal proteins. This noradrenaline-induced stimulation of [14C]tryptophan uptake and its incorporation into [14C]protein is too small an effect to account for the stimulation of melatonin synthesis induced by noradrenaline, however. Thus noradrenaline increased the intracellular content of [14C]tryptophan by only about 70 per cent and the [14C]protein content by only 50–125 per cent, whereas the same concentration of noradrenaline stimulated the synthesis of labelled melatonin from [14C]tryptophan or [3H]tryptophan by 300–700 per cent. In the absence of noradrenaline, about three times as much [14C]tryptophan was incorporated into [14C]indoles as into [14C]protein, while by contrast in the presence of noradrenaline, ten times as much [14C]tryptophan was incorporated into [14C]indoles as into [14C]protein.

Numerous actions of noradrenaline in organs other than the pineal gland are mediated by cyclic AMP (Robison, Butcher and Sutherland 1968). Evidence favouring the possibility that cyclic AMP might also mediate actions of noradrenaline in the rat pineal gland was provided by the finding of Weiss and Costa (1967) that noradrenaline stimulates adenyl cyclase activity in rat pineal homogenates. Accordingly, Shein and Wurtman (1969) and Klein and co-workers (Klein et al. 1970) independently undertook studies to determine whether the stimulation of melatonin synthesis and tryptophan uptake in pineal cultures induced by noradrenaline could be duplicated by cyclic AMP. Addition of cyclic AMP in concentrations as high as 3×10^{-3} M was without effect on either melatonin synthesis or tryptophan uptake. In marked contrast, dibutyryl cyclic AMP (DAMP), a derivative of cyclic AMP which is thought to be more stable to breakdown by the phosphodiesterase that inactivates cyclic AMP, was very effective in stimulating melatonin synthesis from [14C]tryptophan (Shein and Wurtman 1969). Addition of DAMP to the culture medium in concentrations of 3×10^{-3} M or 10^{-3} M was associated with an increase in [14C]melatonin synthesis greater than 300 per cent and an increase in

TABLE IV

EFFECT OF VARIOUS DOSES OF DIBUTYRYL CYCLIC AMP (DAMP) ON PINEAL SYNTHESIS OF [14C]INDOLES AND ON PINEAL CONTENT OF [14C]PROTEIN AND [14C]TRYPTOPHAN

Radioactivity in c.p.m.

DAMP concentration	[14C]melatonin	[14C]serotonin	[14C]5-HIAA	[14C]protein content	[14C]tryptophan content
0*	374 ± 57	348 ± 26	87 ± 31	222 ± 11	449 ± 74
3×10^{-4} M	677 ± 107**	617 ± 78†	51 ± 41	246 ± 25	478 ± 36
1×10^{-3} M	1464 ± 140‡	870 ± 115‡	63 ± 16	230 ± 22	473 ± 35
3×10^{-3} M	1264 ± 55‡	1006 ± 122‡	37 ± 26	193 ± 14	533 ± 81

* Each experimental group included six pineal cultures.
‡ $P < 0.001$, †$P < 0.01$, **$P < 0.05$, differs from controls without DAMP.

(Modified from Shein and Wurtman 1969.)

[^{14}C]serotonin synthesis greater than 200 per cent during a two-day incubation period (Table IV). Addition of DAMP in lower concentration (3×10^{-4} M) caused a smaller but still significant increase in the synthesis of both these [^{14}C]indoles. At all three concentrations, DAMP had no effect on the amounts of [^{14}C]5-HIAA in the media or on the content of [^{14}C]-tryptophan or [^{14}C]protein in the pineals. Klein and associates (Klein *et al.* 1970) also found in their pineal culture system that a DAMP concentration of 2×10^{-1} M markedly stimulated [^{3}H]melatonin synthesis from [^{3}H]-tryptophan during a one-day incubation period. In the roller tube pineal culture system, the time course of the effect of DAMP on the synthesis of pineal [^{14}C]melatonin was shown to be similar to that previously observed for noradrenaline (Shein and Wurtman 1969). As with noradrenaline, the DAMP-induced increase in [^{14}C]melatonin synthesis was apparent after four hours, and persisted throughout two days of incubation.

These findings indicate that DAMP mimics some of the effects of noradrenaline on the pineal organ cultures but not others. DAMP, like noradrenaline, stimulates the synthesis of [^{14}C]melatonin from [^{14}C]-tryptophan. Unlike noradrenaline, DAMP does not stimulate the uptake of [^{14}C]tryptophan or its incorporation into [^{14}C]protein within pineal cells. Accordingly, the findings are compatible with the concept that cyclic AMP mediates the effects of noradrenaline on melatonin synthesis in the pineal but does not mediate the effects of noradrenaline on the uptake of tryptophan by the pineal (Shein and Wurtman 1969).

Klein and his co-workers (Klein, Berg and Weller 1970; Klein and Weller 1970; Berg and Klein 1970) have recently defined one metabolic site at which noradrenaline and DAMP stimulate melatonin synthesis in the rat pineal gland and in doing so have provided further evidence that cyclic AMP mediates the effects of noradrenaline on melatonin synthesis. These investigators have shown that both noradrenaline and DAMP stimulate the activity of the enzyme, N-acetyltransferase, which converts serotonin to N-acetylserotonin. Using a specific radiochemical assay of N-acetyltransferase, Klein and co-workers (Klein and Weller 1970; Klein, Berg and Weller 1970) found that noradrenaline or DAMP treatment results in a seven to tenfold increase in the activity of this enzyme in cultured pineal glands and in a comparable increase in the synthesis of N-[^{14}C]acetylserotonin and [^{14}C]melatonin from [^{14}C]serotonin in the incubation media. *De novo* protein synthesis was implicated in the stimulating effects of both noradrenaline and DAMP on N-acetyltransferase activity and on N-acetylserotonin and melatonin synthesis by the observation that continuous treatment with cycloheximide blocked these effects.

In contrast to the stimulating effect of DAMP on pineal N-acetyl-transferase activity, Berg and Klein (1970) found that DAMP had no effect on the activity of the pineal melatonin-forming enzyme, hydroxyindole-O-methyltransferase (HIOMT), which had previously been thought to be rate-controlling in melatonin synthesis. Earlier, Klein (1969) had found that noradrenaline produced only a small (10 to 20 per cent) increase in HIOMT activity in cultured pineal glands. Klein, Berg and Weller (1970) consider that this noradrenaline-induced increase in HIOMT activity is too small to account for the concomitant seven-to-tenfold stimulation of melatonin synthesis. Accordingly, they conclude that noradrenaline apparently does not control melatonin synthesis by stimulating HIOMT activity via a cyclic AMP mechanism. They propose instead that nor-adrenaline accelerates the enzymic formation of melatonin by the following hypothetical sequence: (i) Noradrenaline stimulates adenyl cyclase and this produces an increase in the intracellular concentration of cyclic AMP; (ii) The increased concentration of cyclic AMP increases the net formation of N-acetyltransferase; (iii) The increased activity of N-acetyltransferase stimulates the formation of N-acetylserotonin and its concentration in the cell; (iv) The increased intracellular N-acetylserotonin concentration enhances the enzymic formation of melatonin by simple mass action. This proposal that noradrenaline controls melatonin synthesis and serotonin content by acting at a single step in the pineal indole pathway is attractive in its simplicity. However, further study will be required to exclude the possibility that noradrenaline may also act at one or more additional metabolic sites in this synthetic pathway (for example, at the level of tryptophan hydroxylase).

Investigators seeking to define the relationship between noradrenaline, adrenergic receptors and adenyl cyclase have suggested that in most and perhaps all tissues the beta adrenergic receptor is adenyl cyclase (Robison, Butcher and Sutherland 1967). In view of the previously described findings which suggest that cyclic AMP mediates the effects of nor-adrenaline on melatonin synthesis in the pineal, Wurtman and Shein (1970, unpublished) undertook to determine by the use of adrenergic blocking agents whether the pineal adrenergic receptors are of the classical alpha or beta type. The alpha blocking agent, phenoxybenzamine, and the beta blocking agent, propranolol, were compared for their capacity to block noradrenaline or DAMP-induced stimulation of melatonin synthesis and noradrenaline-induced stimulation of [^{14}C]tryptophan uptake. It was found that addition of phenoxybenzamine to the nutrient medium in con-centrations of 10^{-4} M, 10^{-5} M or 10^{-6} M was without effect on noradrenaline-induced stimulation of [^{14}C]melatonin synthesis and [^{14}C]tryptophan uptake. In marked contrast, addition of propranolol in concentrations of 10^{-4} M or 10^{-5} M completely blocked the noradrenaline-induced stimulation of [^{14}C]melatonin synthesis but was without effect on the enhancement of [^{14}C]tryptophan uptake by noradrenaline. At a lower dose of 10^{-6} M, propranolol blocked noradrenaline-induced stimulation of [^{14}C]melatonin synthesis to a lesser degree and was still without effect on noradrenaline-enhanced [^{14}C]tryptophan uptake. As was to be expected, in view of the presumed intracellular site of action of DAMP, neither propranolol nor phenoxybenzamine had any effect on DAMP-induced stimulation of [^{14}C]melatonin synthesis. The specific nature of the propranolol blockade of noradrenaline-stimulated [^{14}C]melatonin synthesis

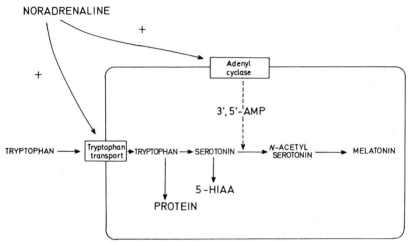

FIG. 1. The effect of noradrenaline on tryptophan metabolism in the pineal. 5-HIAA, 5-hydroxyindole acetic acid. (Modified from Shein and Wurtman 1969.)

was indicated by the fact that, in the absence of noradrenaline, neither propranolol nor phenoxybenzamine had any effect on pineal [^{14}C]melatonin synthesis or on [^{14}C]tryptophan uptake. The finding that the stimulation of [^{14}C]melatonin synthesis by noradrenaline is inhibited by a beta adrenergic blocking agent, but not by an alpha blocking agent, indicates that the pineal receptors for the stimulation of melatonin synthesis are very probably beta adrenergic receptors. In contrast, the "receptors" for the stimulation of tryptophan uptake by noradrenaline are apparently neither classical alpha receptors nor classical beta receptors inasmuch as neither an alpha nor a beta adrenergic blocking agent inhibits this effect of noradrenaline.

The present state of our understanding of the effect of noradrenaline on pineal tryptophan metabolism can be summarized in a schematic form (Fig. 1). Noradrenaline apparently acts (+) on two receptors in the plasma membrane of the pineal parenchymal cell: (*i*) It stimulates tryptophan transport into the cell by acting on a "receptor" which is neither classically alpha nor beta in type. (*ii*) It enhances the activity of adenyl cyclase by acting on a beta receptor and thereby stimulates synthesis of cyclic AMP (3', 5'-AMP). The cyclic AMP thus synthesized then stimulates the activity of the enzyme N-acetyltransferase and thereby accelerates the formation of N-acetylserotonin and melatonin.

SUMMARY

Biochemical and pharmacological studies in rat pineal gland organ cultures have clarified certain of the mechanisms by which the sympathetic innervation to the pineal controls diurnal rhythms in the pineal melatonin and serotonin content which occur *in vivo* in response to environmental lighting. Noradrenaline added to the medium of rat pineal gland cultures stimulates melatonin synthesis from [^{14}C]tryptophan and cellular uptake of labelled tryptophan. Addition of dibutyryl cyclic adenosine monophosphate (DAMP) to the medium of the pineal cultures also stimulates melatonin synthesis but does not enhance tryptophan uptake. Noradrenaline and DAMP both stimulate melatonin synthesis by increasing the activity of the enzyme, N-acetyltransferase, which converts serotonin to N-acetylserotonin. The identical stimulatory effect and site of action of DAMP and noradrenaline on melatonin synthesis in pineal cultures favours the concept that the effect of DAMP reproduces the action of endogenous cyclic AMP in the pineal gland *in situ* produced in response to noradrenaline released upon sympathetic nervous stimulation. The lack of a stimulatory effect of DAMP on [^{14}C]tryptophan uptake in cultured pineal glands indicates that this effect of noradrenaline is not mediated by cyclic AMP. The action of noradrenaline in stimulating melatonin synthesis requires activation of beta adrenergic receptors inasmuch as the stimulation is blocked in pineal cultures by propranolol but not by phenoxybenzamine. The "receptor" in the pineal cell membrane upon which noradrenaline acts to stimulate tryptophan uptake is neither a classical alpha nor beta receptor, since propranolol and phenoxybenzamine both fail to inhibit this effect of noradrenaline in organ culture.

Acknowledgement

The studies reported in the article which were undertaken in our laboratory were supported by U.S. Public Health Service Research Grant NS-06610.

REFERENCES

AXELROD, J., SHEIN, H. M. and WURTMAN, R. J. (1969) *Proc. natn. Acad. Sci. U.S.A.* **62**, 544–549.

BERG, G. R. and KLEIN, D. C. (1970) *Fedn Proc. Fedn Am. Socs exp. Biol.* **29**, 615.

KLEIN, D. C. (1969) *Fedn Proc. Fedn Am. Socs exp. Biol.* **28**, 734.

KLEIN, D. C., BERG, G. R. and WELLER, J. (1970) *Science* **168**, 979–980.

KLEIN, D. C., BERG, G. R., WELLER, J. and GLINSMANN, W. (1970) *Science* **167**, 1738–1740.

KLEIN, D. C. and WELLER, J. (1970) *Fedn Proc. Fedn Am. Socs exp. Biol.* **29**, 615.

PELLEGRINO DE IRALDI, A. and ZIEHER, L. M. (1966) *Life Sci.* **5**, 149–154.

QUAY, W. B. (1963) *Gen. comp. Endocr.* **3**, 473–479.

RAISZ, L. G. (1965) *J. clin. Invest.* **44**, 103–116.

ROBISON, G. A., BUTCHER, R. W. and SUTHERLAND, E. W. (1967) *Ann. N.Y. Acad. Sci.* **139**, 703–723.

ROBISON, G. A., BUTCHER, R. W. and SUTHERLAND, E. W. (1968) *A. Rev. Biochem.* **37**, 149–174.

SHEIN, H. M. and WURTMAN, R. J. (1969) *Science* **166**, 519–520.

SHEIN, H. M., WURTMAN, R. J. and AXELROD, J. (1967) *Nature, Lond.* **213**, 730–731.

TROWELL, O. A. (1959) *Expl Cell Res.* **16**, 118–147.

WEISS, B. and COSTA, E. (1967) *Science* **156**, 1750–1752.

WURTMAN, R. J., AXELROD, J. and KELLY, D. E. (1968) *The Pineal*, pp. 108–140. New York and London: Academic Press.

WURTMAN, R. J., LARIN, F., AXELROD, J., SHEIN, H. M. and ROSASCO, K. (1968) *Nature, Lond.* **217**, 953–954.

WURTMAN, R. J., SHEIN, H. M., AXELROD, J. and LARIN, F. (1969) *Proc. natn. Acad. Sci. U.S.A.* **62**, 749–755.

DISCUSSION

Axelrod: Klein and Weller (1970) have studied the effect of noradrenaline and dibutyryl cyclic AMP (DAMP) on the synthesis of the enzyme *N*-acetyltransferase in organ cultures of the pineal. As Dr Shein said, noradrenaline has very little effect on HIOMT. When noradrenaline was added 20 hours after giving radioactive tryptophan, there was a 10-fold rise in the concentration of *N*-acetyltransferase after 4 hours. This effect is prevented by inhibitors of protein synthesis. Thus, noradrenaline must be synthesizing a new specific protein which is involved in the acetylation step. DAMP will do the same thing as noradrenaline. It would appear therefore that noradrenaline is driving the serotonin rhythm since, as more enzyme is formed, more serotonin will be used up to form *N*-acetylserotonin. But Dr Wurtman has shown that the daily noradrenaline rhythm is an exogenous rhythm, because it is completely abolished by either darkness or light, whereas the serotonin rhythm is endogenous; it persists in darkness. This seems paradoxical.

Shein: This is clearly a paradox, and I have no answer to it. I should like to point to another paradox, that *in vivo*, you and Dr Wurtman have shown that there is a diurnal 2–3-fold variation in the activity of HIOMT.

Most of us had formerly assumed that this was due to the action of nor-adrenaline, perhaps wrongly. Now we find that noradrenaline seems to be mainly concerned with changing the activity of another enzyme, N-acetyltransferase, and the question arises of which factor (or factors) is responsible for the change in the activity of HIOMT. In view of what we have heard about the possibility of cholinergic innervation in the pineal gland, perhaps it would be worthwhile to look in this direction to see whether the HIOMT rhythm is controlled by a cholinergic innervation.

Wurtman: But what is the evidence that HIOMT is not controlled by noradrenaline and that HIOMT is not rate-limiting? I think that in both cases the evidence is inadequate. The evidence that HIOMT is not con-trolled by noradrenaline consists of negative findings, namely that if you take pineals that have been incubated for 48 hours with noradrenaline, homogenize them and assay them for HIOMT activity, you don't find an increase in activity. But what we generally find after homogenizing cultured pineals is a marked decrease in HIOMT activity, which is quite in-compatible with the fact that melatonin synthesis is continuing apace. This probably means that the pineal gets sick; something in the pineal changes so that the amount of HIOMT activity recoverable after incubation *in vitro* is not an estimate of what the enzyme was doing inside the gland. So I would not conclude from our and Dr Klein's inability to show a rise in HIOMT activity that there is no such rise.

I also would not conclude that this is not the step of rate limitation, for several reasons. There is abundant evidence that you can cause 10-fold changes in the activity of an enzyme measured *in vitro* and yet have no change in the rate of that process measured *in vivo*. For example, there is probably ten times more monoamine oxidase in most tissues than is necessary to support normal *in vivo* rates of deamination of noradrenaline. Dr Axelrod and I showed (Wurtman and Axelrod 1963) that monoamine oxidase activity must be inhibited by 90 per cent to produce a change in cardiac noradrenaline metabolism *in vivo*. So the fact that pineal N-acetyltransferase shows 10-fold changes in activity in the presence of noradrenaline may make the enzyme a good candidate for rate-limiting, but it certainly doesn't prove the point. Against the hypothesis that the N-acetyltransferase is limiting are data obtained by Maickel and Miller (1968) showing that rat pineals contain at least ten times as much N-acetyl-serotonin as melatonin. This is compatible with the block in melatonin synthesis being at the terminal step (the O-methylation of N-acetyl-serotonin).

Thirdly, as Dr Shein has pointed out, there is a diurnal rhythm in HIOMT activity *in vivo* which can be exaggerated by keeping animals in continuous light and darkness, and these responses disappear after bilateral superior cervical ganglionectomy. We must certainly *consider* the possibility that non-noradrenergic nerves mediate the photic control of HIOMT activity, but this is really speculation. It is well established that there are noradrenergic neurons in the mammalian pineal; it is only conjectured that the pineal contains cholinergic neurons.

Fourthly, in Dr Shein's and my experiments on dibutyryl cyclic AMP, addition of the adenine nucleotide to the medium caused a big increase in the amount of serotonin that was made and released into the medium—an effect that was not seen with noradrenaline. Hence there seem to be at least three possible rate-limiting steps in melatonin synthesis. To determine which locus is the site of physiological rate limitation we have to develop techniques for incubating pineals with various concentrations of either serotonin or N-acetylserotonin. If N-acetylation is the limiting step, we should be able to drive melatonin synthesis much faster by using high concentrations of N-acetylserotonin than by using similar concentrations of serotonin. This awaits being done. At present I think that dibutyryl cyclic AMP could stimulate melatonin synthesis by acting at any or all of half a dozen enzymic processes, and the fact that we can't show a change in HIOMT activity in homogenates of pineals incubated *in vitro* with noradrenaline or dibutyryl cyclic AMP doesn't particularly upset me. The question which of these steps is physiologically rate-limiting remains open.

Finally, we should consider the implications of the unique localization of HIOMT within the mammalian pineal. Unlike HIOMT, the N-acetylating enzyme is *not* found exclusively in the pineal. McIsaac and Page (1958) have observed that in patients with carcinoid syndrome large amounts of N-acetylserotonin can be released into the urine; hence the N-acetylation of serotonin occurs in other organs besides the pineal (see Schloot *et al.* 1969). One is reminded of the effect of thyroid-stimulating hormone (TSH) on the thyroid. TSH causes a marked increase in the activity of certain lysosomal enzymes that are necessary for degrading thyroglobulin and releasing thyroxin, but it also causes a significant increase in the activity of the enzyme system that traps and oxidizes iodine. It is this latter enzyme system that makes the thyroid the thyroid. In the same sense it seems in June, 1970 that it is HIOMT that makes the pineal biochemically unique.

Shein: I agree with Dr Wurtman that the question remains open of what is the rate-limiting step or steps in melatonin synthesis. However, I think the evidence is fairly good in Klein's culture system that noradrenaline does not markedly influence HIOMT activity. Klein tells me that in his culture system HIOMT remains at approximately the same level for eight hours or more after the initial explantation. Despite this stability of HIOMT activity in his culture system for a period sufficient for noradrenaline to markedly stimulate N-acetyltransferase activity and melatonin synthesis *in vitro*, and sufficient for a 2–3-fold variation in HIOMT activity *in vivo*, Klein can only demonstrate a very small effect of noradrenaline *in vitro* on HIOMT activity. It is, of course, possible that there are necessary co-factors lacking in the *in vitro* system which are present *in vivo*. Nevertheless, I find this very limited effect of noradrenaline on HIOMT activity *in vitro* suggestive of a limited effect of noradrenaline *in vivo* also.

On the effect of dibutyryl cyclic AMP on serotonin synthesis, it is puzzling that DAMP seems to stimulate the synthesis of serotonin (as well as melatonin), whereas noradrenaline seems to stimulate only melatonin synthesis. The data suggest that noradrenaline may be exerting an inhibitory effect on the stimulatory action of cyclic AMP on serotonin synthesis but not on the stimulatory action of cyclic AMP on melatonin synthesis.

Martini: Is there any good evidence that the enzyme that acetylates serotonin is in the pinealocytes and not in the nerve terminals?

Axelrod: It could be in the nerve terminals, but it's certainly in the pinealocytes because in organ culture there are no nerves.

Kordon: Dr Shein, can you really interpret your results in terms of uptake and release from the cells? Can you for instance differentiate between ^{14}C-labelled amines in the tissue and in the culture medium?

Shein: Catron is a monoamine oxidase inhibitor and is not, so far as I know, an inhibitor of re-uptake. We used Catron to inhibit the alternative metabolic pathway of serotonin to 5-hydroxyindole acetic acid and thereby to see whether it would increase the stimulation of serotonin and melatonin synthesis from tryptophan, and so reproduce what we hypothesized about phenylethylamine derivatives other than *l*-noradrenaline, namely that they act primarily by monoamine oxidase inhibition. This is, in fact, what we found. There seemed to be no end-product inhibition by the indoles: none of the indoles—serotonin, melatonin or 5-hydroxyindole acetic acid—had any effect on the synthesis of serotonin or melatonin or 5-hydroxyindole acetic acid from ^{14}C]tryptophan. Nor did any of these indoles have any effect on the uptake of ^{14}C]tryptophan into the cell or its incorporation into protein.

Wurtman: The purpose of this experiment was to see whether serotonin released from nerve endings stimulated pineal cells to increase their rate of serotonin or melatonin synthesis; thus we looked at the effect of "cold" serotonin on the formation of "hot" serotonin from tryptophan by pineal cells. The fact that adding serotonin to the culture had no effect on serotonin synthesis within the pineal cells contrasts with the effect of adding noradrenaline on the synthesis of noradrenaline in, for example, isolated vas deferens (Weiner and Rabadjija 1968). This indicates that while noradrenaline synthesis is very probably controlled by end-product inhibition, serotonin synthesis is probably not influenced by serotonin concentrations. This emphasizes again the danger of making analogies between noradrenaline systems and serotonin systems.

Owman: With regard to the suggestion that noradrenaline in the pineal nerves rather than serotonin is important for indole synthesis *in vivo*, is it possible that in your cultures you already have noradrenaline present from leaking adrenergic nerves driving indole synthesis at a rather high rate which masks any further effect of added serotonin? Or, is it possible that the sensitivity of the culture to serotonin is lower *in vitro* than *in vivo*? The latter part of the question is raised because we found in the thyroid that catecholamines and serotonin, like TSH, could stimulate the formation of colloid droplets in thyroxine-sensitized animals *in vivo*, whereas these effects couldn't be reproduced *in vitro*, apparently owing to a completely different sensitivity of the isolated cells.

Shein: It seems very unlikely that the pineal cultures initially have noradrenaline present (from leaking adrenergic nerves) in a concentration sufficient to drive indole synthesis at a high rate, inasmuch as a further addition of a large dose of noradrenaline is necessary to stimulate the synthesis of melatonin in our *in vitro* system. We have to use as much as 10^{-4} M-noradrenaline. Initially, at the time the pineal organ cultures are set up, there is nothing approaching this concentration of noradrenaline in the cultured pineal glands. Further evidence against a high initial noradrenaline concentration in pineal cultures is provided by Klein's culture system, which is much more sensitive to small concentrations of noradrenaline. In Klein's cultures, addition of 10^{-6} or 10^{-7} M-noradrenaline markedly stimulates melatonin synthesis. Taking together Klein's results and ours, it is highly probable that the stimulatory effects observed are specifically effects of added noradrenaline; it is very unlikely that we are masking the effects of added noradrenaline or serotonin by the presence of noradrenaline that was there initially.

Owman: On the other hand, a large amount of serotonin might be necessary to further enhance the rate of synthesis. The experiment to do would be to denervate the pineals before placing them in organ culture and to see if you find a lowered basal synthesis rate.

Lerner: In the cyclic AMP study, did you use either caffein or theophylline to see if they would produce the expected effects? I agree that it would be good to do the acetylcholine experiment. If one could choose one other substance to test, I would pick histamine. This amine is also present in the pineal gland.

Shein: We did study the effects of theophylline and caffein and we also tried ATP, ADP, AMP and cyclic AMP. Even in high concentrations (3×10^{-3} M) we found that none of these compounds had any effect on melatonin synthesis.

Arstila: It might be wise to check the ATP levels in the pineal gland, and also to use a variety of metabolic inhibitors such as actinomycin D and dinitrophenol in order to get an idea of the viability of the cultured cells. If you culture the whole pineal gland the cells may not be uniformly preserved. There are healthy cells in the outer zone, but in the central areas there may be cells which suffer hypoxic injury and may behave quite differently metabolically from the rest of the cells.

Wurtman: ATP becomes very important, because another pineal enzyme involved in melatonin synthesis, the methionine-activating enzyme, is also ATP-dependent. In an entirely different system, in DOPA-treated animals, we have recently show that the amount of *S*-adenosyl methionine can be limiting in methylation reactions (J. Chalmers, R. J. Baldessarini and R. J. Wurtman, in preparation). So there are several factors which should be added to our 1969 model.

As a general comment, the ability of neurotransmitters such as nor-adrenaline to increase the uptake of amino acid (especially tryptophan) in their receptor cells may be of real importance as a general mechanism of neurotransmitter action. Tryptophan is the limiting amino acid in essentially all cells of the body and thus strongly influences the rates of protein synthesis everywhere. It can thus be conjectured that one way that neurotransmitters work is by increasing the rate of protein synthesis, by increasing tryptophan uptake.

Martini: Rather than incubating the pineals of normal animals, would it be useful to culture "activated" pineals of animals that have been in the dark for a prolonged period?

Axelrod: Klein is doing that experiment now.

REFERENCES

KLEIN, D. C. and WELLER, J. (1970) *Fedn Proc. Fedn Am. Socs exp. Biol.* **29 (2)**, 615.
MAICKEL, R. P. and MILLER, F. P. (1968) *Adv. Pharmac.* **6A**, 71–77.
McISAAC, W. M. and PAGE, I. H. (1958) *Science* **128**, 537.
SCHLOOT, W., TIGGES, F.-J., BLAESNER, H. and GOEDDE, H. W. (1969) *Hoppe-Seyler's Z. physiol. Chem.* **350**, 1353–1361.
WEINER, N. and RABADJIJA, M. (1968) *J. Pharmac. exp. Ther.* **164**, 103–114.
WURTMAN, R. J. and AXELROD, J. (1963) *Biochem. Pharmac.* **12**, 1417–1419.

PINEAL–BRAIN RELATIONSHIPS

Fernando Antón-Tay

Department of Neurobiology, Instituto de Investigaciones Biomédicas,
Universidad Nacional Autonoma, Mexico City

Our present knowledge supports the hypothesis that the mammalian pineal gland is a neuroendocrine transducer (Wurtman and Antón-Tay 1969): it converts a neural input to an endocrine output (melatonin and perhaps other methoxyindoles). The translation step is accomplished by the biosynthesis of melatonin through the action of the enzyme hydroxy-indole-O-methyltransferase (HIOMT) (Axelrod and Weissbach 1961). This enzyme is present in the cytoplasm of the pineal parenchymal cell; it transfers the active methyl group from *S*-adenosyl methionine to the hydroxyindole group in the 5 position of the indole nucleus (Axelrod and Weissbach 1961). In all mammals the pineal gland has been found to be the unique locus of HIOMT (Wurtman and Axelrod 1965). It is assumed that the increase in the activity of HIOMT is followed by an increase in pineal secretory function, and *vice versa* (Wurtman and Antón-Tay 1969).

The input to the pineal gland is provided by the release of noradrenaline at the nerve endings of the postsynaptic fibres from the superior cervical ganglia (Axelrod, Shein and Wurtman 1969). It has been shown that these fibres are the final step of a multisynaptic pathway that carries information generated by the response of retinal photoreceptors to environmental lighting (Moore *et al.* 1968). The activity of HIOMT shows a daily rhythm corresponding to the photoperiod (Axelrod, Wurtman and Snyder 1965). HIOMT activity is lowest at the end of the daily light period and it rises within five hours from the onset of darkness (Axelrod, Wurtman and Snyder 1965). These rhythmic changes disappear immediately when animals are placed under continuous light or darkness: HIOMT activity in rats in light continues to fall independently of the time of day, while that of rats kept in darkness continues to rise for several days. The HIOMT rhythm is also absent among blind animals kept under normal lighting. These data indicate that the daily rhythm in melatonin synthesis is not generated by an endogenous oscillating mechanism which uses the day–night cycle simply as a *Zeitgeber* ("time-giver"). Rather, the pineal rhythm is a direct response to the natural 24-hour cycle of photic input (Wurtman and Axelrod 1965).

Because of the rhythmic change in the activity of pineal function it has been proposed that the mammalian pineal might function as a sort of "biological clock", which delivers time signals generated by light and darkness to centres in the brain that mediate and synchronize other biological rhythms (Wurtman and Axelrod 1965).

There is evidence that the endocrine signal emitted by the pineal is decoded by and can modify the functions of distant target organs. The present paper will describe experimental work that supports the hypothesis that the brain is one of these organs and very likely a major target of the pineal secretions.

BRAIN DISTRIBUTION OF [^{3}H]MELATONIN

Although there is good evidence that melatonin eventually finds its way into the blood (Barchas and Lerner 1964), it is not known whether it is secreted into the blood or into the cerebrospinal fluid (CSF). Circulating melatonin is rapidly metabolized by the liver to 6-hydroxymelatonin (Kopin et al. 1960) and in order to act on the brain it has to cross the blood–brain barrier. Therefore, a different fate of melatonin can be expected when the hormone is injected into the blood from that when it is injected into the CSF. Moreover the biological activity for a given amount will also vary. In order to study these points we have examined the distribution of [^{3}H]melatonin in rat brain after injection into the blood or CSF (Antón-Tay and Wurtman 1969). The animals used were female Wistar rats weighing 160–170 g.

Under light ether anaesthesia one group of rats received 0·774 μCi of [^{3}H]melatonin dissolved in 30 μl of water and injected into the right lateral ventricle; the other group of animals received 5·14 μCi of [^{3}H]melatonin in a final volume of 200 μl by injection into the tail vein. One hour later the rats were killed and their brains dissected and assayed for [^{3}H]melatonin.

More than a hundred times as great a percentage of the administered dose of [^{3}H]melatonin was retained in whole brain, cortex and midbrain after its intraventricular administration as after its intravenous injection. It was also found that [^{3}H]melatonin had selectively localized within the hypothalamus, although the cerebral cortex retained a large percentage of the radioactivity because of its greater weight (Table I). After the intraventricular injection of the hormone the ratio of the hypothalamic to the cortical concentration was about 3·2:1, and after its intravenous administration the ratio was 5·6:1.

TABLE I

REGIONAL DISTRIBUTION OF [³H]MELATONIN IN RAT BRAIN

Region	Weight (mg)	Percentage of administered [³H]melatonin retained (1×10^{-3}) Route of administration		Concentration of [³H]melatonin ($\mu\mu Ci/g$) Route of administration	
		Intra-ventricular	Intra-venous	Intra-ventricular	Intra-venous
Whole brain	1786±40	448·4±96·1	2·17±0·30	2034±511	66±12
Cortex	1092±30	168·2±59·6	1·15±0·18	708±168	55±7
Midbrain	260±20	69·0±13·4	0·82±0·53	1814±293	137±38
Cerebellum	284±12	47·6±3·0	0·82±0·53	1284±128	128±77
Medulla-pons	264±20	42·5±4·4	1·03±0·49	1199±150	198±94
Hypothalamus	80±13	24·4±4·4	0·44±0·13	2300±511	309±64

Groups of six rats received 0·774 μCi of [³H]melatonin intraventricularly, or 5·14 μCi intravenously, and were killed 1 hour later. The right side of the brain was assayed for [³H]melatonin; the left side was dissected into various regions and assayed for [³H]melatonin. Data are presented as mean ± S.E.M.

(From Antón-Tay and Wurtman 1969.)

Thus regardless of the route of administration, melatonin is concentrated in the hypothalamus and the midbrain. This fact is interesting because these are the structures concerned with neuroendocrine functions and also where melatonin produces important biochemical effects. It is therefore very likely that both the neural and endocrine effects are related to the action of melatonin on these areas. Implants of melatonin in the midbrain and hypothalamus block gonadotropin release (Martini, Fraschini and Motta 1968). Because the effects of melatonin on the brain are related to its ability to reach it, the route of administration is important. If the pineal normally secretes melatonin into the CSF, the systemic dose needed to produce a given effect on the brain might be as much as a hundred times greater than the amount of endogenous melatonin that normally produces this effect.

METABOLIC EFFECTS OF MELATONIN ON BRAIN

Not only are the endocrine effects of melatonin probably mediated by the central nervous system; the administration of melatonin also produces distinct effects on EEG activity, sleep and behaviour. The mechanisms underlying both the neural and endocrine effects of melatonin probably involve modifications of the metabolism of central neurotransmitters. Two hours after the intraperitoneal administration of 50 μg/kg of melatonin to rabbits, almost a twofold rise in the hypothalamic concentration of γ-amino butyric acid (GABA) was observed (Table II) and there was a

TABLE II

EFFECT OF VARIOUS INTRAPERITONEAL DOSES OF MELATONIN ON THE
CONCENTRATION OF GABA IN RABBIT HYPOTHALAMUS AND
CEREBRAL CORTEX

Melatonin μg/Kg	GABA (mg/100 g of wet tissue)	
	Cortex	Hypothalamus
0	19±0·26	64±5·2
50	32±1·60*	86±3·1*
100	16±0·95*	54±7·1
250	17±1·18	36±1·6*

* Differs from control group, $P < 0·01$.

significant increase in the concentration in the cerebral cortex (F. Antón-Tay, B. Ortega and R. M. Cruz, unpublished results 1966).

Brain serotonin metabolism is also modified by giving melatonin. The serotonin concentration increases in rat brain one hour after the administration of 500 μg of melatonin. Brains of treated animals contained $0·53 \pm 0·027$ μg of serotonin per gramme of tissue, but those of control rats contained only $0·40 \pm 0·31$ μg per gramme of tissue $(P < 0·01)$ (Antón-Tay *et al.* 1968).

Serotonin is widely distributed in the rat brain and its concentration is not uniform (Dahlström and Fuxe 1964). Brain serotonin is mainly localized in the nerve endings but most of the serotoninergic neurons are in the midbrain; therefore the effects of melatonin on serotonin levels should not be the same for all of the brain regions. In fact when rats were killed 90 minutes after receiving 150 μg of melatonin the concentration of serotonin in the midbrain was 63 ± 13 per cent higher than in control animals. The hypothalamic concentration was also increased but not significantly. The serotonin concentrations in the cerebral cortex, in the olfactory bulb and tubercle remained within control values (Antón-Tay *et al.* 1968).

TABLE III

CHANGES IN SEROTONIN CONTENT OF VARIOUS BRAIN REGIONS IN THE RAT
AFTER MELATONIN ADMINISTRATION

Region	Minutes after melatonin injection			
	0	20	60	180
Midbrain	0·56±0·01	0·65±0·09	0·70±0·05†	0·78±0·07**
Hypothalamus	1·67±0·14	1·87±0·13	2·35±0·27†	1·41±0·05
Cerebral cortex	0·99±0·03	0·85±0·03*	0·84±0·03*	0·97±0·05

Rats received 150 μg of melatonin intraperitoneally. Values are given as μg of serotonin per gramme of tissue ± S.E.M.

* $P < 00·1$, ** $P < 0·02$, † $P < 0·05$.

(From Antón-Tay, Sepulveda and Gonzalez 1970.)

The temporal sequence with which the serotonin concentration changes also differs from one region of the brain to another. Twenty minutes after the administration of 150 μg of melatonin to rats, the serotonin level in the cerebral cortex falls by 50 per cent. Forty minutes later, cerebral serotonin is still depressed but the concentration of the indole in the midbrain and the hypothalamus is rising. After 180 minutes, serotonin in the midbrain is still elevated but cortical and hypothalamic levels are normal (Table III).

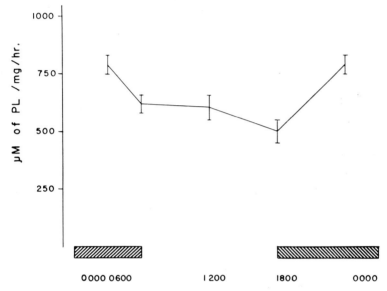

FIG. 1. Daily rhythm in pyridoxal kinase (PL) activity in rat brains. Groups of rats were housed under 12 hours of light per day and killed at 6-hour intervals around the clock (abscissa, time in hours).

There might be several ways by which melatonin produces its effects on brain metabolism. It is possible that one mechanism concerns its ability to increase brain pyridoxal kinase activity (Antón-Tay, Sepulveda and Gonzalez 1970). Pyridoxal kinase catalyses the formation of pyridoxal phosphate in the brain (McCormick and Snell 1959). Pyridoxal phosphate is a cofactor for many reactions; as the prosthetic group of the enzyme aromatic-L-amino acid decarboxylase it is essential for the synthesis of dopamine, serotonin and GABA (Roberts, Rothstein and Baxter 1958).

Ninety minutes after the intraperitoneal administration of 200 μg of melatonin to rats there is a twofold rise in the pyridoxal kinase activity of the brain (in melatonin-treated rats the brain showed 1234 ± 26 units/g, whereas activity in brains in the control group was only 575 ± 29 units/g, $P < 0.001$). When the temporal sequence of changes in pyridoxal kinase

TABLE IV

TEMPORAL SEQUENCE OF CHANGES IN BRAIN PYRIDOXAL KINASE ACTIVITY AFTER INJECTION
OF MELATONIN

Minutes after melatonin injection

	0	45	90	180	360
Pyridoxal kinase activity	633 ± 110	$2786\cdot4\pm244^\star$	$1395\cdot4\pm113^\star$	$1414\pm157^\star$	$692\cdot8\pm52$

Groups of five rats received 200 µg of melatonin intraperitoneally, and were killed after various intervals. Values are given as units of activity per gramme per hour ± S.D.
★ Differs from that of control rats, $P < 0\cdot001$.

after a single dose of 200 µg of melatonin was studied, a good correlation with the change in serotonin levels was found. The peak of activity was measured 45 minutes after the injection of melatonin (Table IV). High levels of activity were still present 90 and 180 minutes later. After 360 minutes enzymic activity returned to normal values. The increases in the activity of this enzyme are related to the dose of melatonin used, and this relationship is maintained with doses ranging from 0·5 mg/kg to 4 mg/kg (Table V).

The mechanism by which melatonin enhances the activity of pyridoxal kinase in the brain *in vivo* very likely involves enhancement of the *de novo* synthesis of the enzyme, since the hormone has no effects *in vitro*.

Moreover, the pretreatment of rats with 2 mg/kg of actinomycin blocks the effects of melatonin (Table VI).

The increases in the concentrations of serotonin and GABA in the brain after melatonin administration may thus be mediated by increases in the activities of 5-hydroxytryptophan and glutamic decarboxylases respectively. Moreover, since pyridoxal phosphate is a cofactor for other decarboxylases and transaminases in the brain, it might be anticipated that increases in the concentration of this cofactor after administration of melatonin would cause changes in several brain functions.

TABLE V

EFFECT OF MELATONIN ON BRAIN PYRIDOXAL KINASE ACTIVITY

Melatonin mg/kg	*Pyridoxal kinase activity*
Control	$100\pm6\cdot7$
0·25	$113\pm19\cdot3$
0·50	$132\pm10\cdot5^\star$
1·0	$184\pm6\cdot1^\star$
2·0	$204\pm16\cdot2^\star$
4·0	$231\pm9\cdot6^\star$

Different doses of melatonin were given intraperitoneally to groups of 5 rats. The activity of pyridoxal kinase was measured 90 minutes later. Values are given as percentage of control activity ± S.D.
★ Differs from control rats, $P < 0\cdot001$.

TABLE VI

EFFECT OF ACTINOMYCIN D ON THE ENHANCEMENT OF BRAIN
PYRIDOXAL KINASE ACTIVITY BY MELATONIN

Group	Pyridoxal kinase activity
Control	680 ± 105
Melatonin	2300 ± 205*
Actinomycin D	600 ± 105
Actinomycin D and melatonin	700 ± 120

Groups of 6 rats received 2 mg/kg of actinomycin D intraperitoneally at zero time. Two hours later 200 µg of melatonin or its diluent was injected intraperitoneally. All animals were killed at the end of the third hour. Values are given as units per gramme per hour $\pm$ s.d.
* Differs from control group, $P < 0 \cdot 001$.

The amount of melatonin secreted by the pineal varies with the photo-period (Axelrod, Wurtman and Snyder 1965), and thus the activity of pyridoxal kinase might not follow this pattern. It was found that brains of rats killed around the clock had different levels of pyridoxal kinase activity: during the light period (lights on from 0600 to 1800 hours) the enzyme activity was low; it started to rise some time after the beginning of the dark period and reached a peak at midnight.

SUMMARY

The mammalian pineal gland is a neuroendocrine transducer. It converts information from the nervous system to an endocrine signal (melatonin). After the injection of [³H]melatonin into the blood or cerebrospinal fluid, the radioactive material was found to be concentrated by the mid-brain and the hypothalamus. These are also the structures in which melatonin increases GABA and serotonin concentrations. After melatonin administration there is also an increase in the activity of brain pyridoxal kinase. It is suggested that the effects of melatonin on the brain are probably mediated by modifications in the amount of pyridoxal phosphate available to the brain.

REFERENCES

ANTÓN-TAY, F., CHOU, C., ANTON, S. and WURTMAN, R. J. (1968) Science 162, 277–278.
ANTÓN-TAY, F., SEPULVEDA, J. and GONZÁLEZ, S. (1970) Life Sci. 9, 1283–1288.
ANTÓN-TAY, F. and WURTMAN, R. J. (1969) Nature, Lond. 221, 474–475.
AXELROD, J., SHEIN, H. M. and WURTMAN, R. J. (1969) Proc. natn. Acad. Sci. U.S.A. 62, 544–549.
AXELROD, J. and WEISSBACH, H. (1961) J. biol. Chem. 236, 211–213.
AXELROD, J., WURTMAN, R. J. and SNYDER, S. H. (1965) J. biol. Chem. 240, 949–955.
BARCHAS, J. and LERNER, A. B. (1964) J. Neurochem. 11, 489–491.
DAHLSTRÖM, A. and FUXE, K. (1964) Acta physiol. scand. 62, suppl. 232, 1.
KOPIN, I. J., PARE, C. M. B., AXELROD, J. and WEISSBACH, H. (1960) Biochim. biophys. Acta 40, 377–378.

MARTINI, L., FRASCHINI, F. and MOTTA, M. (1968) *Recent Prog. Horm. Res.* **24**, 439–496.
MCCORMICK, D. B. and SNELL, E. E. (1959) *Proc. natn. Acad. Sci. U.S.A.* **45**, 1371.
MOORE, R. Y., HELLER, A., BHATNAGAR, R. K., WURTMAN, R. J. and AXELROD, J. (1968)
    Archs Neurol., Chicago **18**, 208–218.
ROBERTS, E., ROTHSTEIN, M. and BAXTER, C. F. (1958) *Proc. Soc. exp. Biol. Med.* **97**, 796.
WURTMAN, R. J. and ANTÓN-TAY, F. (1969) *Recent Prog. Horm. Res.* **25**, 493–514.
WURTMAN, R. J. and AXELROD, J. (1965) *Scient. Am.* **213**, 50–60.

DISCUSSION

Martini: One argument against melatonin being one of the active pineal hormones is that this compound has a very short half-life. Your data indicate that melatonin can be concentrated in several brain structures and remain there for at least 45 minutes. This seems to indicate that the compound may be bound to nervous structures for some time and consequently have a prolonged effect. This is a very important point. A second important point is that the biochemical modifications induced by melatonin survive the half-life of melatonin.

Antón-Tay: The half-life of melatonin in blood is a few minutes (Kopin *et al.* 1961) but we know nothing about its half-life in the cerebrospinal fluid or in brain tissue.

Martini: A further important aspect of your data is that with different doses of melatonin you can produce either an increase or a decrease in the concentration of GABA in the hypothalamus (Table II, p. 216). Behavioural studies made by M. C. Fioretti and myself (see General Discussion, p. 368) have indicated that with intraventricular injections of melatonin you can potentiate the effects of both CNS-inhibiting and CNS-stimulating drugs. This puzzling finding of ours may probably be due to the dose-related effect on GABA which you have just shown.

Antón-Tay: When we injected large doses (e.g. 500 μg) of melatonin and looked at the serotonin content of the brain, the largest doses were not more effective in increasing brain serotonin.

Reiter: In your studies on the uptake of labelled melatonin, were the amygdala and the hippocampus included in the cortical sections?

Antón-Tay: Both the amygdala and the hippocampus were included in the section that we have termed "cortex". Relatively little label was localized in this section.

Reiter: Did you ever check the effect of the age of the animal on the uptake?

Antón-Tay: No. In our experiments we used only female rats weighing 160–170 g.

Reiter: Have you attempted radioautographic localization of the melatonin in the brain? Where specifically in the hypothalamus did it localize?

Antón-Tay: We didn't do this, because we were using [³H]melatonin. For radioautography we would need [¹⁴C]melatonin of greater specific activity.

Mess: Dr Antón-Tay's experiments are crucial in respect of the theory that the target organ, or at least one of the most important target organs, of pineal hormones, is the central nervous system. The fact that labelled material is taken up by another tissue doesn't, however, mean in itself that it is the point of attack of the hormone, because uptake might have several causes. For example, we showed (Mess and Hámori 1965) that ¹³¹I-labelled somatotropic hormone accumulates in greatest amount in the portio principalis of the tubules of the kidney and in the Kupffer's cells of the liver; in other words, uptake here indicated elimination. But comparing Dr Antón-Tay's experiments with other enzyme histochemical studies, his results are one of the most important confirmations of our assumption (Fraschini, Mess and Martini 1968) that within the central nervous system the hypothalamus and the reticular formation of the mesencephalon, that is to say the midbrain, constitute one of the most important points of attack of pineal hormones, which then have secondary effects on the gonad–genital system.

Wurtman: There is a serotoninergic tract that runs from the midbrain to the hypothalamus and elsewhere, with its cell bodies in the raphe nucleus. It is tempting to speculate that melatonin, which is a derivative of serotonin, has some special relationship to this tract. Radioautographic studies on the sites of melatonin localization within the midbrain might be very useful in establishing this relationship.

Herbert: One piece of information that is missing is the way in which the various methoxyindoles cross the "blood–brain barrier". Have you any information on any other substances besides melatonin—methoxytryptophol, for example?

Antón-Tay: No.

Axelrod: I would predict that if the hydroxy group is free it will have trouble getting across the blood–brain barrier. Once it has a non-polar group like a methoxy group, it should get through. If it has an acetyl group on the other end it will also get through, but with a carboxyl group it will have trouble. Methoxytryptophol should get in very easily.

Nir: We have some figures on bufotenine. The difference in its behavioural effect on rats between systemic doses (intraperitoneal) and those injected directly into the lateral cerebral ventricle was at least 2000-fold, and in some parameters even as much as 20 000-fold.

8*

Axelrod: That compound should not get through the blood–brain barrier at all.

Shein: I wonder, Dr Antón-Tay, whether by using doses of melatonin which are optimal for stimulating brain serotonin concentrations and repeating them, say every 4 hours, one would get continued stimulation of serotonin levels in the brain? If this proved possible it would be interesting to study the behavioural effects of these elevated levels of brain serotonin, in view of the theory currently under intensive investigation in Europe that altered brain serotonin concentrations may be implicated in the aetiology of affective disorders in man. It might be interesting to study the effects of this treatment regimen in some of the animal models which have been used to investigate affective states.

Antón-Tay: Yes, I agree. I have made some observations on the effects of chronic administration of melatonin to human volunteers. Melatonin produces a sensation of well-being and in some cases elation. On a few occasions hallucinations were reported. We are now studying the EEG correlates of those changes. (See also General Discussion, p. 363.)

Nir: We have been studying the interrelationship between the pineal gland and the brain by comparing the electrocortical activity of pinealectomized mature female rats with that of sham-operated and intact controls—each animal was used as its own intact control by recording the EEG before and again after operation (either pinealectomy or sham).

Electroencephalogram tracings in pinealectomized rats (Fig. 2) showed a basic electrical activity of permanent regular monorhythmic waves, while those in the intact and sham-operated animals (Fig. 1) were notched, of high amplitude, polyrhythmic and polymorphic. A shift from low frequency (2–3 cycles/second) in the intact and sham-operated rats (Fig. 1) to high frequency (8–11 cycles/second) in the pinealectomized animals (Fig. 2) was observed. The amplitude of the recordings of the pinealectomized rats (Fig. 2) (35–75 μV) was much lower than that of sham-operated and intact controls (50–200 μV) (Fig. 1).

Against this background of basic electrical activity of permanent, symmetrical monorhythmic and monomorphic waves, intermittent sporadic paroxysmal outbursts of slow waves (2–4 cycles/second) with high amplitudes (150–200 μV) of centrocephalic origin were recorded in the pinealectomized rats (Fig. 3).

Thus we see that despite what we heard earlier from Dr Ariëns Kappers that there are no tracts linking the pineal directly to the central nervous system, by removing the pineal we can produce marked electrical changes in the brain. These changes might result from shifts in relative levels of activity in physiologically counterbalanced functional systems. We know

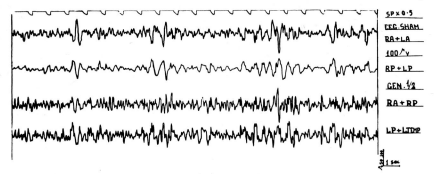

FIG. I (Nir). EEG of sham-operated rat, showing irregular waves of low frequency and high amplitude. Speed record: 0·5 s per mark. RA + LA = right anterior and left anterior frontal electrodes; RP + LP = right posterior and left posterior occipital electrodes; RA + RP = right anterior and right posterior electrodes; LP + L.Temp. = left posterior occipital and left temporal electrodes.

that ablation of the pineal results in hyperactivity of the gonads, due to the increase in gonadotropic hormones, as has been shown by Dr Martini's group (Motta, Fraschini and Martini 1967), and by others, and in high circulating concentrations of oestrogen which accompany the continuous oestrus induced by pinealectomy in female rats. This endocrine shift might be the cause of the hyperactivity of the cortex we recorded.

We obtained additional support for our finding of characteristic changes in the electrical activity of the brain after pinealectomy by studying the brain's electrocortical activity in pinealectomized, sham-operated and intact control female rats receiving lethal doses of pentobarbitone. These experiments demonstrated that the electrophysiological reaction of

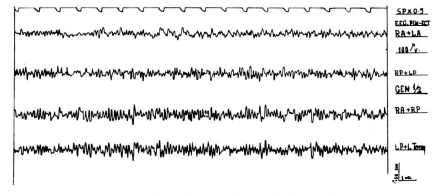

FIG. 2 (Nir). EEG of pinealectomized rat, showing regular mono-rhythmic waves of high frequency and low amplitude. Abbreviations as Fig. I.

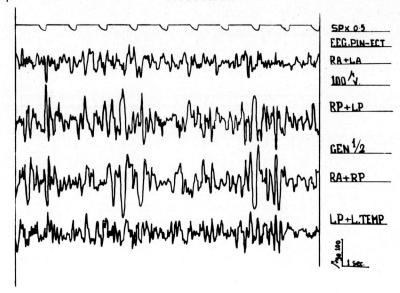

Fig. 3 (Nir). EEG of pinealectomized rat. Intermittent sporadic
paroxysmal outbursts of waves of centrocephalic origin. Abbreviations
as Fig. 1.

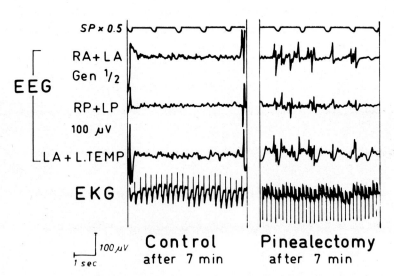

Fig. 4 (Nir). EEGs seven minutes after injection of pentobarbitone. In
the pinealectomized animals spiky wave discharges occur; in the
controls, insignificant changes. Abbreviations as Fig. 1.

the brain (and heart muscle) to lethal doses of pentobarbitone is deferred in the pinealectomized animals. Whereas in the sham-operated and intact controls death occurred within 7–10 minutes, in the pinealectomized rats it was delayed until the fifteenth minute, or even longer. The electro-cortical reactions of the pinealectomized animals differed from those of the controls at all intervals recorded from the time of injection until death occurred. For example, seven minutes after injection, spiky wave discharges were recorded in the pinealectomized animals, whereas in the controls no deviation from the usual polyrhythmic and polymorphic activity was observed (Fig. 4). This phenomenon may be related to the increased excitability of the brain, observed in the form of seizure-like electrocortical discharges, found in pinealectomized female rats.

Kappers: How much time elapsed between pinealectomy and the EEG recordings?

Nir: Recuperation took one to two weeks.

Miline: We have studied the activity of the supraoptic nucleus in adult male rats under the influence of aqueous extracts of the pineal gland and of melatonin. Diuresis was measured in control and treated rats and was found to be augmented by these pineal compounds. After epiphysectomy the activity of the supraoptic nucleus is increased (and diuresis diminished). There is a very intimate functional connexion between the hypothalamus and the pineal gland. The hypothalamus is the strategic point for the action of pineal hormones (Miline 1960). Dr Antón-Tay's data on GABA suggest that the activity of the supraoptic nucleus, the site of secretion of vasopressin, may be influenced by intermediary or inhibitory neurons. It is possible that epiphysectomy produces changes in the inhibitory neurons and the activity of the supraoptic nucleus is increased.

Nir: In our experience pinealectomy does not cause any change in either the ratio between the urinary excretion in dark and light periods or the total output. These experiments were carried out in adult female rats of the Hebrew University's "Sabra" strain and they were followed up for eight weeks after operation.

Miline: In which seasons did you do this?

Nir: The experiments spanned both summer and winter. The difference between our results and Dr Miline's perhaps stems from the fact that we used female rats and his were male, and also from strain variations.

Wurtman: Dr Ramon Piezzi and I have been interested in the roles of serotonin in the pituitary and median eminence, and have found quite large amounts of serotonin in both areas. There was initially some difficulty in proving that the compound with which we were dealing really was serotonin, in as much as previous studies by Björklund and Falck (1969) had demonstrated within mammalian pituitaries a compound that differed chemically from serotonin but had similar fluorescence properties after formaldehyde fixation. Hence it was necessary to confirm the identity of pituitary serotonin using several biochemical techniques.

Within the pituitary, the highest concentration of serotonin was found in the pars intermedia (Piezzi, Larin and Wurtman 1970). One important and unanswered question is whether this serotonin is localized within MSH-secreting cells or in endings of brain axons that impinge on the pars intermedia. Dr Owman tells me he has identified serotoninergic nerves that arise in the hypothalamus and terminate within the pars intermedia.

Dr Piezzi has examined the effects of several specific physiological inputs (melatonin treatment, or dehydration for five days) on the content of serotonin in different portions of the rat pituitary (Table I) (Piezzi and Wurtman 1970). Among rats treated with 150 μg of melatonin intra-peritoneally per day for five days and then killed, there was no change in the serotonin content in the pars distalis or pars nervosa, but there was a sig-nificant *increase* in the pars intermedia. The weight of the pars intermedia and the quantity of protein in the pars intermedia also went up 1·4-fold, so the actual amount of serotonin was about double in melatonin-treated animals compared with control animals. In contrast, dehydration caused a striking *decrease* in the serotonin concentration and content of the pars distalis. There was also a striking decrease in the pars nervosa after five days, but no change in the pars intermedia. So there seems to be selectivity, in that a physiological input that one would expect to be stressful and to cause a big release of vasopressin has a big effect on serotonin in the anterior and posterior pituitary, whereas melatonin, which is known to release MSH from the pars intermedia (Kastin and Schally 1967), has a specific effect on serotonin in this part of the pituitary.

What is the physiological significance of the rise in serotonin in the pars intermedia after giving melatonin? Several thoughts come to mind. It

TABLE I (Wurtman)

SEROTONIN CONTENT OF THE RAT PITUITARY AFTER
TREATMENT WITH MELATONIN AND AFTER DEHYDRATION

Pituitary region	Melatonin	Dehydration
	(μg/mg protein)	
Pars distalis	0·14/0·11*	0·08/0·14**
Pars intermedia	0·36/0·25**	0·23/0·20
Pars nervosa	0·16/0·15	0·08/0·16**

* Treatment/control groups.
** Statistically significant difference.

has been shown (Antón-Tay *et al.* 1968) that systemic treatment with melatonin increases the amounts of serotonin in certain parts of the brain, for example the hypothalamus and the midbrain. Hence it's not altogether surprising that melatonin would cause an increase in the serotonin content of the pars intermedia. We suspect that this material is present in the terminals of neurons located within the hypothalamus. Studies are now under way to correlate the MSH content of the cultured pars intermedia with its serotonin content, in collaboration with Dr Shein and Dr Lerner. We are culturing bits of bovine pituitary and hope to determine whether the time at which serotonin ceases to be present in this tissue (which is about four days) coincides with the time at which MSH ceases to be present. So far, the answer appears to be no. This suggests that the MSH is present in the cells whereas at least part of the serotonin is present within nerve endings.

REFERENCES

Antón-Tay, F., Chou, C., Anton, S. and Wurtman, R. J. (1968) *Science* **162**, 277–278.
Björklund, A. and Falck, B. (1969) *Z. Zellforsch. mikrosk. Anat.* **93**, 254.
Fraschini, F., Mess, B. and Martini, L. (1968) *Endocrinology* **82**, 914–924.
Kastin, A. J. and Schally, A. V. (1967) *Nature, Lond.* **213**, 1238–1240.
Kopin, I. J., Pare, C. M. B., Axelrod, J. and Weissbach, H. (1961) *J. biol. Chem.* **236**, 3072–3075.
Mess, B. and Hámori, J. (1965) *Acta histochem.* **20**, 143–148.
Miline, R. (1960) *Biol. hung.* **1**, 105–130.
Motta, M., Fraschini, F. and Martini, L. (1967) *Proc. Soc. exp. Biol. Med.* **126**, 431–435.
Piezzi, R. S., Larin, F. and Wurtman, R. J. (1970) *Endocrinology* **86**, 1460–1462.
Piezzi, R. S. and Wurtman, R. J. (1970) *Science* **169**, 285–286.

LUTEINIZATION INDUCED BY PINEALECTOMY IN THE POLYFOLLICULAR OVARIES OF RATS BEARING ANTERIOR HYPOTHALAMIC LESIONS

B. Mess, A. Heizer, A. Tóth and L. Tima

Department of Anatomy, University Medical School, Pécs, Hungary

ELECTROLYTIC destruction of the antero-basal region of the hypothalamus of the female rat provokes a syndrome characterized by persistent vaginal oestrus and a polyfollicular (in some cases, polycystic) state of the ovaries. The mechanism of the development of this anovulatory syndrome has been reported (Dey 1941, 1943; Hillarp 1949; Flerkó 1954). Many authors (Van der Werff ten Bosch, Van Rees and Wolthuis 1962; Bradshaw and Critchlow 1966; Tima and Flerkó 1967) agree moreover that lesions of the preoptic and/or suprachiasmatic area destroy the neural mechanism triggering the release of luteinizing hormone (LH). Tima and Flerkó (1967) have shown that the pituitary of rats bearing antero-basal hypothalamic lesions contains sufficient amounts of LH to elicit ovulation. Rats demonstrating this anovulatory syndrome were hypophysectomized and subsequently were injected intraperitoneally with extracts of their own hypophyses. Ovulation occurred within 48 hours after injection. This is clear-cut evidence that the pituitary gland does contain an ovulatory quantum of LH, but because of the lack of the neural trigger mechanism, it is not able to release this hormone. A continuous and permanent level of follicle stimulating hormone (FSH) in the blood might be responsible for the constant oestrous state and the lack of ovulation.

Various data from the literature have established the fact that the pineal gland exerts an inhibitory influence on the gonad–genital system (Kitay 1954; Kitay and Altschule 1954; Wurtman, Altschule and Holmgren 1959; Thiéblot and Blaise 1965). Moszkowska (1966a, b) assumed that the pineal body normally inhibits the synthesis and release of pituitary gonadotropins in three different ways. The so-called F_3 fraction of pineal extract inhibits FSH release by a direct action on the pituitary; serotonin acts through the inhibition of the hypothalamic releasing factors, and melatonin inhibits LH release "in a still unclarified way". In previous investigations performed in the Department of Pharmacology, University of Milan (Mess et al. 1966; Fraschini, Mess and Martini 1968) an increase in the pituitary

LH content of pinealectomized male rats had been demonstrated; moreover the weights of the peripheral reproductive organs were also increased, indicating that the pineal body normally inhibits both synthesis and release of LH. This LH-inhibiting effect of melatonin is mediated through the central nervous system. Implantation of homologous pineal gland or of purified melatonin into the median eminence of the hypothalamus, or into the reticular substance of the mesencephalon, significantly depressed the rise in pituitary LH content induced by castration.

On the basis of the data summarized above, we tried to influence the anovulatory syndrome elicited by suprachiasmatic lesions by removing the pineal gland.

MATERIAL AND METHODS

Nulliparous, mature female rats of our inbred strain (originally Wistar), weighing 150–180 g, were kept on an artificial standard diet. Environmental temperature was 28 ± 1°C and the lighting schedule consisted of 14 hours of light and 10 hours of darkness during the entire experimental period. Animals were given bilateral suprachiasmatic lesions. A direct current of 4–5 mA, applied for 6 seconds, was used for each lesion. Vaginal smears were recorded daily for a two-month period. At the end of the second month, animals showing persistent vaginal cornification were laparotomized in order to verify the polyfollicular state of the ovaries; subsequently pinealectomy was performed by the technique of Grant, Jenner and Willy (1966), modified in our laboratory (Group A).

The recording of daily vaginal smears was continued after pinealectomy. Animals were killed between the 2nd and 23rd day after pinealectomy. Ovaries were fixed in 10 per cent formalin; the frozen sections were stained with Sarlach R-haematoxylin stain and examined histologically. The formation of corpora lutea and thecal luteinization were considered as histological evidence for increased secretion of LH.

In the rats of Group B (operated on in the same way as those in Group A) oviducts were dissected on the second oestrous day following the first dioestrous phase after pinealectomy and the number of tubal ova was counted to provide direct evidence of ovulation.

Rats in Group C (suprachiasmatic lesion and pinealectomy, as in Groups A and B) were treated with melatonin. A daily dose of 30 μg was injected subcutaneously from the day of pinealectomy for a 12-day period. The occurrence of ovulation and luteinization was checked either on the 13th day of treatment with melatonin or 2–3 weeks after withdrawal of this compound.

Sham pinealectomy (Group D) was performed on rats bearing the same type of hypothalamic lesion as animals of the previous groups by allowing a cranial blood loss equivalent to that experienced during pinealectomy.

The exact site and extension of the hypothalamic lesion was checked by histological examination of serial sections of the brain stained with haematoxylin and eosin.

EXPERIMENTAL RESULTS

Vaginal smears of the persistently oestrous rats showed metoestrous and dioestrous phases a few days after pinealectomy. The vaginal cycle was

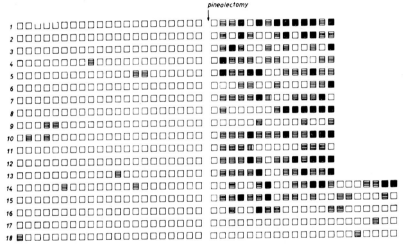

Fig. 1. Changes in vaginal smears following pinealectomy in rats bearing suprachiasmatic lesions. The first recorded day is the 30th day after the hypothalamic lesion. ▥, prooestrus; □, oestrus; ▤, metoestrus; ■, dioestrus.

fairly irregular, although a cyclic tendency was evident. This irregular cycle was continuous until the day of sacrifice. Fig. 1 represents vaginal smears of rats of Group A. The character of the vaginal cycle is fairly similar in all other groups except for the sham-operated one, where persistent vaginal cornification returned after a few days of metoestrous or dioestrous activity in the acute postoperative period.

At autopsy, fresh corpora lutea were found in the majority of cases (Fig. 2c), while a marked thecal luteinization was observed in a few animals (Fig. 2d). Less than one-third of the ovaries had preserved their original polyfollicular state (Fig. 2b).

Two weeks after pinealectomy, corpora lutea were present in 15 out of

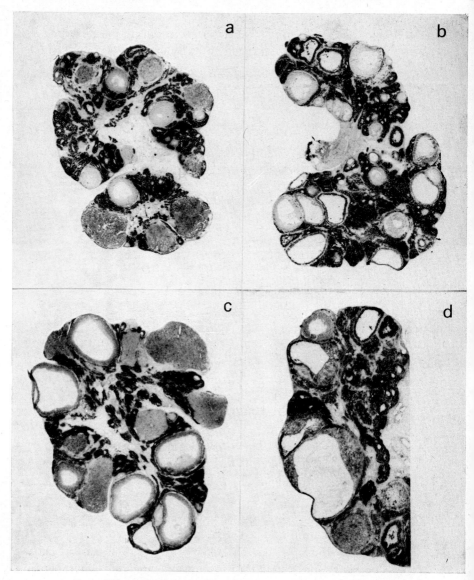

FIG. 2. Histology of the ovaries of rats bearing suprachiasmatic lesions
with or without concomitant pinealectomy.
  (a) Intact control rat. Fresh corpora lutea are evident.
  (b) Polyfollicular ovary of a rat bearing suprachiasmatic lesions.
  (c) Ovary of a rat bearing suprachiasmatic lesions, two weeks after
subsequent pinealectomy. Large fresh corpora lutea are visible.
  (d) Rat of the same group as (c), with marked thecal luteinization.
Sarlach R–haematoxylin stain. × 15.

25 rats and pronounced thecal luteinization was evident in 3 cases (Group A), representing a 72·0 per cent incidence of luteinization (Table I).

The formation of corpora lutea may be the consequence of ovulation, but it is well known that thecal luteinization, or the luteinization of atretic follicles, may also lead to the development of corpora lutea. The histological character of these corpora lutea (Fig. 2c), however, provided some evidence that they developed from ovulated follicles. In order to clarify the real mechanism of formation of corpora lutea in the pinealectomized animals we checked the Fallopian tubes for ova in a subsequent experiment (Group B), as direct evidence for ovulation. Tubal ova were found between the 2nd and 23rd day after pinealectomy in 7 out of the 16 animals of Group B. However, fresh corpora lutea were seen in 11 rats. Thus ovulation occurred in only 43·7 per cent while luteinization nearly reached the level (68·7 per cent) observed in Group A.

The effect of pinealectomy was completely counteracted by giving melatonin (Table I). No formation of corpora lutea or any sign of thecal luteinization was detected in the 16 pinealectomized and melatonin-treated rats of Group C. According to our preliminary data, ovulation and luteinization occurs, however, 2–3 weeks after withdrawal of melatonin.

No corpora lutea were present in the ovaries of the sham-operated animals, and only a very moderate thecal luteinization was observed in a single case (Table I; Group D).

TABLE I

EFFECT OF PINEALECTOMY ON OVULATION AND LUTEINIZATION IN THE POLYFOLLICULAR OVARIES OF RATS BEARING SUPRACHIASMATIC LESIONS

Experimental group	Number of rats	Number of rats showing			Percentage occurrence of	
		Ovulation	Corpora lutea	Thecal luteinization	Ovulation	Luteinization
A Pinealectomy. Killed 14 days after operation	25	not investigated	15	3	not investigated	72·0
B Pinealectomy. Oviducts investigated for tubal ova 2–23 days after operation	16	7	11	0	43·7	68·7
C Pinealectomy + melatonin treatment. Killed 13 days after operation	16	0	0	0	0	0
D Sham-operation. Killed 14 days after operation	7	0	0	1	0	14·3

TABLE II

NUMBER OF TUBAL OVA FOLLOWING PINEALECTOMY IN
RATS BEARING SUPRACHIASMATIC LESIONS

Days after pinealectomy	Number of ova
2	11
5	1
6	9
7	8
7	4
22	8
23	8

The question whether the ovulation observed in Group B can be considered a biologically complete ovulation, or whether only a reduced number of ova were ripened and released, is answered by Table II. The number of tubal ova varied between 4 and 11, which is characteristic for a normal ovulation, and coincides with the size of the litters born in our strain of rats. The probable interpretation of the one exception in Table II where only a single ovum was found in the oviduct will be suggested below.

DISCUSSION

The experiments presented clearly indicate that pinealectomy provokes ovulation and the formation of corpora lutea in the polyfollicular ovaries of rats bearing anterior hypothalamic lesions. Furthermore, these results show that the action of melatonin on the hypothalamo-pituitary-gonad axis might be considered to be one of the factors maintaining anovulatory conditions in rats with anterior hypothalamic lesions.

The blockade of LH mobilization caused by the destruction of the antero-basal hypothalamic area provokes a new "steady state" in the hormonal balance of the female sexual cycle. The new equilibrium is characterized by a continuous predominance of FSH, which is reflected in the polyfollicular state of the ovaries and in the persistent vaginal cornification. This syndrome proved to be fairly well stabilized. Many experimental efforts have been made to elicit luteinization—that is, to provoke LH mobilization in these animals—by progesterone treatment (Greer 1953; Alloiteau 1954); by lowering oestrogen production through subtotal ovariectomy (Flerkó and Bárdos 1961); by bilateral lesions of the premammillary region (Kordon 1966); by unilateral lesions of the premammillary region, or lesions of a more extended area in the middle and posterior part of the hypothalamus (Illei-Donhoffer, Tima and Flerkó 1970). The results of these experiments have proved that luteinization can be provoked in the presence of this syndrome in spite of the irreversible destruction of the so-called LH trigger mechanism in the antero-basal hypothalamus.

The experimental evidence cited in the introduction indicates that the pineal gland may play an active role in the regulation of the hypophysial-gonadal system. One of the most important effects of the pineal body is its influence on the secretion of pituitary gonadotropic hormones, especially LH (Moszkowska 1966a, b; Mess et al. 1966; Fraschini, Mess and Martini 1968). The results of the present study might also be interpreted on the basis of an effect on the secretion of LH. Pinealectomy causes an increased and rapid mobilization of LH which might be sufficient to induce ovulation and the consequent development of corpora lutea in the originally polyfollicular ovaries. It can also be assumed that in some instances when LH mobilization was not intensive or rapid enough to produce ovulation, this slightly increased, or protracted LH mobilization resulted in thecal luteinization only.

Tubal ova were found only in 43 per cent of the pinealectomized animals, while fresh corpora lutea were present in more than 60 per cent (see Table I). This discrepancy might be explained by the occasional occurrence of a slight and protracted mobilization of LH. Another possibility must also be taken into account: the changes in the phases of the vaginal cycle are fairly irregular (see Fig. 1); to determine the exact day of ovulation on the basis of the vaginal smear is therefore not precise or reliable enough. Therefore, it seems very probable that in those cases where no released ova were found in the oviduct and fresh corpora lutea were present in the ovaries, the autopsy was performed too late, the ova already having passed through the oviduct. The second case in Table II supports this latter assumption. In this rat only a single ovum was detected in the Fallopian tube, and it already showed signs of cleavage (a morula with four cells). It seems very probable that most of the ova reached the uterus at the time of investigation and only the last one was still present in the isthmic end of the tuba uterina. A few hours later this animal most likely would belong to the group of rats with fresh corpora lutea without tubal ova.

The signs of increased mobilization of LH (ovulation and luteinization) observed after pinealectomy very probably might be due to specific effects of the decreased level of the hormone-like principles of the pineal gland. Since sham operation failed to provoke luteinization, the effect of a non-specific stress situation can be excluded. On the other hand, the active role of decreased melatonin secretion was indicated by the reversal of the effect of pinealectomy by treatment with melatonin. After withdrawal of this substitution therapy, all the effects of pinealectomy occurred again, within a relatively short time.

Whether the effect of pinealectomy, demonstrated in rats with the anovulatory syndrome, is transitory or permanent has not yet been proved unequivocally. Experiments are now in progress to investigate whether pinealectomy elicits only a short-term output of LH resulting in a single ovulation, or whether pinealectomized rats ovulate again in a cyclic manner. Some preliminary and indirect evidence supports the latter idea. Other experiments have been begun to elucidate the mechanism by which the pineal body influences the female sexual cycle.

SUMMARY

Pinealectomy was performed on female rats bearing lesions in the suprachiasmatic hypothalamic area. The anovulatory syndrome, with persistent vaginal cornification and polyfollicular ovaries, caused by the antero-basal hypothalamic lesion, was influenced profoundly by pinealectomy. An irregular, but evident cyclicity of the vaginal smears returned and fresh corpora lutea were found in the ovaries 2 weeks after pinealectomy. Tubal ova were also demonstrated in the pinealectomized animals, showing that corpora lutea were developed from post-ovulatory follicles. Sham pinealectomy failed to influence the persistent vaginal oestrus and the polyfollicular state of the ovaries.

All these effects of pinealectomy could be counteracted by treatment with melatonin in a daily dose of 30 μg per rat. Withdrawal of melatonin resulted, however, in ovulation and luteinization.

The question remains open whether pinealectomy causes only a single ovulation by means of an acute output of LH or whether pinealectomized rats ovulate again in a cyclic manner.

Acknowledgement

We wish to express our gratitude to the Regis Chemical Company, Chicago, Illinois, for having kindly supplied us with purified melatonin.

REFERENCES

ALLOITEAU, J. J. (1954) *C.r. Séanc. Soc. Biol.* **148**, 223–226.
BRADSHAW, M. and CRITCHLOW, V. (1966) *Endocrinology* **78**, 1007–1014.
DEY, F. L. (1941) *Am. J. Anat.* **69**, 61–87.
DEY, F. L. (1943) *Am. J. Physiol.* **129**, 39–46.
FLERKÓ, B. (1954) *Acta morph. hung.* **4**, 475–492.
FLERKÓ, B. and BÁRDOS, V. (1961) *Acta endocr., Copenh.* **37**, 418–422.
FRASCHINI, F., MESS, B. and MARTINI, L. (1968) *Endocrinology* **82**, 919–924.

GRANT, L., JENNER, F. A. and WILLY, B. (1966) *J. Physiol., Lond.* **182**, 24.

GREER, M. A. (1953) *Endocrinology*, **53**, 380–390.

HILLARP, N. A. (1949) *Acta endocr., Copenh.* **2**, 11–23.

ILLEI-DONHOFFER, Á., TIMA, L. and FLERKÓ, B. (1970) *Acta biol. hung.* **21**, 197–206.

KITAY, J. J. (1954) *Endocrinology* **54**, 114–116.

KITAY, J. J. and ALTSCHULE, M. D. (1954) *The Pineal Gland—A Review of the Physiologic Literature.* Cambridge, Mass.: Harvard University Press.

KORDON, C. (1966) In *La Physiologie de la Reproduction chez les Mammifères*, pp. 458–474, ed. Jost, A. Paris: Centre National de la Recherche Scientifique.

MESS, B., FRASCHINI, F., PIVA, F. and MARTINI, L. (1966) In *Hormonal Steroids*, p. 361, ed. Romanoff, E. B. and Martini, L. Excerpta Medica International Congress Series no. 111. Amsterdam: Excerpta Medica Foundation.

MOSZKOWSKA, A. (1966a) In *Hormonal Steroids*, p. 361, ed Romanoff, E. B. and Martini, L. Excerpta Medica International Congress Series no. 111. Amsterdam: Excerpta Medica Foundation.

MOSZKOWSKA, A. (1966b) *Probl. Actuels Endocr. Nutr.* **10**, 213–228.

THIÉBLOT, L. and BLAISE, B. (1965) In *Structure and Function of the Epiphysis Cerebri* (*Progress in Brain Research* vol. 10), pp. 577–584, ed. Kappers, J. A. and Schadé, J. P. Amsterdam: Elsevier.

TIMA, L. and FLERKÓ, B. (1967) *Endocrinologia experimentalis* **1**, 193–199.

VAN DER WERFF TEN BOSCH, J. J., VAN REES, G. P. and WOLTHUIS, C. L. (1962) *Acta endocr., Copenh.* **40**, 103–110.

WURTMAN, R. J., ALTSCHULE, M. D. and HOLMGREN, U. (1959) *Am. J. Physiol.* **197**, 108–110.

DISCUSSION

Martini: I have been considering recently why people have never thought of the pineal gland as the physiological regulator of the 24-hour rhythmicity of LH release which occurs in female rats. As you know, the classic experiments of J. W. Everett (1964) show that if you give Nembutal before the 2–4 p.m. "critical period" occurring on the day of pro-oestrus you can delay ovulation by one day; LH release (as now shown by radio-immunological assay) will also occur one day later, again between 2 and 4 p.m. If 24 hours later you give a second injection of Nembutal to Nembutal-blocked rats, you usually delay ovulation by another 24-hour period.

Since data which are rapidly accumulating indicate that melatonin has a depressant effect on the central nervous system, and since the 2–4 p.m. "critical period" is the time when melatonin is not present in the body because of the suppressive effect exerted by light on its biosynthesis, one might postulate that the 24-hour periodicity in the release of LH is due to the cyclicity of the formation of melatonin (Fraschini and Martini 1970). I think Dr Mess's data are particularly relevant in this respect because they show quite clearly that if you take the pineal out (and consequently elim-inate the inhibitory effect induced by melatonin) you may induce LH release and ovulation.

Wurtman: One can add several other factors. Dr Kordon and co-workers

(1968) have shown that brain serotonin is especially related to this critical period. The serotonin content of the brain shows a diurnal rhythm and, as Dr Antón-Tay mentioned, the amounts of serotonin in the brain are related to the availability of melatonin.

Reiter: Dr Mess, what is the longest time after pinealectomy that vaginal smears were studied?

Mess: Twenty-three days. During that time irregular cyclicity was continuous.

Reiter: But did they ever become persistently oestrous again in that period?

Mess: No.

Reiter: In essence, then, you could simulate your experimental conditions by putting the animals in continuous light, which would physiologically pinealectomize the animals. Have you tried this?

Mess: No, but it is a good idea; maybe it could be tried in animals with anterior hypothalamic lesions. But I can't agree that continuous light is equivalent to pinealectomy, so I am not sure that it would give the same results as pinealectomy.

Wurtman: I think I would agree with Dr Mess about this. The mechanism by which light affects the pineal involves the inferior accessory optic tracts which run within the medial forebrain bundles for part of their course—hence nerve inputs generated by light do reach the medial forebrain bundles. From there they can go to two places; they can descend through the spinal cord to reach the sympathetic nerves leading to the pineal; they could also be transmitted directly to the medial hypothalamus, where they would influence cells releasing hypophysiotropic hormones. Hence it would be foolhardy to say that *the* only route by which light affects the gonads is via the pineal; I think it more likely that *an* effect of light on the gonads is via the pineal, but additional effects of light on the gonads are probably mediated directly, by the medial forebrain bundle and the medial hypothalamus.

Reiter: I agree entirely that there are undoubtedly effects of constant light on reproduction that are exclusive of any effect on the pineal. I meant that short-term exposure to constant light should, in essence, constitute a physiological pinealectomy. Of course if you maintained the rats in constant light for a long time they would go into constant oestrus anyway.

Herbert: First, I would agree with Dr Martini's comment because it seems to me that if the pineal gland in the rat has a function, a likely one is timing ovulation in relation to light. Secondly, I wonder if Dr Mess's experiments have a bearing on the mechanism of the persistent oestrus produced by anterior hypothalamic lesions? It has always struck me that there is a close parallel between the effects of such lesions and those of constant light. Both result in continuous vaginal cornification, and in either condition ovulation can be induced by progesterone or by vaginal stimulation. I wonder whether one might postulate that these lesions in some way "sensitize" the animals to the action of light, and so when you remove the pineal you reverse the effect?

Mess: I don't think so, because it is well established, despite some contradictions in the literature, that lesions of the anterior hypothalamus switch out the LH trigger mechanism which then provokes continuous FSH secretion and consequently a continuous level of oestrogen in the blood, so the animal is in a state of constant oestrus and shows an anovulatory syndrome, but I don't believe that this would run through the pineal light effect. It is a direct effect running through FSH, elicited by switching off the LH trigger. This syndrome can be *influenced* from the pineal, because pinealectomy has an LH-mobilizing effect. We switched out the LH-mobilizing mechanism with the lesion but we could provoke an acute mobilization of LH by removing the pineal gland, but I don't believe it has anything to do, or only very indirectly, with lighting schedules.

Kordon: The primary effect of your hypothalamic lesions would appear to be to enhance circulating levels of FSH and possibly oestrogen, with the disturbance of LH release as a secondary result (as shown, for example, by the fact that you still found enough LH in the pituitary to promote ovulation in animals with lesions). So you might postulate that the LH-triggering mechanism, which is not blocked directly by the lesion but possibly by the excess oestrogen, is de-inhibited by pinealectomy. Could one not also assume that the thresholds of central structures sensitive to oestrogen are affected by pinealectomy? This could easily be tested by treating the animals with additional oestrogen after pinealectomy, and by investigating whether or not the treatment prevents the restoration of ovulation.

Mess: Our experiments have been done on a relatively limited number of animals so far and many possible aspects of the mechanism have not been investigated yet. I think it is possible that a lesion switching out the so-called oestrogen-sensitive receptor system of the anterior hypothalamus may also have a profound effect on FSH secretion, but I wanted to simplify the mechanism of the lesion producing constant oestrus to one crucial factor only; I pointed out that LH release is blocked because this gave us the first impulse to work with pinealectomy, when we found that pinealectomy mobilized LH. Our experiments in Milan also showed that

there is something wrong with LH release after a lesion of the suprachiasmatic area of the hypothalamus. As to the actual mechanism of the
lesion, the one you mentioned is one of the possibilities, but I believe it to
be more probable that the switching off of the LH trigger is the primary
event, and the effect on FSH secretion is secondary only.

Miline: Dr Mess, are the newly formed corpora lutea that you see after
pinealectomy active? Are they changed in structure, with signs of involution? Can we speak about the liberation of the luteotropic (LTH)
factor in this experiment? Secondly, I have the impression from your
illustrations that the interstitial cells are also hyperplasic after pinealectomy.
Is this so?

Mess: We have never measured the mobilization of luteotropic hormone
by bioassay, but histologically the ovaries look completely normal and in
animals which lived two or three weeks after pinealectomy we often found
several different generations of corpora lutea, very fresh ones and older
ones already showing regressive signs, indicating that it might not be a
single ovulation but two or three more subsequent ovulations. The
interstitial tissue of the ovaries seemed also to be identical in the pinealectomized animals bearing anterior hypothalamic lesions and in the intact
controls. The so-called interstitial glands were perhaps in some instances
more developed in the pinealectomized rats, but this difference was never
significant.

Shein: You verified that the corpora lutea were formed from ovulated
follicles by observing whether there were ova in the Fallopian tubes, but I
was interested to notice that the sequence of development of oestrus and
dioestrus was altered in these animals and I wonder whether you checked
to see if the ova once released were normal and capable of supporting life?
Did you see whether you could get embryos developing? The altered
sequence of development of oestrus and dioestrus suggests the possibility
of altered levels of oestrogen and progesterone, and so makes me wonder
whether the uterus would be sufficiently prepared hormonally to nourish
the fertilized ova properly after implantation.

Mess: They appeared to be completely normal ova and in one case
cleavage was already visible. But I don't know whether viable embryos
would have resulted.

REFERENCES

EVERETT, J. W. (1964) *Physiol. Rev.* **44**, 373–431.
FRASCHINI, F. and MARTINI, L. (1970) In *The Hypothalamus*, pp. 529–549, ed. Martini, L.,
      Motta, M. and Fraschini, F. New York and London: Academic Press.
KORDON, C., JAVOY, F., VASSENT, G. and GLOWINSKI, J. (1968) *Eur. J. Pharmac.* **4**, 169–174.

BIOCHEMICAL FRACTIONS AND MECHANISMS INVOLVED IN THE PINEAL MODULATION OF PITUITARY GONADOTROPIN RELEASE

A. Moszkowska, C. Kordon and I. Ebels

Equipe de recherches neuroendocrinologiques du CNRS, Laboratoire d'Histophysiologie du Collège de France, Paris, France; and Department of Organic Chemistry, State University of Utrecht, The Netherlands

Although experimental results suggested many years ago that the pineal may inhibit growth of the gonads, substantial progress in this field has occurred only in the last ten years, since the pineal began to be considered as one of the central regulating mechanisms in charge of pituitary control rather than as an endocrine organ only. Newer approaches in research on the pineal were made possible by a better understanding of the nervous structures involved in the mechanisms regulating the release of gonadotropins, as well as by technical and methodological progress in the pharmacology of central transmitters and in the biochemistry of pineal material.

The existence of a gonadotropin inhibitory activity in the pineal has now been established beyond doubt. However, in spite of the fact that these antigonadotropic effects of the gland may be very important in particular endocrine states, it should be emphasized that pineal mechanisms are not able to account entirely for the regulation of gonadotropic functions. Pinealectomized animals always exhibit at least some normal gonadotropic responses; we therefore have to assume that the epiphysis is at the most capable of a complementary, modulating influence on the activity of the central structures primarily responsible for pituitary regulation.

This situation makes it somewhat difficult to determine the precise physiological significance of pineal mechanisms. Methodological considerations add further difficulties to such attempts, particularly in experiments involving treatment with pineal extracts. Many substances present in the central nervous system have pharmacological or non-specific effects when supplied directly to receptor sites or structures where they would not be available under normal conditions. This is of course especially true of the pineal, since the pathways by which epiphysial products may reach ventral brain structures or the pituitary are still completely unknown.

We shall first review here the most recent demonstrations of pineal involvement in gonadotropin regulation. We shall then discuss the role of substances or fractions derived from the pineal in the secretion of gonadotropic hormones, with particular reference to the way in which these compounds may interfere with the physiological control of the pituitary.

EVIDENCE FOR THE INHIBITORY EFFECT OF THE PINEAL ON PITUITARY GONADOTROPIN SECRETION

Older experiments on the stimulatory effects of pinealectomy have not always been very convincing; some authors have even reported contradictory results, possibly because the observations were not made under similar experimental conditions or in comparable species (see the reviews by Kitay and Altschule 1954; Wiener 1968; Kappers 1969; Reiter and Fraschini 1969).

Clear-cut evidence for the inhibition of gonadotropic functions by the pineal was first obtained from the pinealectomy of seasonal breeders like the hamster, in which the intervention induces marked alterations in gonadal weight (Czyba, Girod and Durand 1964; Hoffman and Reiter 1965; Girod, Durand and Czyba 1967). At the same time it could be shown that even polycyclic animals like the rat may show important responses to the ablation of the pineal (Moszkowska and Scemama 1968a, b; Reiter et al. 1968). However, this effect can only be obtained in polycyclic species when the hormonostatic feedback processes which regulate the secretion of gonadotropins are no longer intact. These mechanisms can be partially disconnected by postnatal treatment with testosterone, a procedure which has been shown to decrease the sensitivity of the nervous system to steroid feedback (Barraclough and Haller 1970) and to render gonadotropic functions more dependent upon external factors (Kordon and Hoffmann 1967; Hoffmann, Kordon and Benoit 1968). In these conditions, normal hormonostatic mechanisms no longer seem able to compensate for variations in the stimulatory input of the hypothalamic areas regulating gonadotropin secretion; consequently, such variations become much more apparent than under normal conditions and result in clear-cut gonadal responses (Hoffmann, Kordon and Benoit 1968).

For instance, male or female rats kept in the dark after postnatal testosterone treatment show only a very weak development of the gonads (Hoffmann, Kordon and Benoit 1968). However this lack of gonadal stimulation may be counteracted by postnatal pinealectomy; this then results in marked stimulation of gonadal weight and activity, by comparison with unoperated controls (Figs. 1 and 3) (Moszkowska and Scemama 1968a; Reiter *et al.* 1968) and in important structural changes in the gonads of male (Fig. 2) as well as of female rats (Fig. 4).

More discrete effects of pinealectomy have also been observed in mice; in this species, precocious ablation of the epiphysis results in hyperplasia (but without noticeable hyperactivity) of the testicular interstitial cells (Lombard-des-Gouttes 1967). This effect has not been reproduced in the normal rat (Moszkowska 1967b), although in that case the intervention was reported to affect the gonadotropin content of the pituitary (Fraschini, Mess and Martini 1968). In the strain of rats used in our laboratory (Wistar), precocious pinealectomy affected the gonadotropin content of the pituitary only during a short period of prepubertal life; later differences in pituitary activity between pinealectomized and sham-operated animals could no longer be detected, in either normal or castrated animals (Table I) (Lombard-des-Gouttes 1970).

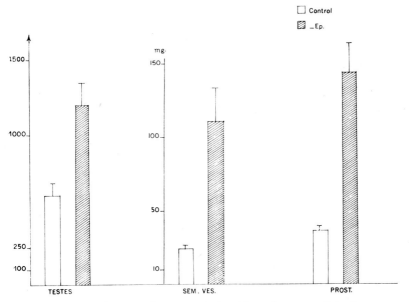

FIG. 1. Weight in mg of testes, seminal vesicles and prostate of pinealectomized or sham-operated male rats pretreated with testosterone
propionate (2 mg subcutaneously) 5 days after birth and kept in the dark
from 21 days of age. The rats were pinealectomized 10 days after birth
and sacrificed at the age of 60 days. Notice the marked weight increase
of the gonads and particularly the accessory glands.

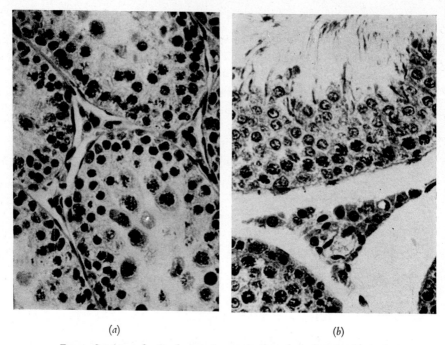

(a)   (b)

FIG. 2. Sections of testes from testosterone-treated rats kept in the dark
(same conditions of treatment as in Fig. 1).   (a) Sham-operated; (b)
pinealectomized.   Notice the recovery of spermatogenesis and the
development of seminiferous tubules and of the interstitial tissue after
removal of the epiphysis. Haemalum-eosin-saffran stain.   × 562.

TABLE I

PITUITARY GONADOTROPIN CONTENT AFTER PINEALECTOMY IN NORMAL OR
CASTRATED MALE RATS

Hormonal activity assayed by evaluation of uptake of ^{32}P in the immature testis (see Gogan
1968), a test mainly affected by LH activity.

*Relative pituitary gonadotropin content**

Age (days)	Number of animals	Pinealectomized		Pinealectomized and castrated	
		Average ratio	Confidence limits**	Average ratio	Confidence limits**
12	6	1·06	0·90–1·26	1·11	0·59–2·12
21	6	1·56†	1·17–2·21	1·60†	1·06–2·50
40	6	1·22†	1·09–1·43	1·19	0·89–1·60
50	6	1·12	0·88–1·52	1·01	0·80–1·50
80	6	1·23	0·99–1·63	1·08	0·70–1·66

*Gonadotropic activity in normal or castrated pinealectomized male rats over gonadotropic
activity in corresponding unpinealectomized controls.
**For a probability of 95 per cent.
† Difference significant at $P < 0·05$.

(From Lombard-des-Gouttes 1970.)

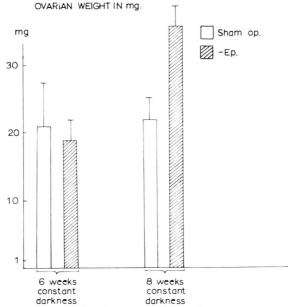

OVARIAN WEIGHT IN mg.

☐ Sham op.

▨ −Ep.

6 weeks
constant
darkness

8 weeks
constant
darkness

Fig. 3. Ovarian weight of pinealectomized or sham-operated female rats treated with testosterone as in Fig. 1, after 6 or 8 weeks in constant darkness. After 8 weeks, pinealectomy significantly enhances ovarian growth.

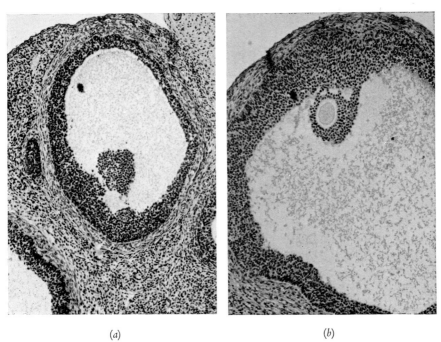

(a)   (b)

Fig. 4. Section of ovaries from testosterone-treated rats kept in the dark (same conditions of treatment as in Fig. 1). (a) Sham-operated; (b) pinealectomized. Notice the important follicular growth induced by the operation. Haemalum-eosin-saffran stain. ×112 (From Kordon, Moszkowska and Ebels 1970.)

EFFECT OF TREATMENT WITH VARIOUS PINEAL FRACTIONS

The pineal contains high levels of monoamines, particularly catechol-amines and indoleamines, but its glandular structure makes it capable of elaborating other secretion products besides central nervous mediators. Since treatment with extracts of the whole pineal are able to inhibit gonadotropin release from the pituitary *in vivo* and *in vitro* (Moszkowska 1955, 1965a, b), it was of interest to fractionate such crude extracts and to localize the fractions inhibiting release of gonadotropins.

Chromatographic fractionation

Our fractionation procedures have been described in detail in various publications (Ebels 1967; Moszkowska and Ebels 1970; Ebels, Moszkowska and Scemama 1970). Here we shall only summarize the main separation steps which yield active fractions.

After gel filtration on Sephadex G-25 (Fine) of an extract of sheep pineal powder, two fractions with a gonadotropic modulating activity have been obtained: fraction F2 and fraction F3. The Sephadex G-25 fraction F3 may be further purified on Sephadex G-10 in 0·2 M-pyridine—0·05 M-acetic acid buffer at pH 5·8; an active fraction with a molecular weight below 700 can be obtained by this procedure, which increases the specific activity of the fraction about 100 times by comparison with that of the crude extract.

The activity of the Sephadex G-25 fraction F2 can be accumulated by chromatography on the weak cation exchanger Amberlite IRC-50, XE-64, further separated on an anion exchanger Dowex 1X 2, and finally eluted from this column with 0·01 M-collidine-acetate buffer at pH 4·0.

Evaluation of the biological activity of pineal fractions

In vitro *studies*. The fraction F3 described above inhibits the release of gonadotropin from incubated rat pituitaries in a very similar way to that described previously after treatment *in vitro* with crude pineal extract. From 0·4 to 2·0 mg per half-pituitary significantly decreases the activity of the incubation medium in a gonadotropin assay modified (Ebels, Moszkowska and Scemama 1965) from the technique of Steelman and Pohley (1953), thus pointing to a major effect of the fraction on FSH excretion (Fig. 5). That fraction F3 is inhibiting the excretion of gonadotropins from the gland, and not interfering with the biological activity of the already released hormone, is shown by the fact that it is inactive when incubated together with purified FSH (Fig. 5).

The opposite effects of fraction F2 have been discussed in detail in other

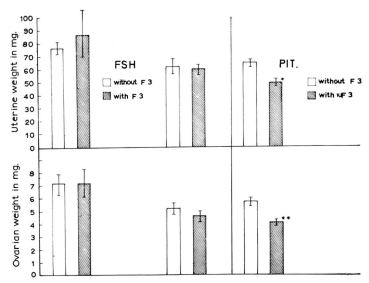

FIG. 5. Effect *in vitro* of the pineal fraction F3 on gonadotropic activity of purified FSH and of the incubation medium of rat pituitaries. The pineal factor affects the release of gonadotropin from the gland, and not the biological activity of the hormone simply incubated with it. This suggests an active inhibition of release and not an inactivation of the released material.

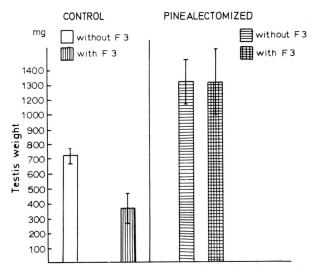

FIG. 6. Effect of chronic treatment *in vivo* with the pineal fraction F3 on testicular weight in testosterone-treated rats kept in the dark. F3 reduced growth of the testes in sham-operated but not in pinealectomized rats. The inhibitory activity of the fraction thus seems mainly present in conditions where the initial turnover of gonadotropic hormones is rather low.

reviews and will not be considered here (Moszkowska, Ebels and Scemama 1965).

In vivo *studies*. Chronic treatment with F3 for 14 days at a rate of three injections of 0·3 mg per week inhibits the growth of the gonads and accessory glands in the male rat (Fig. 6). Surprisingly, treatment with F3 is only effective in intact animals and not in pinealectomized rats; that is, in our testosterone-pretreated preparation, in conditions where the turnover of gonadotropins in the pituitary is much higher than in intact animals.

Discussion

The evaluation of F3 activity *in vitro* shows that this fraction is able to inhibit gonadotropin release from the pituitary directly. This action may be a physiological one, in spite of the relatively large amounts of the substance which proved necessary to block FSH secretion (the dose per pituitary corresponds to about 160 sheep pineal glands); however, this figure is possibly overestimated, since the biochemical yield of our fractionation procedure is rather poor; moreover, the substance has proved to be very labile, and poorly soluble in water, ethyl alcohol or acetone, and was recovered in the dry residue after extraction.

In vitro, F3 mainly affects the release of FSH, as we have seen. This effect does not therefore seem to account for the whole inhibitory activity of the pineal, which also affects the liberation of LH (Moszkowska 1951, 1955, 1965a, b, 1967a, b; Thiéblot et al. 1954). That F3 is only *one* pineal factor among several is further substantiated by the incomplete inhibition of gonadotropins exhibited by this fraction *in vivo*. We therefore have to consider the effect of other pineal substances, in particular indoleaminergic material. We may recall in this respect that fraction F3 is very likely not to contain melatonin or 5-methoxytryptophol, since it does not migrate through the Sephadex G-10 column at the same rate as these substances (Moszkowska and Ebels 1970).

EFFECTS OF TREATMENT WITH VARIOUS SYNTHETIC EPIPHYSIAL SUBSTANCES
In vitro *studies*

Unlike our F3 fraction, indoleamines (serotonin, melatonin or 5-methoxytryptophol) have no direct action on gonadotropin secretion from the pituitary (Moszkowska 1965a, b; Kordon and Moszkowska 1967; Moszkowska and Ebels 1970). Serotonin (5-HT), but not melatonin, affects the hypophysial response *in vitro* only when the gland is activated by adding hypothalamic fragments to the incubation medium (Moszkowska

1965*b*), which suggests that the primary action of serotonin is on hypothalamic tissue rather than on the pituitary.

In vivo *studies*

Chronic treatment with serotonin in young rats of either sex for prolonged periods of time (from 21 to 60 days of age) reduces pituitary and testicular weight; the size of the testicular tubules seems to be affected more than the interstitial tissue or the accessory organs. Furthermore, delayed vaginal opening is induced by the treatment (Moszkowska 1965*a*). Monoamine oxidase inhibitors like nialamide, when given together with

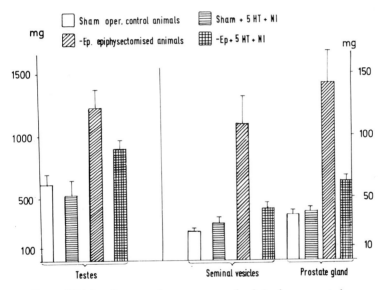

FIG. 7. Weight of testes and accessory sex glands in sham-operated or pinealectomized rats with or without the administration of nialamide and serotonin (5-HT) (Moszkowska and Ebels 1970).

serotonin to prevent it being rapidly metabolized, have been shown to potentiate these effects (Moszkowska, unpublished results). Similar results could also be obtained in testosterone-treated, pinealectomized rats kept in the dark as described above (Fig. 7) (Moszkowska and Ebels 1970). These experiments are in good agreement with observations showing that treatment with serotonin (Corbin and Schottelius 1961; O'Steen 1964; Moszkowska 1965*a*, *b*, 1970), or with melatonin (Wurtman, Axelrod and Chu 1963; Moszkowska 1965*b*; Fraschini, Mess and Martini 1968; Mess *et al.* 1966; Motta, Fraschini and Martini 1967), as well as with serotonin

precursors (Psychoyos 1966; Kordon *et al.* 1968) interferes with gonadotropin release, even in acute conditions.

In pinealectomized, testosterone-treated animals, 5-methoxytryptophol
does not interfere with the release of gonadotropin (Moszkowska and
Ebels 1970).

MODE OF ACTION OF THE PINEAL ON THE HYPOTHALAMUS

The effects of direct treatment with 5-HT, as reported above, cannot
easily be attributed to a pineal-mediated action, however. When introduced into the general circulation, the amine does not cross the blood-

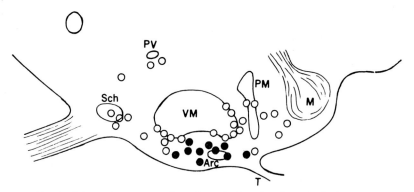

FIG. 8. Schematic representation of a sagittal section through the hypothalamus showing the sites where stimulation of extraneuronal release
of endogenous 5-HT (by direct microinjection of drugs) inhibits ovulation in the immature rat pretreated with serum gonadotropin. Black
circles, effective microinjection sites; open dots, ineffective sites; Arc,
arcuate nucleus; M, medial mammillary nucleus; PM, premmamillary
area; PV, paraventricular nucleus; Sch, suprachiasmatic nucleus; T,
pituitary stalk; VM, ventromedial nucleus. (From Kordon 1969.)

brain barrier and can thus reach only a few ventral structures, in particular
the median eminence (Lichtensteiger and Langemann 1966); this observation is substantiated by experiments showing that increased endogenous
release of 5-HT affects the release of gonadotropin only when induced in
the median eminence region (Fig. 8) (Kordon 1969; Kordon and Vassent
1968). Systemically administered 5-HT is thus more likely to affect
directly hypothalamic mechanisms regulating pituitary functions, rather
than the pineal involvement in these mechanisms. We may recall in this
respect that the medio-basal region of the hypothalamus is able to synthesize 5-HT *in situ*, as shown by the fact that pooled fragments of median
eminence can incorporate [³H]tryptophan into [³H]5-HT *in vitro* (Fig. 9)
(Hamon *et al.* 1970). That such incorporation is specific for 5-HT neurons

was demonstrated by *in vivo* studies made after the destruction of serotonin-ergic cell bodies (Pujol *et al.* 1969).

We therefore investigated whether pinealectomy would cause changes indirectly in the amine content of the hypothalamus, which contains most of the nervous structures responsible for gonadotropic control. The hypothalamus and other brain structures were carefully dissected out from

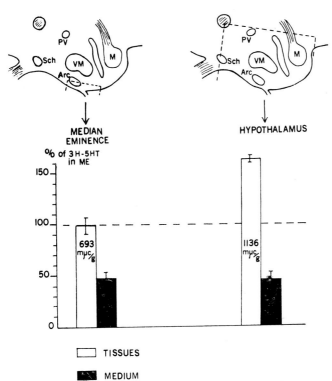

FIG. 9. Amount of tritiated serotonin [³H]-5HT, expressed as counts per minute, synthesized from [³H]tryptophan in the tissue (white bars) and released into the incubation medium (black bars) in pooled fragments of entire hypothalamus or of median eminence. Although the rate of synthesis is greater in the whole hypothalamus, a readily detectable amount of labelled amine is formed in the isolated median eminence. (Abbreviations as in Fig. 8.)

young castrated female rats, as well as from sham-operated or pinealecto-mized castrated litter mates. In this experiment, castration and pinealec-tomy were performed on 10-day-old animals; they were sacrificed 20 days later. The hypothalamuses from two animals were pooled, extracted and analysed for serotonin according to the method described by Bogdanski and co-workers (1956). Extracts of the remainder of the brain were analysed in the same way, after removal of the cerebellum.

TABLE II

SEROTONIN CONTENT OF THE HYPOTHALAMUS AND OTHER BRAIN STRUCTURES
AFTER PINEALECTOMY

Group	Number of rats	Serotonin content*	
		Hypothalamus	Rest of brain**
Sham-operated	12	100·0 ± 17·8	100·0 ± 2·6
Pinealectomized	13	43·1 ± 11·9†	110·1 ± 4·7

*Expressed as percentage of the sham-operated ± S.E.M.
**Brain after removal of hypothalamus and cerebellum.
†Difference from controls significant at $P < 0.001$.

(From Javoy et al. 1970.)

The results indicate that pinealectomy induces a very sharp decrease in endogenous serotonin in the hypothalamus over the time period of our experiments (Javoy et al. 1970) (Table II). In contrast, the serotonin content of other brain structures does not seem to be different in pinealectomized and intact animals. Pinealectomy thus seems to decrease sharply the 5-HT content of the hypothalamus; this result is in good agreement with the fact that 5-HT is inhibitory to gonadotropin release, and may provide an explanation for the disinhibited gonadotropic state found in pinealectomized animals. However, this action of the pineal on the 5-HT content of the hypothalamus is not likely to be a simple, direct action in which the low 5-HT content in pinealectomized subjects could be accounted for by the disappearance of a pineal 5-HT supply to the hypothalamus; it is more probably mediated by a modulation of the turnover of the amine in central serotoninergic cell bodies.

The serotonin-depleting effect of pinealectomy, which could partly account for the physiological effects of the ablation of the pineal gland, would thus rather seem to be dependent upon an indirect effect of pineally elaborated substances on serotoninergic metabolism within the hypothalamus itself. It is interesting that this pineal effect on the diencephalon is a selective one, since the amounts of 5-HT in the rest of the central nervous system do not appear to be affected by the absence of the pineal. More work is required to assess which pineal substance is involved in this regulating mechanism. A tempting hypothesis would be to involve melatonin in this effect (Wurtman and Axelrod 1965, 1966), since this hormone has been shown to be taken up selectively in the basal hypothalamus (Antón-Tay and Wurtman 1969), and, moreover, to be able to increase 5-HT in this region of the brain when administered systemically (Antón-Tay et al. 1968)—the opposite effect to the one we have described after a pinealectomy-induced fall in the melatonin supply to the hypothalamus.

CONCLUSIONS

Although no formal conclusion may be drawn yet about the mode of intervention of the pineal in the processes regulating gonadotropin release, we see that the role of this organ appears more complex than was originally proposed. Various fractions, and not only indoleaminergic compounds, seem to be involved in the modulation exerted by the pineal over neuro-endocrine regulation. The importance of the pineal appears to be critical chiefly in particular hormonal conditions, as for instance around the onset of puberty, in the unstable equilibrium re-set necessary for the wide cyclic variations in gonadotropin levels observed in seasonal breeders (Gogan 1968), or in experimental conditions where normal hormonostatic feedback mechanisms have been disrupted.

At any rate, various coexisting modes of pineal influence on the pituitary have to be considered. Non-indoleaminergic fractions have different effects on gonad stimulation from fractions containing indoleamines, and these effects have their main impact at different levels. F3 seems primarily to interfere with the secretion of FSH, by a direct action on pituitary release mechanisms. F2 appears to have opposite effects at the same level (Moszkowska, Ebels and Scemama 1965). Indole compounds* have no effects *in vitro*; their activity can only be demonstrated *in vivo*, and there they interfere mainly with the regulation of LH release.

It may therefore be hypothesized that F3 affects the pituitary directly, reaching it by the general circulation. More experiments are required, in particular when our extraction procedures have been improved to give an increased yield of purified F3, before we can say that this is a physiological regulating mechanism.

Other fractions, and possibly the indoleaminergic compounds elaborated in the pineal, act directly on the nervous structures in charge of pituitary regulation. Such an action could imply a supply of pineal substances to the hypothalamus by intraventricular transport, since synthetic forms of substances present in the pineal and injected intraventricularly may be actively concentrated in the medio-basal hypothalamus (Antón-Tay and Wurtman 1969). No formal demonstration of such transport has been given yet, so that its physiological significance is still a matter of speculation. Nevertheless, the idea that pineal products may specifically affect the metabolism of central nervous mediators in determined systems of neurons may provide interesting working hypotheses for future research in pineal physiology.

* The possibility that synthetic indole compounds found effective in inhibiting gonado-tropin release may exist in a different biochemical form within the pineal under physiological conditions cannot be completely excluded.

9*

SUMMARY

The involvement of the pineal in the regulation of the release of pituitary gonadotropins appears particularly relevant in certain endocrine states. In the rat, for instance, pinealectomy produces discrete but transient effects on the gonads; however, in certain experimental situations, the effects of the pineal can be made more apparent. This is also the case in other species such as seasonal breeders where the hormonostatic feedback mechanisms are less rigidly regulated.

Such effects of pinealectomy are reviewed and discussed. They raise various problems about the mode of action of the pineal: what are the pineal substances involved, and where is their primary impact on the complex structures which regulate pituitary secretion? Two different types of pineal factors seem to account for the anti-gonadotropic activity of the pineal. Chromatographic fractionation of pineal extracts yields purified fractions of molecular weight about 700 which act directly on the pituitary to antagonize the release of gonadotropic hormones *in vitro*, particularly FSH. Indoleaminergic material, which is not active on the pituitary itself, interferes with the hypothalamic regulation of LH secretion.

The hypothalamic mediation observed in the latter case, as well as data stressing the importance of endogenous serotonin in the control of LH release, led us to study the effects of pinealectomy on serotonin in the hypothalamus. Pinealectomy strikingly reduced serotonin levels in the hypothalamus in immature castrated female rats but not in other central structures. The possible ways in which the pineal influences pituitary functions are discussed in the light of these results and of data from other authors showing that a pineal indoleamine, melatonin, is able to increase hypothalamic serotonin.

REFERENCES

ANTÓN-TAY, F., CHOU, L., ANTON, S. and WURTMAN, R. J. (1968) *Science* **162**, 277.
ANTÓN-TAY, F. and WURTMAN, R. J. (1969) *Nature, Lond.* **221**, 474.
BARRACLOUGH, C. E. and HALLER, E. W. (1970) *Endocrinology* **86**, 542.
BOGDANSKI, D. S., PLETSCHER, A., BRODIE, B. B. and UDENFRIEND, S. J. (1956) *J. Pharmac. exp. Ther.* **117**, 82.
CORBIN, A. L. and SCHOTTELIUS, A. (1961) *Am. J. Physiol.* **201**, 1176.
CZYBA, J. C., GIROD, M. and DURAND, N. (1964) *C.r. Séanc. Soc. Biol.* **158**, 744.
EBELS, I. (1967) *Biol. Med., Paris* **56**, 305.
EBELS, I., MOSZKOWSKA, A. and SCEMAMA, A. (1965). *C.r. hebd. Séanc. Acad. Sci., Paris, Sér. D* **260**, 5126.
EBELS, I., MOSZKOWSKA, A. and SCEMAMA, A. (1970) *J. Neuro-visc. Rel.* **32**, 1–10.
FRASCHINI, F., MESS, B. and MARTINI, L. (1968) *Endocrinology* **82**, 914.

GIROD, C., DURAND, N. and CZYBA, J. C. (1967) *C.r. Séanc. Soc. Biol.* **161,** 1575.

GOGAN, F. (1968) *Gen. comp. Endocr.* **11,** 316.

HAMON, M., JAVOY, F., KORDON, C. and GLOWINSKI, J. (1970) *Life Sci.* **9,** 167.

HOFFMAN, R. A. and REITER, R. J. (1965) *Science* **148,** 1609.

HOFFMANN, J., KORDON, C. and BENOIT, J. (1968) *Gen. comp. Endocr.* **10,** 109.

JAVOY, F., JEANNE-ROSE, M., SCEMAMA, A., KORDON, C. and MOSZKOWSKA, A. (1970) *Life Sci.* in press.

KAPPERS, J. A. (1969) *J. Neuro-visc. Rel.* suppl. 9, 140.

KITAY, J. I. and ALTSCHULE, M. D. (1954) *The Pineal Gland: A Review of the Physiologic Literature.* Cambridge, Mass.: Harvard University Press.

KORDON, C. (1969) *Neuroendocrinology* **4,** 129.

KORDON, C. and HOFFMANN, J. (1967) *C.r. Séanc. Soc. Biol.* **161,** 1262.

KORDON, C., JAVOY, F., VASSENT, G. and GLOWINSKI, J. (1968) *Eur. J. Pharmac.* **4,** 169.

KORDON, C. and MOSZKOWSKA, A. (1967) In *Neurosecretion,* p. 140, ed. Stutinsky, F. Berlin: Springer.

KORDON, C. and VASSENT, G. (1968) *C.r. hebd. Séanc. Acad. Sci., Paris, Sér. D* **266,** 2473.

LICHTENSTEIGER, W. and LANGEMANN, H. (1966) *J. Pharmac. exp. Ther.* **151,** 400.

LOMBARD-DES-GOUTTES, M. N. (1967) *C.r. hebd. Séanc. Acad. Sci., Paris, Sér. D* **264,** 2141.

LOMBARD-DES-GOUTTES, M. N. (1970) Thèse de Sciences, Université de Paris.

MESS, B., FRASCHINI, F., PIVA, F. and MARTINI, L. (1966) In *Hormonal Steroids,* p. 361, ed. Romanoff, E. B. and Martini, L. Excerpta Medica International Congress Series no. 111. (Abstracts.) Amsterdam: Excerpta Medica Foundation.

MOSZKOWSKA, A. (1951) *C.r. Séanc. Soc. Biol.* **145,** 843.

MOSZKOWSKA, A. (1955) *Revue Suisse Zool.* **62,** 198.

MOSZKOWSKA, A. (1965a) *Revue Suisse Zool.* **72,** 145.

MOSZKOWSKA, A. (1965b) In *Structure and Function of the Epiphysis Cerebri (Progress in Brain Research* vol. 10), pp. 564–575, ed. Kappers, J. A. and Schadé, J. P. Amsterdam: Elsevier.

MOSZKOWSKA, A. (1967a) *Biol. Med., Paris* **56,** 403.

MOSZKOWSKA, A. (1967b) *Rev. Eur. Endocr.* **4,** 351.

MOSZKOWSKA, A. (1970) In *Colloque International sur la Photorégulation de la Reproduction chez les Oiseaux et les Mammifères,* p. 569. Publication no. 172. Paris: Centre National de la Recherche Scientifique.

MOSZKOWSKA, A. and EBELS, I. (1970) *J. Neuro-visc. Rel.* **31,** suppl. 1, 83.

MOSZKOWSKA, A., EBELS, I. and SCEMAMA, A. (1965) *C.r. Séanc. Soc. Biol.* **159,** 2298.

MOSZKOWSKA, A. and SCEMAMA, A. (1968a) *C.r. Séanc. Soc. Biol.* **162,** 636.

MOSZKOWSKA, A. and SCEMAMA, A. (1968b) *Archs Anat. Histol. Embryol.* **51,** 475.

MOTTA, M., FRASCHINI, F. and MARTINI, L. (1967) *Proc. Soc. exp. Biol. Med.* **126,** 431.

O'STEEN, W. K. (1964) *Endocrinology* **77,** 937.

PSYCHOYOS, A. (1966) *C.r. hebd. Séanc. Acad. Sci., Paris, Sér. D* **263,** 986.

PUJOL, J. F., BOBILLIER, P., BUGUET, A., JONES, B. and JOUVET, M. (1969) *C.r. hebd. Séanc. Acad. Sci., Paris, Sér. D* **268,** 100.

REITER, R. J. and FRASCHINI, F. (1969) *Neuroendocrinology* **5,** 219.

REITER, R. J., SORRENTINO, Y. C., HOFFMANN, J. C. and RUBIN, P. M. (1968) *Neuroendocrinology* **3,** 246.

STEELMAN, S. L. and POHLEY, F. M. (1953) *Endocrinology* **53,** 604.

THIÉBLOT, L., SIMONNET, H., BATAILLE, L. and MELIK, T. (1954) *J. Physiol., Paris* **46,** 539.

WIENER, H. (1968) *N.Y. St. J. Med.* **68,** 1019.

WURTMAN, R. J. and AXELROD, J. (1965) In *Structure and Function of the Epiphysis Cerebri (Progress in Brain Research* vol. 10), pp. 520–528, ed. Kappers, J. A. and Schadé, J. P. Amsterdam: Elsevier.

WURTMAN, R. J. and AXELROD, J. (1966) *Probl. actuels Endocr. Nutr.* **10,** 189.

WURTMAN, R. J., AXELROD, J. and CHU, E. W. (1963) *Science* **141,** 277.

DISCUSSION

Wurtman: When one talks about serotonin or noradrenaline or dopamine in the hypothalamus, one is really talking about two separate anatomical loci. Serotonin can be in the hypothalamus because it is in the nerve endings of neurons that ascend from the mesencephalon or because it is in cell bodies and perhaps nerve endings of tracts which are entirely within the hypothalamus. We have found quite large amounts of serotonin in the median eminence (Piezzi, Larin and Wurtman 1970), which confirms what you have found about synthesis of serotonin in the median eminence. The serotonin in the median eminence most likely derives from small serotoninergic tracts of cell bodies that are themselves within the hypothalamus. So if melatonin has an effect on hypothalamic serotonin it could either come about, as you have suggested, because melatonin is acting on neurons whose cell bodies are down in the raphe nucleus, or because melatonin is acting on neurons which are entirely contained within the hypothalamus. I suspect it's doing both, and in fact Dr Antón-Tay's data on the time course of the effect of melatonin on brain serotonin showed clearly that the changes in the hypothalamus differ from both the cortical changes (which represent, I think, serotonin in nerve endings) and the changes in the mesencephalon (which represent serotonin in cell bodies). This suggests that both kinds of structures store serotonin within the hypothalamus.

Owman: There are certainly possibilities that these effects can be brought about both on cell bodies and on terminals located in the hypothalamus. Previous histochemical mappings of serotoninergic and other aminergic neurons in the brain are not complete, in the sense that several of the systems contain too low amounts of the amine to be visible under normal conditions. We have made a number of lesions in the hypothalamus and have apparently transected hitherto unknown aminergic tracts, because under conditions when the tract is transected and the transmitter piles up proximally, with the fluorescence technique you can reveal previously invisible aminergic cell bodies located in, for example, the posterior hypothalamic nucleus (A. Björklund, B. Falck, Ch. Owman and K. A. West, to be published).

Kordon: It would be very useful if people who have made hypothalamic lesions and have found either pharmacological or neuroendocrine effects could compare their results.

Martini: I was impressed by the studies in which you showed that pinealectomy induces an increase of serotonin in the median eminence region of the hypothalamus. Would it be possible to see whether pinealectomy also modifies stores of serotonin in the mesencephalon, which is the region in which the cell bodies of the ascending serotoninergic pathways are located?

Kordon: This was the reason why we assayed the serotonin content of other brain structures as well. However, under our experimental conditions (21 days after precocious pinealectomy), we found no difference between controls and operated animals elsewhere than in the hypothalamus. The serotonin content of the midbrain should perhaps be investigated at shorter intervals after pinealectomy.

Kappers: What is the chemical nature of the F3 fraction? Could it possibly be a polypeptide?

Kordon: The only available evidence is that the molecular weight of the fraction is under 700 and that it does not migrate as melatonin or 5-methoxytryptophol do (it migrates rather like dopamine). We do not know yet whether or not it is a polypeptide.

Wurtman: Dr Lerner has been looking at other compounds in the pineal. Are there any other families of compounds that might be reasonable candidates for Dr Kappers' compound?

Lerner: We have never looked at peptides; only at relatively small molecules.

Martini: The evidence that dopamine might be the releaser of the LH-releasing factor from the hypothalamic neurons which produce it is based on Dr Moszkowska's and Dr Kordon's findings as well as on the *in vitro* evidence by H. P. G. Schneider and S. M. McCann (1969). R. Fiorindo and I have incubated rat median eminence tissue, anterior pituitary tissue and dopamine in a system similar to that used by Schneider and McCann. As an index of the secretion of the LH-releasing factor we measured LH in the medium after a few hours of incubation. We never found that dopamine really releases LH-releasing factor in this system. Consequently we decided to study whether other CNS mediators might be involved. Acetylcholine proved to be an extremely efficient releaser of LH-releasing factor in the media in which median eminence tissue was incubated together with the anterior pituitary. We did not get any release of LH by incubating acetylcholine with anterior pituitary tissue in the absence of the median eminence. We could counteract the effect of acetylcholine added to the combined median eminence–anterior pituitary system by adding atropine and potentiate it by adding inhibitors of acetylcholinesterases.

Kordon: Your point about a possible cholinergic involvement in the regulation of LH release is certainly very important; it is further substantiated by recent data from Swedish authors (B. Meyerson, personal communication) which suggest a role of median eminence acetylcholine in gonadotropin control. But I think the effects of receptor-blocking drugs are not always conclusive in this respect, because we have no indication that the neurovascular junctions within the median eminence really respond to neurotransmitters in the same way that true synapses do.

REFERENCES

PIEZZI, R. S., LARIN, F. and WURTMAN, R. J. (1970) *Endocrinology* **86,** 1460–1462.
SCHNEIDER, H. P. G. and McCANN, S. M. (1969) *Endocrinology* **85,** 121–132.

MECHANISMS OF INHIBITORY ACTION OF PINEAL PRINCIPLES ON GONADOTROPIN SECRETION

F. Fraschini, R. Collu* and L. Martini

Department of Pharmacology, University of Milan, Italy

Many publications have recently demonstrated that the pineal gland exerts an inhibitory effect on the reproductive system (Wurtman 1967; Wurtman, Axelrod and Kelly 1968; Mess 1968; Fraschini 1969; Reiter and Fraschini 1969; Fraschini and Martini 1970). This inhibition seems to be exerted through a number of substances synthesized by the gland, namely melatonin (5-methoxy-N-acetyltryptamine), 5-methoxytryptophol, 5-hydroxytryptophol and serotonin (5-hydroxytryptamine) (Wurtman, Axelrod and Kelly 1968; Fraschini and Martini 1970).

The initial purpose of our research was to study whether this inhibitory activity was due to suppression of pituitary gonadotropin secretion. We also wanted to find out whether this inhibitory action was exerted directly on the pituitary gland, or through the nervous structures that regulate pituitary functions. We have also tried to collect data supporting the hypothesis that the normal route taken by endogenous pineal substances is through the cerebrospinal fluid (CSF). To explore these points we have implanted minute amounts of pineal indoles in the central nervous system and measured the resulting gonadotropin levels in the pituitary and in the peripheral blood. We have also injected the same substances into the CSF, by way of an intraventricular cannula. We have finally studied the effects of giving pineal indoles on the time of appearance of puberty and on ovulation in mature rats, events which both depend on pituitary gonadotropins (Ramirez and Sawyer 1965, 1966; Martini *et al.* 1968; Monroe *et al.* 1969).

BRAIN IMPLANTS OF PINEAL INDOLES

This method was chosen for two main reasons. First, to explore whether pineal principles inhibit gonadotropins by acting on the pituitary gland, or whether they need the mediation of nervous structures controlling the secretion of pituitary gonadotropins. Secondly, we wanted to overcome the difficulties which arise from using indole compounds which do not

* Fellow of the Medical Research Council of Canada.

readily cross the blood–brain barrier when injected peripherally (Wurtman, Axelrod and Kelly 1968).

Median eminence implants

Figure 1 summarizes the effects of median eminence implants of indoles and methoxyindoles on pituitary follicle stimulating hormone (FSH) stores. Implants have been made in adult male rats of the Sprague-Dawley strain three weeks after castration and have been left *in situ* for 5 days.

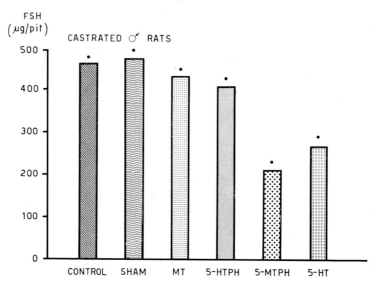

Fig. 1. Effect of implants of indole and methoxyindole derivatives in the median eminence on pituitary FSH content of castrated male rats. Abbreviations: MT, melatonin, 5-HTPH, 5-hydroxytryptophol; 5-MTPH, 5-methoxytryptophol; 5-HT, 5-hydroxytryptamine (serotonin). Each column represents the mean (with the standard error) of three assays performed on three different pools of pituitary glands (nine or ten pituitaries per pool). Results are expressed as FSH content per pituitary since there were no significant variations in pituitary weights in the different groups of animals. (From Fraschini 1969.)

5-Methoxytryptophol and serotonin significantly reduce pituitary FSH stores as measured by bioassay (Steelman and Pohley 1953), whereas melatonin and 5-hydroxytryptophol have no action whatsoever. 5-Methoxytryptophol implanted directly into the pituitary gland has no effect on pituitary FSH stores, whereas serotonin even seems to increase them (Fig. 2). These results apparently indicate that two pineal principles, 5-methoxytryptophol and serotonin, may control FSH secretion, probably by activating special receptors localized in the median eminence.

Figure 3 shows the luteinizing hormone (LH) levels measured by bio-assay (Parlow 1961) after implanting pineal indoles in the median eminence of castrated male rats. As in the previous experiment, the implants have been left *in situ* for 5 days. Serotonin and 5-methoxytryptophol do not modify pituitary stores of LH, while melatonin and 5-hydroxytryptophol significantly reduce the pituitary content of this gonadotropin. The

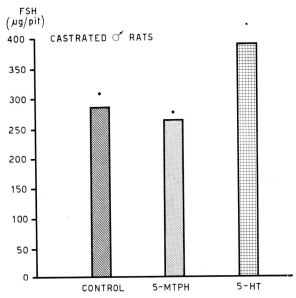

Fig. 2. Effect of implants of methoxytryptophol and 5-hydroxytrypt-amine (serotonin) in the anterior pituitary on pituitary FSH content of castrated male rats. Abbreviations: 5-MTPH, methoxytryptophol; 5-HT, 5-hydroxytryptamine. Each column represents the mean (with the standard error) of three assays performed on three different pools of pituitary glands (nine or ten pituitaries per pool). Results are expressed as FSH content per pituitary since there were no significant variations in pituitary weights in the different groups of animals. (From Fraschini and Martini 1970.)

implantation of melatonin in the cerebral cortex or in the anterior pituitary itself (Fig. 4) has no effect on pituitary stores of LH. The results obtained with melatonin and 5-hydroxytryptophol implants into the median eminence seem to indicate that either the release of LH has been activated, or the synthesis of the hormone has been inhibited. The data summarized in Table I show that plasma levels of LH, as measured according to Parlow's procedure (Parlow 1961), are reduced in animals bearing implants of melatonin in the median eminence. The low pituitary and plasma levels of LH are thus due to an inhibition of the synthesis of LH and not to an activation of its release.

Table I

EFFECT OF IMPLANTS OF MELATONIN INTO THE MEDIAN EMINENCE (ME)
AND THE CEREBRAL CORTEX (CC) ON PLASMA LH LEVELS OF CASTRATED MALE RATS

Groups*	Percentage ovarian ascorbic acid depletion	Plasma LH
ME-sham (7)	21·4±1·7**	present
ME-melatonin (12)	5·1±0·9	absent
CC-melatonin (10)	24·7±2·8	present

* Number of rats in parentheses.
** Values are means ± S.E.

The results obtained with 5-hydroxytryptophol directly implanted into the median eminence are in contrast with the results obtained by Farrell, McIsaac and Powers (1966), which have shown that this compound has no effect on the endocrine system. It must be emphasized, however, that in Farrell's experiments 5-hydroxytryptophol was given systemically; that is, by a route which probably does not allow easy access of the compound to the brain (Wurtman, Axelrod and Kelly 1968). Obviously this factor is not involved when 5-hydroxytryptophol is implanted directly into the central nervous system.

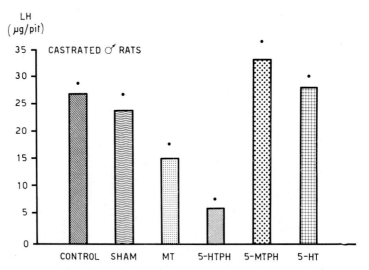

Fig. 3. Effect of implants of indole and methoxyindole derivatives in the median eminence on pituitary LH content of castrated male rats. Abbreviations: MT, melatonin; 5-HTPH, 5-hydroxytryptophol; 5-MTPH, 5-methoxytryptophol; 5-HT, 5-hydroxytryptamine (serotonin). Each column represents the mean (with the standard error) of three assays performed on three different pools of pituitary glands (four or five pituitaries per pool). Results are expressed as LH content per pituitary since there were no significant variations in pituitary weight in the different groups of animals. (From Fraschini, Mess and Martini 1968.)

It is interesting to underline the fact that the two indole derivatives which control LH secretion (melatonin and 5-hydroxytryptophol) seem both to operate at the median eminence level. This suggests that the median eminence has at least two types of receptors sensitive to pineal compounds. One type, which appears to be involved in the control of LH secretion, is sensitive to changing levels of melatonin and 5-hydroxytryptophol. The

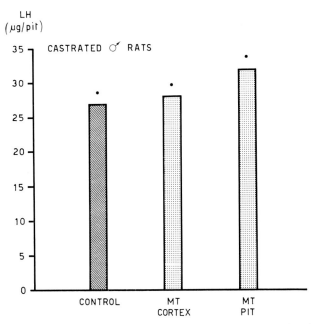

FIG. 4. Effect of implants of melatonin in the cerebral cortex and in the anterior pituitary on pituitary LH content of castrated male rats. Abbreviations: PIT, pituitary; MT, melatonin. Each column represents the mean (with the standard error) of three assays performed on three different pools of pituitary glands (four or five pituitaries per pool). Results are expressed as LH content per pituitary since there were no significant variations in pituitary weights in the different groups of animals. (From Fraschini and Martini 1970.)

other, which apparently regulates FSH secretion, seems to be sensitive to changing levels of 5-methoxytryptophol and serotonin.

From these results one may draw the following conclusions. First of all, the pineal gland appears to control pituitary gonadotropin secretion through at least two different humoral channels. Melatonin and 5-hydroxytryptophol inhibit LH secretion, while serotonin and 5-methoxytryptophol inhibit FSH secretion. Secondly, the effects of pineal indoles and methoxyindoles on gonadotropin secretion seem to be exerted through specific brain receptors rather than directly on pituitary cells. Lastly, since methoxyindoles (i.e. melatonin and 5-methoxytryptophol) can be synthesized only by the pineal gland, at least in mammalian species, they are probably more important than serotonin and 5-hydroxytryptophol as pineal regulators of pituitary activity.

Midbrain implants

The implantation of melatonin in the midbrain of castrated male rats has been shown to induce a significant decrease of pituitary levels of LH (Fig. 5).

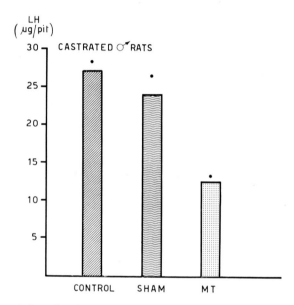

FIG. 5. Effect of implants of melatonin (MT) in the reticular formation of the midbrain. Each column represents the mean (with the standard error) of three assays performed on three different pools of pituitary glands (four or five pituitaries per pool). Results are expressed as LH content per pituitary since there were no significant variations in pituitary weights in the different groups of animals. (From Fraschini *et al.* 1968.)

From these data one can conclude that the receptors sensitive to melatonin are also localized in the midbrain. These observations are particularly interesting since the demonstration by Antón-Tay and Wurtman (1969) that melatonin, administered intravenously or injected in the lateral ventricles of the brain, is selectively concentrated in the midbrain. Its intraperitoneal administration has been shown also to be followed by a significant increase in midbrain serotonin (Antón-Tay *et al.* 1968). Since serotoninergic axons, arising from cell bodies in the midbrain, provide a major input to the hypothalamus via the medial forebrain bundle (Dahlström and Fuxe 1964), it is possible that melatonin exerts part of its action through a serotoninergic pathway.

INTRAVENTRICULAR ADMINISTRATION OF PINEAL INDOLES

Having demonstrated that the pineal principles act through specific receptors localized in the median eminence and in the midbrain, we then tried to establish whether these substances can also be effective after intraventricular administration, which probably reproduces the physiological route of secretion of the pineal principles. Preliminary data from our laboratory show that 90 minutes after intraventricular administration of melatonin to normal adult male rats, pituitary LH stores are significantly decreased while FSH stores are unchanged. By contrast, after intraventricular administration of serotonin, pituitary levels of FSH are significantly decreased. It is remarkable that also in these experiments, melatonin depressed only LH stores, while serotonin was able to depress only FSH stores. These results are similar to those obtained with brain implants.

The results obtained with this method of administration allow us to suggest that the physiological route of secretion and of transport of pineal principles is probably through the CSF. This is also supported by recent anatomical findings (Wurtman, Axelrod and Kelly 1968; Sheridan, Reiter and Jacobs 1969).

EFFECT OF METHOXYINDOLES ON PUBERTY AND OVULATION

Having demonstrated that pineal principles when implanted in the brain or injected into a lateral ventricle inhibit the secretion of pituitary gonadotropins, we decided to study whether these same principles play a physiological role in the onset of puberty and in the control of ovulation.

Puberty

In a first set of experiments we have explored the effect of methoxyindoles on the onset of puberty. The few data available seem to indicate that sexual maturation (a complex process requiring the interaction of gonads, pituitary gland and neuroendocrine mechanisms) may be influenced by the pineal gland. Pinealectomy induces early vaginal opening in the rat (Wurtman 1967), whereas the administration of pineal extracts has the opposite effect (Kitay and Altschule 1954). Wurtman, Axelrod and Chu (1963) and Motta, Fraschini and Martini (1967) have also found that subcutaneous injections of melatonin delay vaginal opening and decrease ovarian weight in rats. Serotonin has also been shown by Botros and

Robson (1960) to induce a delay in sexual maturation of female mice. In addition, drugs which inhibit the catabolism of serotonin by blocking the enzyme monoamine oxidase (e.g. iproniazid), markedly delay sexual maturation (Botros and Robson 1960; Setnikar, Murmann and Magistretti 1960). The puberty-delaying effect of serotonin and of melatonin seems to be exerted through the central nervous system. Corbin and Schottelius (1961) have observed a delay of sexual development of normal female rats after intraventricular injections of serotonin.

In our experiments on sexual maturation, the parameter investigated was the time of vaginal opening. The two methoxyindoles shown by our previous experiments to exert a specific inhibitory effect on pituitary gonadotropin activity (melatonin on LH, and 5-methoxytryptophol on FSH) have been used in the experiments to be described here. Experimental rats were stereotaxically implanted with cannulae, permanently cemented to the skull, which allowed the long-term injection of substances into one of the lateral ventricles of the brain (Hayden, Johnson and Maickel 1966).

Animals were operated on on the 23rd day of age. Starting from the 25th day of age, daily injections were given in the morning through the needle with a Hamilton syringe. Pineal methoxyindoles were dissolved in a few drops of methanol, diluted in saline (0·9 per cent) and then injected in a daily amount of 80 μg/20 μl per rat. Body weight and the perineum were checked every morning, and the injections terminated when canalization of the vagina was established. The animals were autopsied at either 46 (5-methoxytryptophol-treated) or 56 days of age (melatonin-treated) and the weight of endocrine organs was recorded.

Table II shows the effects of intraventricular administration of melatonin and 5-methoxytryptophol on the vaginal opening time (VOT). A highly statistically significant difference exists between the VOT of methoxyindole-treated animals and that of the two groups of controls

TABLE II

EFFECT OF INTRAVENTRICULAR INJECTIONS OF MELATONIN AND
5-METHOXYTRYPTOPHOL ON THE TIME OF VAGINAL OPENING

Groups	Number of rats	Days
Untreated controls	65	$36·0\pm0·44$*
Saline	36	$37·0\pm0·98$
Melatonin 80 μg/rat/day§	15	$40·7\pm1·30$**†
5-Methoxytryptophol 80 μg/rat/day§	14	$40·3\pm1·00$**‡

* Values are means ± S.E.
** $P \leqslant 0·0005$ vs. untreated controls.
† $P \leqslant 0·025$ vs. saline.
‡ $P \leqslant 0·05$ vs. saline.
§ Treatment begun on 25th day of age.

TABLE III

EFFECT OF INTRAVENTRICULAR INJECTIONS OF MELATONIN ON THE WEIGHT OF ENDOCRINE
ORGANS OF FEMALE RATS KILLED ON THE 56th DAY OF AGE

Groups*		Final body weight g	Anterior pituitary mg	Adrenals mg	Ovary mg	Uterus mg
Untreated controls	(30)	173·0 ±3·26**	8·51±0·18	60·80±1·19	70·36±3·61	272±24
Saline	(15)	171·40±7·80	8·14±0·48	61·20±2·73	64·50±5·02	217±20†
Melatonin 80 µg/rat/day§	(15)	175·60±5·70	8·93±0·36	63·70±2·37	61·84±5·54	227±23‡

* Number of rats in parentheses.
** Values are means ± S.E.
† P≤0·025 vs. untreated controls.
‡ P≤0·05 vs. untreated controls.
§ Treatment begun on 25th day of age.

(untreated and treated with the vehicle, 6 per cent methanol in saline). When the weights of the endocrine organs of melatonin-treated rats are compared with those of saline-treated animals, no significant difference can be found (Table III). However, a significant difference exists between the weights of the uteri of the untreated control group and those of the two groups receiving intraventricular injections.

The effect of 5-methoxytryptophol administration on the weights of endocrine organs is shown in Table IV. The ovarian weights of saline and methoxyindole-treated animals are significantly lower than those of controls. No difference exists between the ovarian weights of the two groups of intraventricularly injected animals. Uterine weights of 5-methoxytryptophol-treated and of saline-treated rats are lower than those of untreated controls, but the differences are not significant.

Our results, obtained by administering melatonin directly into a lateral ventricle of the brain, confirm the data on the puberty-retarding activity

TABLE IV

EFFECT OF INTRAVENTRICULAR INJECTIONS OF 5-METHOXYTRYPTOPHOL ON THE WEIGHT OF
ENDOCRINE ORGANS OF FEMALE RATS KILLED ON THE 46th DAY OF AGE

Groups*		Final body weight g	Anterior pituitary mg	Adrenals mg	Ovary mg	Uterus mg
Untreated controls	(35)	169·7±5·1**	8·0 ±0·29	50·50±1·81	61·4 ±3·63	234±70
Saline	(21)	163·3±3·4	7·21±0·26	55·44±2·68	48·43±4·77†	187±17
5-Methoxy-tryptophol 80 µg/day‡	(14)	164·6±3·7	7·44±0·48	55·60±2·40	45·85±3·47†	168±26

* Number of rats in parentheses.
** Values are means ± S.E.
† P≤0·025 vs. untreated controls.
‡ Treatment begun on 25th day of age.

of this compound previously reported by Wurtman, Axelrod and Chu (1963) and by ourselves (Motta, Fraschini and Martini 1967) using, respectively, the intraperitoneal and the subcutaneous routes. Furthermore they show that the other pineal methoxyindole, 5-methoxytryptophol, can also delay the VOT, when given intracerebrally. This compound has been found inactive on this parameter by McIsaac, Taborsky and Farrell (1964) when injected subcutaneously.

The delay in VOT can thus be obtained by the administration of melatonin through either a peripheral (Wurtman, Axelrod and Chu 1963; Motta, Fraschini and Martini 1967) or an intraventricular route, while 5-methoxytryptophol apparently needs to be injected intraventricularly to produce the same effect.

Since sexual maturation has been shown to depend on modifications of pituitary and circulating levels of both LH and FSH (Martini *et al.* 1968), events or substances that modify the secretion of these hormones are likely either to hasten or delay puberty. The fact that melatonin and 5-methoxytryptophol when given independently may retard the appearance of puberty, leads one to suggest that the onset of sexual maturation requires a balanced secretion of the two gonadotropins. When either is suppressed, puberty is delayed.

Our data indicate that a decrease in uterine or ovarian weight may be obtained with both methoxyindoles, but that this is not statistically different from the decrease observed in saline-treated animals. These data do not agree with earlier results showing the existence of a clear-cut difference in uterine and ovarian weight between methoxyindole-treated and saline-treated animals (Wurtman, Axelrod and Chu 1963; McIsaac, Taborsky and Farrell 1964; Motta, Fraschini and Martini 1967). The reason for the reduction of uterine and ovarian weight in animals receiving intraventricular injections of saline solution cannot be explained at the present time.

Ovulation

In the last series of experiments we have tried to obtain a direct proof of the participation of pineal principles in the control of ovulation. Some workers suggested that pinealectomy enhances the ovulatory response following the administration of gonadotropins to immature rats (Dunaway 1966; Dunaway and O'Steen 1966, 1967) and that melatonin and 5-methoxytryptophol have an inhibitory effect on copulation-induced ovulation in rabbits (Farrell, McIsaac and Powers 1966; Farrell, Powers and Otani 1968). Since we had demonstrated that melatonin is able to inhibit the secretion of pituitary LH (which is probably the major ovulatory gonadotropin in the rat), the logical next step was to try to inhibit ovulation by administering this principle. Since the liberation of ovulatory amounts of LH occurs in the rat around the so-called "critical period" of the day of prooestrus (which in our strain of rats and with the lighting conditions of our animal quarters is from 2 p.m. to 4 p.m.) (Everett, Sawyer and Markee 1949; Monroe *et al.* 1969), we decided to administer melatonin around this time. Since the half-life of melatonin is only about 30 minutes (Kopin *et al.* 1961) and the "critical period" lasts about 2 hours, a single injection of melatonin would probably have been insufficient to block ovulation. Melatonin was therefore injected every hour for 4 hours beginning approximately 60 minutes before the "critical period".

Adult female rats were implanted with a permanent cannula in one of the lateral ventricles, enabling us to inject melatonin without anaesthesia and to avoid the well-known blocking effect of anaesthetics on ovulation (Everett, Sawyer and Markee 1949; Everett and Sawyer 1950). After implantation of the cannulae, the oestrous cycles of these rats were carefully checked. Only animals showing at least two regular 4-day cycles were used. The animals were killed the day after the injection of melatonin and ovulation was checked by counting the ova in the Fallopian tubes under a microscope (×40). Results of these experiments are shown in Table V.

Nineteen rats received a total amount of melatonin varying from 100 to 500 μg per rat per day around the "critical period". In seven rats ovulation was completely blocked. In the 12 rats that ovulated, and which constitute 63 per cent of the treated animals, a mean number of 5 ova was found. Eight rats were injected intraventricularly with saline solution. All ovulated and the mean number of ova was 11·7. These results indicate that melatonin completely blocks ovulation in a certain number of rats; in those in which ovulation is not blocked completely the mean number of ova is significantly lower. A group of 11 rats was treated subcutaneously with a total amount of 800 to 1200 μg per rat per day of melatonin around

TABLE V

EFFECT ON OVULATION OF INTRAVENTRICULAR (i.v.t.) AND SUBCUTANEOUS (s.c.) INJECTIONS OF MELATONIN AROUND THE "CRITICAL PERIOD" IN MATURE RATS

Groups	Number of rats treated	Number of rats ovulating	Percentage of rats ovulating	Average number of ova per rat	Number of rats not ovulating
Saline (i.v.t.)	8	8	100	11·7	0
Melatonin (i.v.t.) 100–500 μg/rat	19	12	63	5·0	7
Melatonin (s.c.) 800–1200 μg/rat	11	11	100	10·1	0

the "critical period". All of them ovulated, and the mean number of ova was not significantly different from that of the saline-treated animals.

Figure 6 shows the relationship between the mean number of ova found in the Fallopian tubes and the amounts of melatonin injected intraventricularly. The data in this figure are derived from those summarized in Table V. An inverse relationship seems to exist between the amounts of melatonin and the mean number of ova recovered. It is interesting to

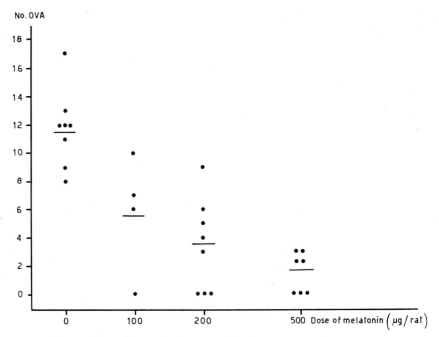

FIG. 6. Effect of increasing amounts of melatonin, injected intraventricularly, on ovulation of female mature rats. Doses of melatonin: 100, 200 and 500 µg/rat. Melatonin was dissolved in few drops of methanol and then diluted in 20 µl of saline (0·9 per cent). Each point represents the number of ova found in the Fallopian tubes of the injected animals. The zero point of the abscissa indicates the number of ova found in the Fallopian tube of saline-treated rats.

notice that in a certain number of rats ovulation was completely blocked even with the lowest amounts of melatonin.

These results thus show that melatonin can exert an inhibitory action on the ovulation of mature rats when injected intraventricularly. It seems essential that the intraventricular injections of melatonin be given around the "critical period". In fact, we have treated a certain number of rats with melatonin some time before the "critical period" without obtaining any blockade of ovulation.

The negative results obtained when melatonin is administered subcutaneously suggest once again that the physiological route of secretion of melatonin is probably through the CSF.

The inhibitory action of melatonin on ovulation can be explained by the fact that this compound blocks the secretion of LH by acting on specific brain receptors, as shown by the data previously discussed. However, another hypothesis cannot be excluded. Recent data have shown in effect that melatonin, when injected intravenously into newborn chickens (Barchas, Da Costa and Spector 1967) or implanted in small amounts into the preoptic area of cats, can produce sleep (Marczynski et al. 1964). In addition, intraventricular and intraperitoneal administrations of melatonin prolong the sleeping effect of pentobarbitone (Barchas 1968; Fioretti et al. 1968). This sedative effect of melatonin has also been documented by electrophysiological techniques, which show the appearance of slow and high voltage waves on the EEG and a decrease of the periods of paradoxical sleep (Hishikawa, Cramer and Kuhlo 1969; Lerner and Case 1960; Marczynski et al. 1964; Supniewski, Misztal and Marczynski 1961). On the basis of these data one might postulate that melatonin, acting as a sedative, might block ovulation through an inhibitory effect exerted on neuronal pathways involved in the control of the ovulatory processes. According to this hypothesis the mode of action of melatonin would not be very different from that of barbiturates and other sedatives (Everett, Sawyer and Markee 1949).

CONCLUSIONS

In conclusion, our data show that pineal principles, when implanted in the central nervous system or injected into the cerebrospinal fluid, have an inhibitory action on the secretion of pituitary gonadotropins. In addition our data suggest that pineal principles, when administered into the cerebrospinal fluid (a route which probably mimics what happens in physiological conditions), may modify major neuroendocrine events such as the onset of puberty and ovulation.

SUMMARY

Recent evidence suggests that indoles and methoxyindoles, synthesized in the pineal gland, exert an inhibitory influence on the secretion of pituitary gonadotropins in the rat. On the basis of previous data it has been postulated that the pineal gland suppresses the release of the two gonadotropins through two different humoral messengers: melatonin specifically inhibits the secretion of LH, while methoxytryptophol specifically reduces the output of FSH. Evidence has also been obtained which indicates that the inhibitory effect of pineal principles is exerted on special receptors sensitive to methoxyindole compounds. These receptors are localized in the hypothalamus and in the midbrain. The suggestion has been put forward that pineal principles may reach these receptors after being secreted into the cerebrospinal fluid. More recent experiments have shown that daily injections of melatonin or 5-methoxytryptophol through a needle permanently implanted in the lateral ventricle of 25-day-old female rats delay vaginal opening. It has also been shown that intraventricular injections of melatonin, made through a permanently implanted needle around the "critical period" of the day of prooestrus, block ovulation in a high percentage of adult female rats.

Acknowledgements

The work described in this paper was supported by Grant No. 67-530 of the Ford Foundation, New York. This support is gratefully acknowledged.

Thanks are due to Mr R. Nebuloni for his skilful technical assistance.

REFERENCES

ANTÓN-TAY, F. and WURTMAN, R. J. (1969) *Nature, Lond.* **221**, 474–475.
ANTÓN-TAY, F., CHOU, C., ANTON, S. and WURTMAN, R. J. (1968) *Science* **162**, 277–278.
BARCHAS, J. (1968) *Proc. west. Pharmac. Soc.* **11**, 22–31.
BARCHAS, J., DA COSTA, F. and SPECTOR, S. (1967) *Nature, Lond.* **214**, 919–920.
BOTROS, M. and ROBSON, J. M. (1960) *J. Endocr.* **20**, x.
CORBIN, A. and SCHOTTELIUS, B. A. (1961) *Am. J. Physiol.* **201**, 1176–1180.
DAHLSTRÖM, A. and FUXE, K. (1964) *Acta physiol. scand.* **62**, suppl. 232, 1.
DUNAWAY, J. F. (1966) *Anat. Rec.* **154**, 340.
DUNAWAY, J. F. and O'STEEN, W. K. (1966) *Tex. Rep. Biol. Med.* **24**, 503–512.
DUNAWAY, J. F. and O'STEEN, W. K. (1967) *Tex. Rep. Biol. Med.* **25**, 525–529.
EVERETT, J. W. and SAWYER, C. H. (1950) *Endocrinology* **47**, 198–218.
EVERETT, J. W., SAWYER, C. H. and MARKEE, J. E. (1949) *Endocrinology* **44**, 234–250.
FARRELL, G., McISAAC, W. M. and POWERS, D. (1966) *Program 48th Meeting of the Endocrine Society*, p. 98. Philadelphia: Lippincott.
FARRELL, G., POWERS, D. and OTANI, T. (1968) *Endocrinology* **83**, 599–603.
FIORETTI, M. C., BARZI, F., BECECCO, D. and FRASCHINI, F. (1968) *Annali Med. Perugia* **59**, 669–673.
FRASCHINI, F. (1969) In *Progress in Endocrinology (Proc. III Int. Congr. Endocrinology)*, pp. 637–644, ed. Gual, C. Excerpta Medica International Congress Series no. 184. Amsterdam: Excerpta Medica Foundation.
FRASCHINI, F. and MARTINI, L. (1970). In *The Hypothalamus*, pp. 529–549, ed. Martini, L., Motta, M. and Fraschini, F. New York and London: Academic Press.
FRASCHINI, F., MESS, B. and MARTINI, L. (1968) *Endocrinology* **82**, 919–924.
FRASCHINI, F., MESS, B., PIVA, F. and MARTINI, L. (1968) *Science* **159**, 1104–1105.
HAYDEN, J. F., JOHNSON, L. R. and MAICKEL, R. P. (1966) *Life Sci.* **5**, 1509–1515.
HISHIKAWA, Y., CRAMER, H. and KUHLO, W. (1969) *Expl Brain Res.* **7**, 84–94.

KITAY, J. I. and ALTSCHULE, M. D. (1954) *The Pineal Gland—A Review of the Physiologic Literature.* Cambridge, Mass.: Harvard University Press.

KOPIN, I. J., PARE, C. M. B., AXELROD, J. and WEISSBACH, H. (1961) *J. biol. Chem.* **236**, 3072–3075.

LERNER, A. B. and CASE, H. D. (1960) *Fedn Proc. Fedn Am. Socs exp. Biol.* **19**, 590–592.

MARCZYNSKI, T. J., YAMAGUCHI, N., LING, G. M. and GRODZINSKA, L. (1964) *Experientia* **20**, 435–437.

MARTINI, L., CARRARO, A., CAVIEZEL, F. and FOCHI, M. (1968) In *Pharmacology of Reproduction*, pp. 13–30, ed. Diczfalusy, E. and Kovarikova, A. Oxford: Pergamon Press.

MCISAAC, W. M., TABORSKY, R. G. and FARRELL, G. (1964) *Science* **145**, 63–64.

MESS, B. (1968) *Int. Rev. Neurobiol.* **2**, 171–198.

MONROE, S. E., REBAR, R. W., GAY, V. L. and MIDGLEY, A. R., JR. (1969) *Endocrinology* **85**, 720–724.

MOTTA, M., FRASCHINI, F. and MARTINI, L. (1967) *Proc. Soc. exp. Biol. Med.* **126**, 431–435.

PARLOW, A. F. (1961) In *Human Pituitary Gonadotropins*, pp. 300–326, ed. Albert, A. Springfield: Thomas.

RAMIREZ, V. D. and SAWYER, C. H. (1965) *Endocrinology* **76**, 1158–1168.

RAMIREZ, V. D. and SAWYER, C. H. (1966) *Endocrinology* **78**, 958–964.

REITER, R. J. and FRASCHINI, F. (1969) *Neuroendocrinology* **5**, 219–255.

SETNIKAR, I., MURMANN, W. and MAGISTRETTI, M. J. (1960) *Endocrinology* **67**, 511–520.

SHERIDAN, M. N., REITER, R. J. and JACOBS, J. J. (1969) *J. Endocr.* **45**, 131–132.

STEELMAN, S. L. and POHLEY, F. M. (1953) *Endocrinology* **53**, 604–616.

SUPNIEWSKI, J., MISZTAL, S. and MARCZYNSKI, T. J. (1961) *Dissnes. Pharm. Warsz.* **13**, 205–217.

WURTMAN, R. J. (1967) In *Neuroendocrinology*, vol. 2, pp. 19–59, ed. Martini, L. and Ganong, W. F. New York: Academic Press.

WURTMAN, R. J., AXELROD, J. and CHU, E. W. (1963) *Science* **141**, 277–278.

WURTMAN, R. J., AXELROD, J. and KELLY, D. E. (1968) *The Pineal.* New York and London: Academic Press.

DISCUSSION

Reiter: We have attempted to inhibit ovulation induced by PMS (pregnant mares' serum) in 28-day-old rats with melatonin given subcutaneously (total of 400 μg). We had great difficulty in inhibiting ovulation when we gave melatonin just prior to endogenous LH release (Reiter, Monaco and Donofrio 1969). We did not do the other experiment of putting melatonin into the cerebrospinal fluid.

Singer: As most studies on the influence of the pineal gland on gonadal function have been confined to females, I should like to describe some studies which Dr Kinson and I have done on male rats which may be of interest. Generally speaking, if pinealectomy was performed when the animals were between 5 and 6 weeks of age (about 100 g) and body and organ weights studied 30 or more days after pinealectomy, we were unable to show any effect on the weight of testis, seminal vesicles or prostate.

On the other hand, if pinealectomy was performed at age 28 days (i.e. one day after descent of the testis in these animals) and the animals studied

two weeks later (at day 42), we found that the combined weight of seminal
vesicles and prostate was significantly raised (Kinson and Singer 1969).
The testes of these animals were examined histologically by Professor
D. Lacy (St Bartholomew's Hospital, London) who found mature sperm
present only in the pinealectomized animals. These observations could be
described as precocious puberty. The animals sacrificed at a later date,
namely 30, 90 and 180 days after pinealectomy, all had mature sperm in
the tubules and it was not possible to distinguish between the pinealectomized and intact controls (unpublished data).

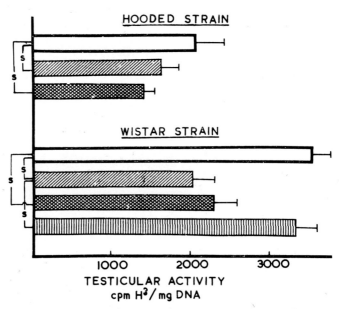

FIG. 1 (Singer). Effect of light restriction on the incorporation of tritiated
thymidine into testicular DNA in Hooded and Wistar rats.

☐   Control L:D 16:8;   ▨   "Dark" L:D 1:23;

▦   Melatonin;   ▥   L:D 1:23 and pinealectomy.

In another study (Kinson and Robinson 1970), Dr Kinson and Miss
Robinson studied the effect of light restriction (1 hour of light per day)
on the incorporation of [^{3}H]thymidine into testicular DNA in two
strains of rat, Hooded and Wistar (Fig. 1). The experiment was started
when the animals were 25 days old and continued for 24 days. Light
restriction inhibited the uptake of thymidine in both strains although the
effect was somewhat greater in Wistar rats. Melatonin, 20 µg/day (lighting
conditions 12:12 L:D, melatonin given 4 hours after light was turned on)

had a similar inhibitory effect. In the Wistars, the effect of pinealectomy on the response to light restriction was also studied. In this case the effect of light restriction was prevented, suggesting that the effect of light on thymidine uptake by the testis is mediated by the pineal gland.

Since moving to Ottawa Dr Kinson has pursued these studies. He has kindly given me two figures summarizing his work. In the first study he followed the weight of the prostate of young rats for 8 weeks, starting at 25 days of age, using two different lighting conditions. When the animals were kept in darkness (2 hours light per day) the weight of the prostate was significantly reduced at the 4th and 7th week compared with animals

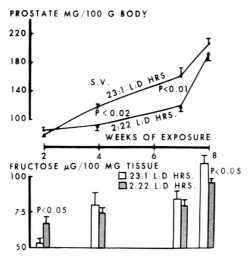

FIG. 2 (Singer). Effect of environmental lighting on the weight and fructose content of the prostate in young rats.

kept in the light for 23 hours per day (Fig. 2). The weight of the seminal vesicles was reduced only at the 4th week. The fructose content of the prostate, which is an indirect index of androgen production, was slightly reduced at 4 and 7 weeks, but significantly reduced at 8 weeks, when the effects on weight were wearing off. The results at 2 weeks were anomalous and cannot be explained.

In his final experiment Dr Kinson studied the effect of daily administration of melatonin on the weight and fructose content of the prostate (Fig. 3). Injections of 50 μg per day were started at 25 days and continued for 8 weeks. Lighting conditions were 12:12 L:D and the injections were given two hours before the lights were turned off. From the 4th to 8th week of treatment the weight of the prostate was significantly reduced in the melatonin-treated animals; by the 8th week the weight of the seminal vesicles was significantly reduced. There was a significant drop in the fructose content of the prostate after 8 weeks.

All these experiments support the view that the pineal gland has an inhibitory effect on both FSH and LH in the male animal, and that melatonin has an inhibitory effect on LH secretion.

Reiter: In my opinion, pinealectomy only advances puberty and does not cause a true gonadal hypertrophy. "Hypertrophy" is the development of an abnormally large organ and I don't think this happens; when you

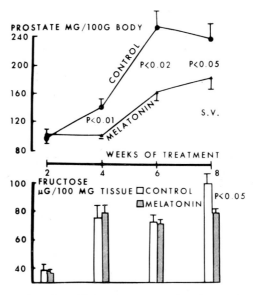

FIG. 3 (Singer). Effect of daily injections of melatonin (50 μg per day) on the weight and fructose content of the prostate in young rats.

remove the pineal gland at a crucial point before puberty you merely get precocious sexual development. Pinealectomy after adulthood rarely causes a significant increase in the weight of the reproductive organs, and if it does, I think it's a premature growth of the reproductive organs to their definitive size; this enlargement is transient since the gonads of the control animals eventually attain the same size. Take as an example the work of Motta, Fraschini and Martini (1967); they obtained a significant hypertrophic response in adult pinealectomized rats which weighed 245 g. They found a modest testicular enlargement and a more pronounced increase in the size of the accessory sex organs within two weeks. I suspect

that they measured the enlargement at just the right interval after pinealectomy and that, if they had waited longer, this difference would have
disappeared.

Axelrod: A word of caution on the administration of melatonin: if one
injects it once a day the effective dose lasts for just a few minutes, and this
might explain the lack of effect after subcutaneous injection, because it is
rapidly metabolized in the liver (Kopin *et al.* 1961). Melatonin given
intraventricularly remains a little longer and this is why you are getting an
effect. I'm sure it's coming out of the brain just as easily as it gets into the
brain. One should inject melatonin in such a way that it is effectively
perfused into the body over the entire 24 hours.

Reiter: We have always felt that that was so. Single daily injections of
melatonin probably have such modest effects because it disappears very
rapidly. This is possibly emphasized by the recent paper of Rust and Meyer
(1970) who implanted pellets of beeswax containing melatonin into
weasels and got very dramatic gonadal atrophy at about 8 weeks. I
presume that under these conditions there was a slow, sustained release of
melatonin. Yet, we have done a similar experiment in rats and observed a
very modest delay in puberty.

Herbert: On the basis of the evidence we have heard here, it is very
difficult to assign a role to the pineal in the timing of puberty in rats,
because the alteration observed after experimental treatment is only two
or three days. To take up the point about administering melatonin: do
we have any idea of the amount of melatonin secreted by the pineal,
perhaps into the cerebrospinal fluid, on which to base our ideas of dosage?

Wurtman: We really have no idea of the amount. The best one can do is
to assume that the enzymes synthesizing melatonin that are rate-limiting
are maximally active, and calculate what the amount synthesized could be.
The important point here, as Dr Antón-Tay mentioned, is that if melatonin
is secreted into the cerebrospinal fluid, and if its uptake into the brain is
what counts, then it is necessary to give at least a hundred times as much of
the compound by systemic routes to get the same effect as produced by
melatonin secreted physiologically. The amounts that are generally given
systemically to experimental animals are of the order of 1 mg/kg. A hun-
dredth part of this brings you down to levels which are compatible with the
amounts the pineal probably can make. I shall refer again to the problem
of input–output relations, which is the big issue in the pineal (see p.
387). It would be very nice if one could provide the physiological input to
the pineal and have a direct chemical measure of the rate of output in response to this input. But one can at least say that the amounts of melatonin
used in the studies described here are not incompatible with the amounts

that the pineal could make, if one assumes that melatonin is normally released into the cerebrospinal fluid.

Martini: Let me comment once again on the question of the half-life of melatonin. If you take a completely different model, namely the effect of oestrogens on the uterus, you may note that oestrogens are necessary for initiating the biochemical processes which lead to an increase of uterine weight as a consequence of new protein synthesis. However, once this process is triggered, oestrogens are no longer needed. There is no evidence against the possibility that melatonin might operate in the same way.

Axelrod: Oestrogen is a hit-and-run drug, whereas melatonin has to be around all the time. You are assuming that melatonin is just like oestrogen, but oestrogen is an exception rather than the rule. Drugs generally have to be present all the time with a very few exceptions, such as oestrogens or dicoumarol. I would assume that melatonin is acting like most other chemicals and has to be present all the time.

REFERENCES

KINSON, G. A. and ROBINSON, S. (1970) *J. Endocr.* **47**, 391.

KINSON, G. A. and SINGER, B. (1969) In *Abstracts of III Int. Congr. Endocrinology*, abst. 448, ed. Gual, C. Excerpta Medica International Congress Series no. 157. Amsterdam: Excerpta Medica Foundation.

KOPIN, I. J., PARE, C. M. B., AXELROD, J. and WEISSBACH, H. (1961) *J. biol. Chem.* **236**, 3072–3075.

MOTTA, M., FRASCHINI, F. and MARTINI, L. (1967) *Proc. Soc. exp. Biol. Med.* **126**, 431.

REITER, R. J., MONACO, L. and DONOFRIO, R. J. (1969) *Am. Zool.* **9**, 1087.

RUST, C. C. and MEYER, R. K. (1970) *Science* **165**, 921–922.

PINEAL PRINCIPLES AND THE CONTROL OF ADRENOCORTICOTROPIN SECRETION

Marcella Motta, O. Schiaffini*, F. Piva† and L. Martini

Department of Pharmacology, University of Milan, Italy

Evidence that the pineal gland exerts a regulatory influence on several endocrine functions is rapidly growing (Wurtman, Axelrod and Kelly 1968; Mess 1968; Reiter and Fraschini 1969; Fraschini and Martini 1970). However, only a few data are available to indicate that the pineal gland and its secretory products (melatonin, 5-methoxytryptophol, 5-hydroxy-tryptophol, etc.) might intervene in the control of the activity of the pituitary–adrenal axis. In addition, the data in this area are conflicting and controversial.

Adrenal ascorbic acid concentrations have been shown to be reduced after pinealectomy (Asagoe and Hamamoto 1959); pinealectomized animals also secrete an increased amount of corticosterone (Kinson and Singer 1967; Kinson, Wahid and Singer 1967; Kinson, Singer and Grant 1968). These results might suggest that the pineal gland normally exerts a tonic inhibitory influence on the secretion of adrenocorticotropin (ACTH). In agreement with this interpretation, Reiter, Hoffman and Hester (1966) have found that the chronic activation of the pineal gland (induced by exposure to short daily photoperiods, or by the removal of the eyes) is followed by a significant regression of adrenal size in the hamster. How-ever, pinealectomy is not regularly followed by adrenal hypertrophy; increase in adrenal weight has been reported to occur after the operation by Wurtman, Altschule and Holmgren (1959) and by Fraschini, Mess and Martini (1968), but not by Roth (1964) or by Kinson, Singer and Grant (1968).

The results obtained after administering purified or synthetic pineal principles are also contradictory. Barchas and co-workers (1969) have reported that in the rat, acute or chronic subcutaneous administration of melatonin does not modify plasma levels of corticosterone and of ACTH, and anterior pituitary stores of ACTH; in addition, a surgical stress is

* Ford Foundation Fellow, on leave of absence from the Department of Neuroendocrin-ology, Institute of Physiology, Medical School, Buenos Aires, Argentina.
† Ford Foundation Fellow.

followed by a comparable increase in plasma corticosterone levels in untreated and in melatonin-treated animals. At variance with these findings, Fraschini, Mess and Martini (1968) have found that intrahypo-thalamic implants of melatonin bring about a significant reduction of adrenal weight in adult castrated male rats. Finally, a report has appeared which suggests that acute administration of melatonin may significantly increase the production of corticosterone in intact rats (Gromova, Kraus and Krecek 1967). This last observation seems to support the finding of Narang, Singh and Turner (1967) that increased adrenal weight follows prolonged treatment with melatonin.

Because of these inconsistencies, we decided to make a comprehensive study of the effects that pineal indoles and methoxyindoles might exert on the pituitary–adrenal axis of the rat. Since previous work in this laboratory had indicated that the endocrine effects of pineal principles are mediated by specific receptors present in the brain (Martini 1969; Fraschini and Martini 1970), in the experiments to be reported here pineal principles were injected directly into the cerebrospinal fluid (CSF) of one of the lateral ventricles, through a chronically implanted cannula. In some experiments, dopamine and noradrenaline were also introduced into the CSF.

METHODS

All experiments were performed in normal adult male rats of the Sprague-Dawley strain, weighing 180–200 g. They were caged in standard conditions, in rooms with controlled temperature and humidity. Lights were on 14 hours per day, from 6.30 a.m. to 8.30 p.m. The rats were fed with a standard pellet diet; water was given *ad libitum*. In all experimental animals a microcannula was introduced into one of the lateral ventricles under pentobarbitone (3 mg/100 g body weight intraperitoneally) anaes-thesia. A Stoelting stereotaxic apparatus was used. In all instances the intracerebral cannulae were placed in position two days before giving the intraventricular injections of pineal principles or of catecholamines; these were administered without anaesthesia. All principles were dissolved in 30 μl of a 0·9 per cent saline solution containing 10 per cent of methanol. Control animals were injected intraventricularly with 30 μl of the saline–methanol mixture. Experiments were designed in a way to permit the sacrifice of all animals at the same time of the day, around 12 noon, in order to avoid the interference of the diurnal corticosterone cycle (Critch-low *et al.* 1963; Mangili, Motta and Martini 1966). Plasma levels of corticosterone were measured by the procedure of Guillemin and co-workers (1959), as modified by Fraschini and co-workers (1964).

RESULTS AND DISCUSSION

Figure 1 shows that 60 minutes after the intraventricular injection of a large dose of melatonin (165 μg/rat) the concentrations of plasma corticosterone in rats in resting conditions are significantly lower than those found in the control group receiving only the vehicle intraventricularly (group indicated as Saline). The effect of melatonin disappears 120 minutes after treatment, and is not apparent 30 minutes after the intraventricular injection. The results of this preliminary experiment have been interpreted as indicating that intraventricular injections of melatonin may inhibit the pituitary–adrenal axis. We also concluded that the effect of melatonin

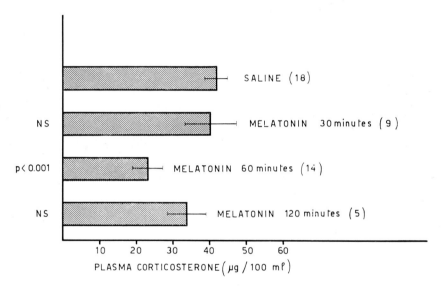

FIG. 1. Effect of intraventricular injections of melatonin (165 μg/rat) on plasma corticosterone concentrations of normal male rats.

needs some time to be established, and that it is not of long duration. This pilot experiment suggested that, in all subsequent trials, a time interval of one hour should be adopted between intraventricular injections and sacrifice of the animals.

Figure 2 confirms, on a larger number of animals, the finding that intraventricular injections of 165 μg per rat of melatonin are followed, in one hour, by a significant drop of plasma corticosterone levels in non-stressed rats. It also shows that one does not need to give these large amounts of the compound in order to block the pituitary–adrenal axis. A very significant reduction of plasma corticosterone concentrations can be observed, in animals in resting conditions, one hour after the intraventricular administration of 5 μg per rat of melatonin. Melatonin is not the only compound of pineal origin capable of inhibiting the pituitary–adrenal axis of the rat; both 5-hydroxytryptophol and 5-methoxytryptophol are able to mimic the effect of melatonin when given intraventricularly in sufficient amounts.

Noradrenaline and dopamine are also able to reduce plasma levels of corticosterone in non-stressed rats, when injected intraventricularly at the dose of 5 μg per rat (Fig. 3). These findings seem to support the hypothesis that a central adrenergic system might tonically inhibit the secretion of ACTH*. The finding that dopamine is able to inhibit the pituitary–

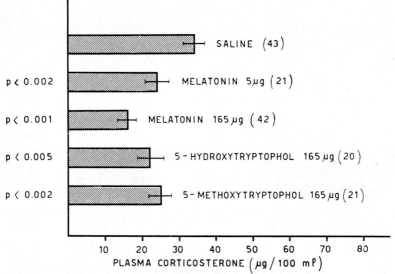

FIG. 2. Effect of intraventricular injections of pineal indoles and methoxy-indoles on plasma corticosterone concentrations of normal male rats.

* The idea that inhibitory adrenergic pathways might be involved in the control of ACTH secretion was proposed by Giuliani, Motta and Martini (1966). They had observed that treatment with the catecholamine depletor, reserpine, could antagonize the inhibitory activity exerted by high doses of dexamethasone on the pituitary–adrenal axis. This hypothesis has been substantiated by recent evidence. Van Loon and co-workers (1969) and Van Loon and Ganong (1969) have reported that intravenous injections of *l*-dopa, a precursor of dopamine and of noradrenaline, inhibit stress-induced ACTH secretion in the dog. The inhibitory activity of the compound is increased by pretreatment with monoamine oxidase inhibitors. Bhattacharya and Marks (1969) have shown in the rat that the administration of an inhibitor of monoamine oxidase, pargyline, and the centrally-active adrenergic drug, amphetamine, lowers resting levels of corticoid secretion and reduces stress-induced activation of the pituitary–adrenal axis. Similar effects of amphetamine in monkeys (Harwood and Bigelow 1960) and in dogs (Lorenzen and Ganong 1967) have also been reported. Carr and Moore (1968) and Krieger and Rizzo (1969) have observed that treatment with a specific inhibitor of catecholamine biosynthesis (α-methyl-tyrosine) increases plasma levels of adrenal corticoids in the rat and cat respectively. The increase in corticoid output appears to be correlated with the degree of depletion of brain catecholamines; repletion of hypothalamic catecholamines with *l*-dopa brings adrenal activity back to normal (Scapagnini et al. 1971).

adrenal axis seems particularly relevant, because of the observation reported by Steiner, Pieri and Kaufmann (1968) that this compound strongly reduces the electrical activity of the hypothalamic neurons which are also inhibited by adrenal corticoids. However, it must be recalled that the data reported here, obtained by injecting small amounts of dopamine intraventricularly, are at variance with those of King and Thomas (1968) and King (1969), who have found that rather large doses of dopamine given intraperitoneally or subcutaneously are able to reduce adrenal ascorbic acid and to increase plasma corticosterone in the rat. The discrepancy

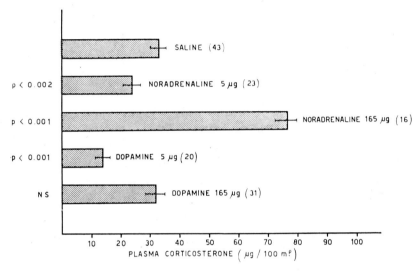

FIG. 3. Effect of intraventricular injections of noradrenaline and dopamine on plasma corticosterone concentrations of normal male rats.

between the two groups of results is probably due to the fact that systemic injections of dopamine exert peripheral effects, which can account for a non-specific activation of the pituitary–adrenal axis. Intracerebral treatment with dopamine has no systemic effect.

Figure 3 also indicates that the effects of the two catecholamines on the pituitary–adrenal axis are quite different when the two compounds are injected intraventricularly in higher doses. Injection of 165 μg per rat of noradrenaline gives a significant stimulation of corticosterone secretion; the same amount of dopamine apparently has no effect. A possible inter-pretation of the activating effect of large amounts of noradrenaline might be that this catecholamine preferentially accumulates in the nerve endings of the nervous pathways inhibiting ACTH secretion. When these nerve

TABLE I

EXPERIMENTAL SCHEME FOR STUDY OF EFFECT OF INHIBITORS OF ACTH SECRETION IN
STRESSED ANIMALS

Time (minutes)	0	20	30	60
Treatment	Melatonin or dopamine	Pentobarbitone	Histamine	Decapitation and blood collection for measurement of plasma corticosterone
Doses	5 µg and 165 µg/rat	3 mg/100 g body weight	400 µg/100 g body weight	
Route of administration	Intraventricular	Intraperitoneal	Intravenous	

terminals are saturated, noradrenaline might also be concentrated in adrenergic neurons which activate the secretion of ACTH. However, the possibility that these very high doses of noradrenaline might also have systemic peripheral effects cannot be disregarded.

After showing that both pineal principles and catecholamines may reduce plasma concentrations of corticosterone of animals in resting conditions, we thought it of interest to study whether the same compounds might inhibit ACTH secretion in rats exposed to an effective stressing procedure. In order to submit all animals to a stress of comparable intensity, we injected a standard dose of histamine intravenously (400 µg/100 g body weight) (Mangili et al. 1965). The scheme followed in these experiments is outlined in Table I. Animals were first injected, through the brain cannula, with either melatonin or dopamine. Controls received the saline–methanol mixture intraventricularly. Thirty minutes after the intraventricular administrations, histamine was injected under pentobarbitone anaesthesia. Animals were killed as usual one hour after the intracerebral injections (30 minutes after exposure to histamine stress).

Table II shows clearly that animals treated with histamine and receiving only the vehicle intraventricularly (group indicated as Histamine) have plasma levels of corticosterone which are significantly higher than those found in the group of controls receiving saline solution intravenously and

TABLE II

EFFECT OF INTRAVENTRICULAR INJECTION OF MELATONIN ON HISTAMINE-INDUCED ACTIVATION
OF THE PITUITARY–ADRENAL AXIS OF MALE RATS

Groups*		Plasma corticosterone (µg/100 ml)	Significance (P)
Saline (48)		$27 \cdot 67 \pm 2 \cdot 01$†	
Histamine 400 µg/100 g body weight (37)		$46 \cdot 25 \pm 2 \cdot 02$	$< 0 \cdot 001$ vs. saline
Histamine + melatonin 5 µg	(12)	$37 \cdot 67 \pm 4 \cdot 96$	$< 0 \cdot 05$ vs. histamine
Histamine + melatonin 165 µg	(19)	$40 \cdot 38 \pm 2 \cdot 67$	$< 0 \cdot 05$ vs. histamine

* Number of rats in parentheses.   † Values are means ± S.E.

TABLE III

EFFECT OF INTRAVENTRICULAR INJECTION OF DOPAMINE ON HISTAMINE-INDUCED ACTIVATION
OF THE PITUITARY–ADRENAL AXIS OF MALE RATS

Groups*		Plasma corticosterone (μg/100 ml)	Significance (P)
Saline	(48)	27·67 ± 2·01†	
Histamine 400 μg/100 g body weight	(37)	46·25 ± 2·02	< 0·001 vs. saline
Histamine + dopamine 5 μg	(9)	33·69 ± 3·99	< 0·005 vs. histamine
Histamine + dopamine 165 μg	(12)	37·43 ± 1·95	< 0·02 vs. histamine

* Number of rats in parentheses.   † Values are means ± S.E.

the saline–methanol mixture intraventricularly (group indicated as Saline). In animals in which histamine has been injected after the intracerebral treatment with either the low or the high dose of melatonin, plasma corticosterone concentrations do not reach the high values found in animals given the stressing drug without pineal principles. A certain degree of activation of the pituitary–adrenal axis is still present; however, the difference between the corticosterone titres of the animals receiving histamine after melatonin and those receiving histamine without melatonin protection is statistically significant.

The results obtained in similar experiments in which dopamine was given intraventricularly are summarized in Table III. The data indicate that intraventricular injections of this catecholamine are also able partially to inhibit the effect of histamine on the pituitary–adrenal axis. It is interesting to recall in this connexion that some unpublished data from Ganong's laboratory prove that intraventricular injections of dopamine are able to inhibit the ACTH-activating effect of a surgical stress in the dog (Van Loon, personal communication) and the afternoon rise of plasma corticosterone levels in the rat (Scapagnini, personal communication).

The data obtained in the stressed animals thus confirm the findings in animals in resting conditions. They indicate not only that melatonin and dopamine may intervene in an inhibitory fashion in the mechanisms controlling ACTH secretion, but also that these agents must be considered strong inhibitors of the pituitary–adrenal axis.

Because of the strong blocking action exerted by catecholamines on the pituitary–adrenal axis, the question was asked whether the similar effect exerted by melatonin might be mediated through an activation of the postulated adrenergic ACTH-inhibiting pathway. To answer this question, it was decided to repeat the histamine–melatonin and the histamine–dopamine experiments in animals in which cerebral stores of catecholamines had been depleted by the previous administration of reserpine. The drug (Serpasil, CIBA) was given intraperitoneally, in a

TABLE IV

EFFECT OF INTRAVENTRICULAR INJECTION OF MELATONIN ON HISTAMINE-INDUCED ACTIVATION
OF THE PITUITARY–ADRENAL AXIS OF MALE RATS PRETREATED WITH RESERPINE (200 μg/100g
BODY WEIGHT)

Groups*		Plasma corticosterone (μg/100 ml)	Significance (P)
Saline	(18)	22·08±2·66**	
Histamine 400 μg/100 g body weight	(23)	42·28±2·68	<0·001 vs. saline
Histamine + melatonin 5 μg	(7)	60·94±4·41	<0·001 vs. histamine
Histamine + melatonin 165 μg	(14)	38·85±4·10	NS vs. histamine

* Number of rats in parentheses.   ** Values are means ± s.e.

dose of 200 μg/100 g body weight, 24 hours before submitting the animals
to the experimental procedure summarized in Table I. This dose of
reserpine has been shown to induce a very significant and long-lasting (up
to 7 days) decrease in brain catecholamines (Carr and Moore 1968).

As shown in Table IV, histamine is still very effective as a stimulus for
the adrenal gland in animals pretreated with reserpine. This result agrees
with the findings by Van Peenen and Way (1957) and by Carr and Moore
(1968). If one compares the percentage increase in plasma corticosterone
induced by histamine in animals not receiving reserpine with that in
animals pretreated with reserpine, it appears that histamine is more effective in rats in which cerebral stores of catecholamines have been depleted.
This interpretation is supported by the observation made by Hall and
Marks (1968) that carbachol injected intraventricularly is a more powerful
stimulator of ACTH secretion in rats pretreated with reserpine than in
untreated animals. These findings again support the view that ACTH
secretion is normally kept under an inhibitory tone by a central adrenergic
mechanism. When this inhibition is eliminated, stressing procedures are
no longer counterbalanced and may become more effective.

In animals pretreated with reserpine, intraventricular injections of
melatonin do not reduce the stressing effect of histamine (Table IV). This
is the opposite of what had been previously observed in animals not
pretreated with reserpine.

TABLE V

EFFECT OF INTRAVENTRICULAR INJECTION OF DOPAMINE ON HISTAMINE-INDUCED ACTIVATION
OF THE PITUITARY–ADRENAL AXIS OF MALE RATS PRETREATED WITH RESERPINE (200 μg/100 g
BODY WEIGHT)

Groups*		Plasma corticosterone (μg/100 ml)	Significance (P)
Saline	(18)	22·08±2·66†	
Histamine 400 μg/100 g body weight	(23)	42·28±2·68	<0·001 vs. saline
Histamine + dopamine 5 μg	(15)	33·73±3·07	<0·02 vs. histamine
Histamine + dopamine 165 μg	(16)	38·47±3·90	NS vs. histamine

* Number of rats in parentheses.   † Values are means ± s.e.

In a similar experiment (Table V) in which dopamine was administered intraventricularly and histamine was given intravenously to animals pre-treated with reserpine, it was found that the catecholamine is still able to antagonize the stimulatory effect of histamine on the pituitary–adrenal axis. A similar finding has recently been reported by Hall and Marks (1968). These observations may be taken as further evidence of the existence of an adrenergic system inhibiting ACTH secretion*.

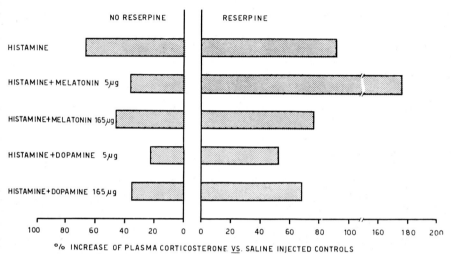

FIG. 4. Effect of intraventricular injections of melatonin and dopamine on histamine-induced activation of the pituitary–adrenal axis of normal male rats treated or not treated with reserpine. Values of plasma cortico-sterone levels are expressed as the percentage increase compared to saline-injected control rats.

* Two adrenergic systems are possible candidates for such a role: (1) the intrahypothalamic dopaminergic system of the tubero-infundibular region; and (2) the noradrenergic system which has its nerve terminals in the hypothalamus and whose cell bodies are mainly localized in the midbrain (Fuxe and Hökfelt 1969). In favour of the tubero-infundibular dopaminergic system is the finding reported here that dopamine inhibits ACTH secretion in reserpinized animals also; it is known that reserpine does not influence the uptake of dopamine in this region (Fuxe, Hamberger and Malmfors 1966, 1967). Data indicating that adrenalectomy is followed by an increase of amine storage (Akmayev and Donath 1966), and that treatment with high doses of corticoids induces a depletion of catecholamines (Akmayev and Donath 1966) and an increased activity (Fuxe and Hökfelt 1969) in these dopaminergic neurons, also suggest a role for this intrahypothalamic system. However, the bulk of evidence seems to emphasize the major role of the noradrenergic fibres impinging on the hypothalamus. The terminals of these fibres show an increased rate of amine turnover (Kety et al. 1967; Fuxe and Hökfelt 1967; Corrodi, Fuxe and Hökfelt 1968; Javoy, Glowinski and Kordon 1968; Bliss, Ailion and Zwanziger 1968; Simmonds 1969) and a depletion of amine stores (Maynert and Levi 1964; Bliss, Ailion and Zwanziger 1968) under the influence of different types of stresses or after adrenalectomy. Furthermore complete transection at midbrain level, interrupting the noradrenergic input to the hypothalamus (Fuxe and Hökfelt 1969), induces permanent activation of the pituitary–adrenal axis (Fraschini et al. 1964). Chronic hypersecretion of ACTH is also found in animals submitted to a complete "hypothalamic deafferentation" according to Halasz' technique (Halasz 1969). This operation, which eliminates all inputs to the hypothalamus, also interrupts adrenergic afferents.

Figure 4 summarizes the experiments involving histamine stress (the figure is derived from data presented in Tables II-V). The graphic representation shows clearly (1) that histamine is more effective in reserpinized rats than in untreated animals; (2) that melatonin does suppress the effect of histamine in animals not receiving reserpine, but is completely ineffective after depletion of brain catecholamines; and (3) that dopamine is able to reduce the activating effect of histamine in animals either treated or not treated with reserpine.

CONCLUSIONS

Several conclusions may be drawn from these results. First of all, it appears that both pineal indoles (5-hydroxytryptophol) and pineal methoxyindoles (melatonin, 5-methoxytryptophol) are able to suppress the pituitary–adrenal axis of animals in resting conditions. This finding may be relevant with regard to the diurnal rhythm which is observed in the activity of the pituitary–adrenal axis of the rat. It is known that in this species, plasma concentrations of corticosterone (Critchlow et al. 1963; Mangili, Motta and Martini 1966) and of ACTH (Retiene et al. 1968; Retiene 1970) as well as hypothalamic stores of the corticotropin-releasing factor (David-Nelson and Brodish 1969) are significantly higher in the afternoon than in the morning. One might speculate that the increased function of the hypothalamic–pituitary–adrenal axis observed in the afternoon is due to the reduced production of inhibiting methoxyindoles in the pineal gland, as a consequence of the suppression of hydroxyindole-O-methyltransferase activity during the light period (Wurtman, Axelrod and Kelly 1968).

The fact that melatonin counteracts the effect on ACTH secretion exerted by histamine, which is a potent stressful stimulus, suggests that pineal principles might also intervene in maintaining the homeostasis of the pituitary–adrenal axis when this is disturbed by exogenous influences. In this connexion it would be important to know whether stressful stimulation modifies the biosynthesis and release of pineal indoles and methoxyindoles.

The observation that melatonin loses its ability to interfere with the stimulating effect of histamine on ACTH secretion in rats deprived of brain catecholamines, coupled with the finding that dopamine is an inhibitor of histamine stress both in untreated and in reserpine-treated animals, raises the possibility that the effect of melatonin on the pituitary–adrenal axis might be mediated by the activation of a central adrenergic pathway normally inhibiting ACTH secretion. This aspect might be further clarified by studying whether treatment with melatonin results in changes in the stores or in the turnover rates of brain catecholamines. Alterations in brain serotonin content after treatment with melatonin have been reported (Antón-Tay *et al.* 1968). Finally, one might point out that the demonstration that melatonin influences the pituitary–adrenal axis after having been added to the CSF may be taken as evidence in favour of the possibility that pineal principles are physiologically released into the CSF rather than into the blood (Sheridan, Reiter and Jacobs 1969; Wurtman, Axelrod and Kelly 1968; Wurtman 1970; Fraschini and Martini 1970).

SUMMARY

The possible participation of pineal principles and of catecholamines in the control of the pituitary–adrenal axis has been studied in adult male rats. It has been shown that in non-stressed animals melatonin (5-methoxy-N-acetyltryptamine), 5-methoxytryptophol and 5-hydroxytryptophol significantly decrease plasma corticosterone concentrations after acute injection into the lateral cerebral ventricles. Plasma corticosterone is also reduced in animals in resting conditions after the intraventricular injection of small amounts of dopamine and noradrenaline. Intraventricular injections of melatonin and of dopamine are also able to counteract the increase in plasma corticosterone induced by the intravenous administration of histamine. After treatment with reserpine, melatonin loses its ability to inhibit the stressing effect of histamine, while dopamine is still active. It is concluded that principles synthesized in the pineal gland may block the activity of the pituitary–adrenal axis both in resting conditions and after exposure to stress. Since melatonin is not effective when brain catecholamines have been depleted, it is possible that pineal principles operate by activating an adrenergic pathway inhibiting the pituitary–adrenal axis.

Acknowledgements

The work described in this paper was supported by Grant No. 67–530 of the Ford Foundation, New York. This support is gratefully acknowledged. Thanks are due to Miss Paola Assi and to Mr L. Guadagni for their skilful technical assistance.

REFERENCES

AKMAYEV, I. G. and DONATH, T. (1966) *Z. Zellforsch. mikrosk. Anat.* **74,** 84–91.
ANTÓN-TAY, F., CHOU, C., ANTON, S. and WURTMAN, R. J. (1968) *Science* **162,** 277–278.
ASAGOE, Y. and HAMAMOTO, A. (1959) *Yonago Acta med.* **3,** 192–198.
BARCHAS, J., CONNER, R., LEVINE, S. and VERNIKOS-DANELLIS, J. (1969) *Experientia* **25,** 413–414.
BHATTACHARYA, A. N. and MARKS, B. H. (1969) *Proc. Soc. exp. Biol. Med.* **130,** 1194–1198.

BLISS, E. L., AILION, J. and ZWANZIGER, J. (1968) *J. Pharmac. exp. Ther.* **164,** 122–134.

CARR, L. A. and MOORE, K. E. (1968) *Neuroendocrinology* **3,** 285–302.

CORRODI, H., FUXE, K. and HÖKFELT, T. (1968) *Life Sci.* **7,** 107–112.

CRITCHLOW, V., LIEBELT, R. A., BAR-SELA, M., MOUNTCASTLE, W. and LIPSCOMB, H. S. (1963) *Am. J. Physiol.* **205,** 807–815.

DAVID-NELSON, M. A. and BRODISH, A. (1969) *Endocrinology* **85,** 861–866.

FRASCHINI, F. and MARTINI, L. (1970) In *The Hypothalamus*, pp. 529–549, ed. Martini, L., Motta, M. and Fraschini, F. New York and London: Academic Press.

FRASCHINI, F., MESS, B. and MARTINI, L. (1968) *Endocrinology* **82,** 919–924.

FRASCHINI, F., MANGILI, G., MOTTA, M. and MARTINI, L. (1964) *Endocrinology* **75,** 765–769.

FUXE, K., HAMBERGER, B. and MALMFORS, T. (1966) *J. Pharm. Pharmac.* **18,** 543–544.

FUXE, K., HAMBERGER, B. and MALMFORS, T. (1967) *Eur. J. Pharmac.* **1,** 334–341.

FUXE, K. and HÖKFELT, T. (1967) In *Neurosecretion*, pp. 165–177, ed. Stutinsky, F. Berlin: Springer-Verlag.

FUXE, K. and HÖKFELT, T. (1969) In *Frontiers in Neuroendocrinology*, 1969, pp. 47–96, ed. Ganong, W. F. and Martini, L. London and New York: Oxford University Press.

GIULIANI, G., MOTTA, M. and MARTINI, L. (1966) *Acta endocr., Copenh.* **51,** 203–209.

GROMOVA, E. A., KRAUS, M. and KRECEK, J. (1967) *J. Endocr.* **39,** 345–350.

GUILLEMIN, R., CLAYTON, G. W., LIPSCOMB, H. S. and SMITH, J. D. (1959) *J. Lab. clin. Med.* **53,** 830–832.

HALASZ, B. (1969) In *Frontiers in Neuroendocrinology*, 1969, pp. 307–342, ed. Ganong, W. L. and Martini, L. London and New York: Oxford University Press.

HALL, M. M. and MARKS, B. H. (1968) *Pharmacologist* **10,** 225.

HARWOOD, C. T. and BIGELOW, W. M. (1960) *Pharmacologist* **2,** 9.

JAVOY, F., GLOWINSKI, J. and KORDON, C. (1968) *Eur. J. Pharmac.* **4,** 103–104.

KETY, S. S., JAVOY, F., THIERY, A. M. and GLOWINSKI, J. (1967) *Proc. natn. Acad. Sci. U.S.A.* **58,** 1249–1254.

KING, A. B. (1969) *Proc. Soc. exp. Biol. Med.* **130,** 445–447.

KING, A. B. and THOMAS, J. A. (1968) *J. Pharmac. exp. Ther.* **159,** 18–21.

KINSON, G. and SINGER, B. (1967) *J. Endocr.* **37,** xxxvii–xxxviii.

KINSON, G. A., SINGER, B. and GRANT, L. (1968) *Gen. comp. Endocr.* **10,** 447–449.

KINSON, G., WAHID, A. K. and SINGER, B. (1967) *Gen. comp. Endocr.* **8,** 445–454.

KRIEGER, D. T. and RIZZO, F. (1969) *Am. J. Physiol.* **217,** 1703–1707.

LORENZEN, L. C. and GANONG, W. F. (1967) *Endocrinology* **80,** 889–892.

MANGILI, G., MOTTA, M. and MARTINI, L. (1966) In *Neuroendocrinology*, vol. 1, pp. 297–370, ed. Martini, L. and Ganong, W. F. New York and London: Academic Press.

MANGILI, G., MOTTA, M., MUCIACCIA, W. and MARTINI, L. (1965) *Eur. Rev. Endocr.* **1,** 247–253.

MARTINI, L. (1969) *Gen. comp. Endocr.* suppl. 2, 214–226.

MAYNERT, E. W. and LEVI, R. (1964) *J. Pharmac. exp. Ther.* **143,** 90–95.

MESS, B. (1968) *Int. Rev. Neurobiol.* **2,** 171–198.

NARANG, G. D., SINGH, D. V. and TURNER, C. W. (1967) *Proc. Soc. exp. Biol. Med.* **125,** 184–188.

REITER, R. J. and FRASCHINI, F. (1969) *Neuroendocrinology* **5,** 219–255.

REITER, R. J., HOFFMAN, R. A. and HESTER, R. J. (1966) *J. exp. Zool.* **162,** 273–268.

RETIENE, K. (1970) In *The Hypothalamus*, pp. 551–568, ed. Martini, L., Motta, M. and Fraschini, F. New York and London: Academic Press.

RETIENE, K., ZIMMERMAN, E., SCHINDLER, W. J., NEUENSCHWANDER, J. and LIPSCOMB, H. S. (1968) *Acta endocr., Copenh.* **57,** 615–622.

ROTH, W. D. (1964) *Am. Zool.* **4,** 53–57.

SCAPAGNINI, U., VAN LOON, G. R., MOBERG, G. P. and GANONG, W. F. (1971) *Neuroendocrinology* in press.

SHERIDAN, M. N., REITER, R. J. and JACOBS, J. J. (1969) *J. Endocr.* **45,** 131–132.

Simmonds, M. A. (1969) *J. Physiol., Lond.* **203**, 199–210.

Steiner, F. A., Pieri, L. and Kaufmann, L. (1968) *Experientia* **24**, 1133–1134.

Van Loon, G. R. and Ganong, W. F. (1969) *Physiologist* **12**, 381.

Van Loon, G. R., Hilger, L., Cohen, R. and Ganong, W. F. (1969) *Fedn Proc. Fedn Am. Socs exp. Biol.* **28**, 438.

Van Peenen, P. F. D. and Way, E. L. (1957) *J. Pharmac. exp. Ther.* **120**, 261–267.

Wurtman, R. J. (1970) In *The Hypothalamus*, pp. 153–165, ed. Martini, L., Motta, M. and Fraschini, F. New York and London: Academic Press.

Wurtman, R. J., Altschule, M. D. and Holmgren, U. (1959) *Am. J. Physiol.* **197**, 108–110.

Wurtman, R. J., Axelrod, J. and Kelly, D. E. (1968) *The Pineal.* New York and London: Academic Press.

DISCUSSION

Kordon: Your data are very interesting, Dr Motta, but I don't agree with some of your conclusions. What you consider as "basal" corticosterone levels appear to me rather high, compared with the values usually reported (between 0 and 10 μg/100 ml plasma); shouldn't levels of 12 μg or more, as reported in your experiments, rather be considered as stress values, possibly due to the presence of your implanted cannulas?

On the other hand, effects of a direct monoamine supply into the ventricles should be interpreted with caution. There is probably no more than 1 μg of noradrenaline in the whole rat brain; when you inject 165 μg or even 5 μg of the amine into the ventricle, you certainly affect the whole equilibrium of the central nervous system and run the risk of inducing many unspecific effects. This may further account for some discrepancies between your results and some others, which suggested that correlations between catecholaminergic systems and ACTH control are more complex than you postulate. In particular, both stimulation and inhibition of the extraneuronal release of catecholamines result in a transient increase in corticosterone blood levels; however, both treatments are unable to block the responses to sound or electrical stresses (Carr and Moore 1968; Kordon 1970). From these results the authors concluded that the involvement of noradrenergic structures in ACTH control was unlikely to be a direct one.

Motta: You are right in pointing out that the plasma levels of corticosterone in our groups of controls are rather high. The reason for this is probably that all animals in our experiments have a chronically implanted cannula in the brain; in addition, they are given the intraventricular injections of the vehicle without anaesthesia. You may be right in saying that our controls are exposed to a mild chronic stress.

Kordon: Did you ever pretreat your animals with daily saline injections, in order to attenuate the stressing effect of the experimental injection?

Motta: No, we did not try this procedure. This might be a good idea for further experiments.

Owman: As a general point relating to the stress introduced by implanting a cannula into the ventricle, we have made continuous recordings (closed system, Statham P23AC transducer) of intracranial pressure in rabbits. We found that just the implantation of the cannula into the lateral ventricle causes a five-fold increase in the intracranial pressure which persists for about 30 hours (Edvinsson *et al.* 1970).

Fiske: Dr Motta has suggested that the pineal may be involved in the regulation of adrenal cortical secretion. We too, have been interested in this possibility and have followed the effect of superior cervical ganglionectomy on the diurnal corticosterone rhythm in Sprague Dawley female rats of the Charles River strain. Our results indicate that characteristic daily changes in corticosterone levels are maintained after ganglionectomy, a procedure which blocks diurnal responses of the pineal. Since this might simply have reflected an adrenal rhythm established prior to ganglionectomy, the photoperiod was reversed and three weeks later the corticosterone levels were checked again. Although this study has not been completed, it appears that ganglionectomized, as well as sham-operated controls, show a reversal in corticosterone levels in response to a change in the photoperiod. These results indicate that the pineal is not essential for the maintenance of the rise and fall in plasma corticosterone which occurs in response to the photoperiod.

Wurtman: Professor S. Feldman of the Hebrew University (personal communication) finds that after bilateral lesions in the inferior accessory optic tract (the pathway that mediates the effects of light on the pineal and also on the medial forebrain bundle), the ability of a flash of light to cause corticosterone secretion is lost. Hence it appears that the same retinal projection mediates the effects of light on adrenocortical function and pineal function. One cannot conclude from this that the effect of light on adrenocortical function necessarily involves the pineal; it may do so, but it might also result from direct effects on the medial hypothalamus (see p. 238).

Singer: As Dr Motta's paper has not dealt with the influence of pineal principles on aldosterone secretion, it might be of value to review some studies which Dr Kinson and I have done in the rat on the influence of the pineal gland on the secretion rates of both aldosterone and corticosterone. I should point out that our experiments dealt with the *long-term* effect of pinealectomy or administration of melatonin and that secretion rate was determined from estimations in adrenal vein blood; and that in order to obtain this blood a great deal of surgical stress was produced. Thus what we were probably measuring in our experiments was the *maximum secretory capacity* of the gland.

Our study of the pineal gland stemmed from our interest in the factors which regulate the secretion of aldosterone. We undertook these studies at a time when *both stimulatory and inhibitory* effects on the adrenal cortex had been reported using pineal extracts or substances isolated from the pineal gland. As it was not certain that substances extracted from the gland were being secreted in sufficiently great amounts to have their reported effect, or if they were having an effect, whether the stimulatory and inhibitory substances cancelled each other out, we used a different approach. We decided to remove the pineal gland to see what effect this operation, without further treatment, had on the secretion rate of adrenocortical hormones. We also wished to know if the pineal gland was involved in any way in the adrenal response in aldosterone secretion to such stimuli as dietary sodium deficiency or the response to application of a renal artery clip, which normally produces hypertension. More recently we have studied the effect of chronic administration of melatonin in intact rats.

I should like briefly to summarize our results. All experiments were performed on male animals of the Wistar strain. Unless otherwise stated, when pinealectomy was performed it was done on animals between 5 and 6 weeks of age weighing approximately 100 g. Aldosterone and corticosterone secretion rates were determined by measuring these hormones in adrenal vein blood collected under anaesthesia under standard conditions. A *single* sample, collected over 15 minutes (in more recent studies 10 minutes) was obtained from each animal. The steroid content was determined using a modification of the double isotope method of Kliman and Peterson (1960). The secretion rate of these steroids was determined from these values and expressed as μg/kg body wt per adrenal per hour. We did not attempt to correct for the concentration of these steroids *entering* the adrenal gland as in both cases the values would have been negligible compared with those *leaving* the gland. Please note that the secretion rate of corticosterone is considerably higher than that of aldosterone.

In our first experiment we studied the effect of pinealectomy on adrenal cortical hormone secretion in experimental renal hypertension (Kinson, Wahid and Singer 1967). The animals were pinealectomized at 100 g body weight. After 10 days we placed a clip on one renal artery and *20* days after this (i.e. 30 days after pinealectomy) adrenal vein blood was collected. The blood pressure was determined indirectly, every week, using an ankle cuff and photocell. Fig. 1 shows the results of studies on six groups of animals. There were two groups of intact animals, one of which was "sham-clipped" and the other was "clipped" (i.e. a silver clip was placed on one renal artery). A similar pair of groups were also sham-pinealectomized, while a third pair were pinealectomized. Examination of the aldosterone secretion rates of the "non-clipped" animals shows clearly that 30 days after pinealectomy the aldosterone secretion rate was raised, while sham-pinealectomy had no effect. Application of a renal artery clip resulted in hypertension in intact, sham-pinealectomized and pinealectomized animals. The onset and intensity of hypertension was the same in all groups. Neither sham-pinealectomy nor pinealectomy

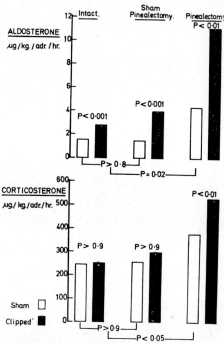

FIG. 1 (Singer). Effect of pinealectomy on adrenal cortical hormone secretion in experimental renal hypertension in rats.

affected the blood pressure in the "non-clipped" animals. In the intact and sham-pinealectomized animals, application of a renal artery clip increased aldosterone production. In the pinealectomized animals, a similar increase occurred but in this case the values in both the sham-clipped and clipped animals were higher than in the other sets. Application of a renal artery clip in normal and sham-pinealectomized rats did not affect the secretion rate of corticosterone. In the pinealectomized rats, the sham-clipped animals secreted significantly increased amounts of corticosterone, and in this case, unlike the other two sets, application of a renal artery clip resulted in an increase in corticosterone production.

These results suggest that the presence of the pineal gland is not necessary in order to produce the response to application of a renal artery clip
with respect to hypertension and aldosterone secretion. They also suggest
that the pineal gland probably has some inhibitory effect on the secretion
of both hormones, since in its absence the secretion rates of both hormones
are increased, at least as determined in the surgically stressed animals 30
days after pinealectomy.

The next point we studied was the effect of dietary sodium deficiency
(Kinson and Singer 1967). Dietary salt restriction was started 10 days

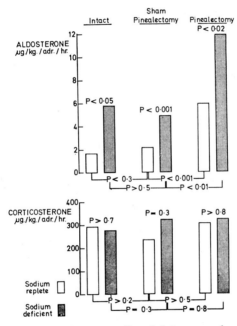

Fig. 2 (Singer). Effect of dietary sodium deficiency on adrenal cortical
hormone secretion in pinealectomized, sham-pinealectomized and
normal rats.

after pinealectomy and was continued for *one* week. At the end of this time
(i.e. 17 days after pinealectomy) we collected adrenal vein blood and
measured the adrenal hormone content as before (Fig. 2). Again, six
groups of animals were studied, including two groups of intact animals
one of which was sodium replete and the other sodium deficient. A similar
pair of groups were sham-pinealectomized, while the third pair were
pinealectomized. The diet resulted in a significant increase in aldosterone
secretion in *all* sodium-deficient animals. However, pinealectomy itself
resulted in an increase in aldosterone production, even in the sodium

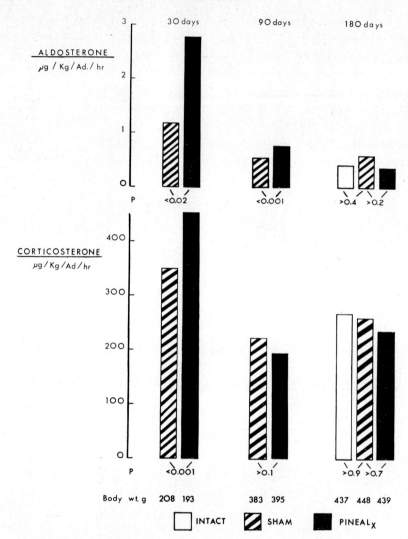

FIG. 3 (Singer). Effect of pinealectomy on the secretion rates of adrenal cortical hormones at 30, 90 and 180 days after pinealectomy.

replete animals, and the effect of dietary sodium deficiency was super-imposed on this, resulting in an extremely high final value. Neither the diet nor the surgery (i.e. sham-pinealectomy or pinealectomy) influenced the secretion rate of corticosterone.

Thus it appears that the presence of the pineal gland is not necessary for demonstrating an effect of sodium deficiency on the secretion of aldosterone. Also it appears that at 17 days after pinealectomy, aldosterone secretion was raised, but not that of corticosterone, whereas in the previous study, made 30 days after pinealectomy, the secretion rates of both hormones were raised. Thus it seemed to us that the time course of the effect of pinealectomy was different for each hormone. We therefore undertook a long-term study on the effect of pinealectomy on the secretion rates of these hormones. This time we used more carefully controlled conditions; we used litter mates and controlled lighting (12:12) and constant temperature (21 °C) (Kinson, Singer and Grant 1968).

Secretion rates of aldosterone and corticosterone were estimated from adrenal vein blood collected at the times indicated in Fig. 3. At 30 days after pinealectomy the secretion rates of both aldosterone and corticosterone were significantly elevated compared with sham-pinealectomized controls, thus confirming our earlier study. At 90 days aldosterone secretion was still elevated, but the difference was not as dramatic, while corticosterone secretion was no longer elevated. (Note the decrease in secretion rates with age when values are expressed as μg/kg per adrenal per hour.) By 180 days neither aldosterone nor corticosterone secretion rates were significantly raised in the pinealectomized animals, compared with either intact or sham-pinealectomized control animals.

In the three studies on the effect of pinealectomy on adrenocortical function just described, it would appear that the pineal gland may exert an inhibitory effect on adrenocortical function which can be demonstrated most clearly 30 days after pinealectomy in young males, although it does not appear to modify significantly the adrenal response either to the application of a renal artery clip with subsequent production of hypertension or to dietary sodium deficiency.

Although aldosterone secretion was found to be significantly raised from the 17th to the 90th day after pinealectomy while corticosterone secretion was significantly elevated only on the 30th day, this does not rule out the possibility that the effect was mediated by ACTH, as the different zones of the adrenal cortex may well respond differently, over the course of time, to changes in ACTH stimulation. The work of Martini's group had suggested that ACTH secretion was inhibited by melatonin, as implantation of melatonin into the median eminence results in adrenal atrophy. Our own studies on the effects of ablation did not provide any direct information on this point. We therefore decided, more recently, to explore the effect of chronic administration of melatonin in intact animals to determine whether this substance was responsible for the apparent inhibitory influence of the pineal gland on the adrenal cortex. We undertook these experiments rather reluctantly, as we were aware of the difficulty in interpreting negative results. In this type of experiment a negative result might be due to the use of the wrong dosage, site or frequency of injection, time of day of injection, lighting conditions or, of course, the wrong pineal principle.

Nevertheless, we did two experiments. In both we used male Wistar rats. Daily injections of melatonin were started when the animals were 26 days old, and these injections were continued for 30 days. Natural lighting conditions were used and injections were given at 10 a.m. In the first experiment we gave 20 μg per day of melatonin in 0·1 ml of 10 per cent alcohol, intraperitoneally. (Stock solutions were prepared using absolute alcohol. Dilutions were made up approximately every 3 days.) The last injection was given on the day before adrenal vein blood was collected. In this experiment no evidence of an inhibitory, or stimulatory, effect of melatonin on the secretion rates of either aldosterone or corticosterone was found.

We tried a second experiment in which we used 10 times as much melatonin (200 μg per day) and reduced the volume of solvent by one half (from 0·1 ml in the first experiment to 0·05 ml in the second). In this experiment we gave our final injection one hour before induction of anaesthesia in preparation for collecting adrenal vein blood. Again, even with this dose of melatonin, we found no evidence of a significant influence on the secretion rate of these two hormones.

One possible explanation for our negative results which I have not mentioned is that the effect of melatonin can only be demonstrated in unstressed animals. However, in view of the fact that we were able to demonstrate an effect of the *chronic* absence of the pineal gland in surgically stressed animals I think it reasonable to expect that the *chronic* administration of biologically effective doses of melatonin would have an effect in surgically stressed animals.

Another possibility, which we haven't explored, is that in order to demonstrate an effect of melatonin in our system it may be necessary first to remove the pineal gland; that is, it may not be possible to demonstrate an effect of melatonin in an animal already secreting its normal complement of this substance.

Finally I should say that although our experiments suggest that the pineal gland may have an inhibitory effect on the adrenal cortex via ACTH, we have found no evidence that it is involved in the adrenal responses in aldosterone secretion which are seen after either sodium deficiency or the production of experimental renal hypertension, which are probably mediated by the renin–angiotensin mechanism.

Nir: We have investigated the interrelationship between the pineal gland and the activity of the adrenal cortex by studying the effect of

TABLE I (Nir)

THE EFFECT OF PINEALECTOMY ON BLOOD CORTICOSTERONE LEVELS OF
FEMALE RATS UNDER VARIOUS CONDITIONS OF LIGHT FOR 10 DAYS

(Plasma corticosterone values given in μg per cent ± S.E. of the mean)

Light exposure	Pinealectomized	Sham-operated
Continuous light	15·1±3·3	14·6±2·0
Continuous darkness	16·9±4·2	8·6±1·6
Alternating light and darkness	9·1±2·5	6·5±0·9

constant light and constant darkness on blood corticosterone levels in pinealectomized and control rats.

Pinealectomized, sham-operated and intact 22-day-old female rats were exposed to constant light, darkness, or an alternate light–dark schedule (lights on from 7 a.m. to 7 p.m.). After 10 or 30 days the rats were killed by decapitation and their blood corticosterone determined.

Table I shows the effect of pinealectomy on blood corticosterone concentrations in rats after 10 days' exposure to the various conditions of light. It can be seen that pinealectomy increases blood corticosterone in rats kept in alternating light and dark. This increase, however, reaches significant levels only in the animals exposed to continuous darkness. No difference whatsoever was found between the pinealectomized and sham-operated control animals exposed to continuous light.

It can be further seen from Table I that continuous light significantly increased the blood corticosterone concentrations in the sham-operated controls compared with those of their counterparts kept in alternating light and continuous darkness. In the pinealectomized group the difference between blood corticosterone concentrations of the animals exposed to various conditions of light is obliterated.

Thus it appears that the increased concentrations of blood corticosterone produced by pinealectomy and those brought about by exposure to continuous light are effected by the same mechanism.

Table II demonstrates what happens in the animals after 30 days' exposure to these same lighting conditions. The difference between the pinealectomized and sham-operated control rats, so marked in the animals kept in

TABLE II (Nir)

THE EFFECT OF PINEALECTOMY ON BLOOD CORTICOSTERONE LEVELS OF FEMALE
RATS UNDER VARIOUS CONDITIONS OF LIGHT FOR 30 DAYS

(Plasma corticosterone values given in μg per cent ± S.E. of the mean)

Light exposure	Pinealectomized	Sham-operated	Intact
Continuous light	24·5±2·2*	23·9±2·0*	20·7±3·1*
Continuous darkness	11·0±1·1	11·2±1·1	9·8±1·4
Alternating light and darkness	10·1±1·1	10·5±1·0	11·3±1·2

* $P < 0.01$.

continuous darkness, has completely disappeared and no difference exists between pinealectomized and control groups exposed to any form of lighting.

Continuous light, however, still acts as a stress factor and the blood corticosterone concentrations of all groups of rats—pinealectomized, sham-operated and intact controls—are significantly higher than those of the animals kept in alternating light and darkness.

Our results appear to differ from those of Dr Singer, who saw no effect of pinealectomy after 17 days but obtained one after 30 days.

Miline: My co-worker Dr Devečerski has studied the morphology of the adrenal gland after pinealectomy in male adult rats (Devečerski 1965). He observed hyperplasia of the zona fasciculata and the zona reticularis, especially in rats sacrificed 2–3 months after removal of the pineal. Succinic dehydrogenase, ATPase and non-specific esterase activities were augmented; mitochondria were very polymorphic and increased in number. Lipofuscin granules in the zona reticularis were also increased. Intramedullary sympathetic ganglion cells were binucleate and increased in number; the periadrenal brown tissue was also very hyperplasic. Succinic dehydrogenase was increased there also.

Before melatonin was discovered and available, we had studied the influence of red light (long wavelength light) on the pineal gland and on the adrenal glands of immature rabbits. We found involution in the pineal glands but accelerated sexual maturation (Miline 1949). The adrenal cortex showed hyperplasia of the zona fasciculata and zona reticularis. Thus atrophy of the pineal gland was correlated with hyperplasia of the zona fasciculata and the androgenic zone—the zona reticularis.

We studied the effect of darkness in immature rabbits. Sexual maturation was very retarded and depressive changes occurred in the zona reticularis and also hyperplasia of the pineal gland. In adult male rats the supraoptic nuclei are very reactive in the light and very much depressed after continuous darkness (Miline 1957; Fiske and Greep 1959). This is one connexion between the hypothalamic centre and the target organs.

From these results, we conclude that the influence of the pineal on the activity of the adrenals and gonads passes through the hypothalamo-hypophysial complex.

Carr, A. and Moore, R. (1968) *Neuroendocrinology* **3**, 285.
Deverčerski, V. (1965) *Histofiziološke odlike nadbubrežne žlezde nakon epifizektomije.* Thesis, Medical Faculty, Novi Sad.
Edvinsson, L., Nielsen, K. C., Owman, Ch. and West, K. A. (1970) *J. appl. Physiol.* in press.

FISKE, V. M. and GREEP, O. R. (1959) *Endocrinology* **64,** 175–185.

KINSON, G. A. and SINGER, B. (1967) *Neuroendocrinology* **2,** 273.

KINSON, G. A., SINGER, B. and GRANT, L. (1968) *Gen. comp. Endocr.* **10,** 447.

KINSON, G. A., WAHID, A. K. and SINGER, B. (1967) *Gen. comp. Endocr.* **8,** 445.

KLIMAN, B. and PETERSON, R. E. (1960) *J. biol. Chem.* **235,** 1639.

KORDON, C. (1970) In *Neuroendocrinologie*, ed. Benoit, J. and Kordon, C. Paris: Centre National de la Recherche Scientifique.

MILINE, R. (1949) *Med. Prog.* **3,** 86–92.

MILINE, R. (1957) In *Pathophysiologia Diencephalica*, pp. 159–164, ed. Curri, S. B., Martini, L. and Kovac, W. Vienna: Springer.

THE ROLE OF THE PINEAL GLAND IN THE CONTROL BY LIGHT OF THE REPRODUCTIVE CYCLE OF THE FERRET

J. HERBERT

Department of Anatomy, University of Birmingham *

INTRODUCTION

Light and the annual breeding season of the ferret

FEMALE ferrets kept in daylight come into oestrus once a year, in the spring, a finding which, by itself, suggests that this annual cycle may be correlated with some change in the environment. Furthermore, ferrets transferred across the equator from England to South Africa change the onset of their breeding season by about six months, whereas those kept near the equator may breed at any time of the year (Bedford and Marshall 1942). Under normal conditions, oestrus continues without interruption for about 20 weeks provided that the animal is unmated.

The ferret was the first mammalian species in which the effect of artificial light on oestrus was demonstrated (Bissonnette 1932). Much of the experimental work on this species is of doubtful quality because of the small numbers of animals used, or because individual animals were given several different light treatments; but some conclusions seem justified. Oestrus can be induced during winter by exposing ferrets during the autumn to artificial light, given either as an extra ration at the end of the normal period of daylight ("evening illumination") (Bissonnette 1932) or by putting them into wholly artificial light with a photoperiod greater than about twelve hours per day ("long days"). Under these conditions females may breed during December or January whereas, in England, oestrus usually begins during late March or April.

The optimum length of artificial long days seems to be 14 hours, since photoperiods greater or less than this (including continuous light) induce oestrus less rapidly (Hammond 1952). The stimulating effect of a given photoperiod is greater the later it is given in the period of anoestrus (Marshall 1963a). Although "short days" (i.e. photoperiods less than twelve hours) do not accelerate oestrus if given as a single dose, the same

---

* Present address: Department of Anatomy, University of Cambridge.

amount given in subdivided doses within the 24-hour period is highly effective (Hammond 1951; Hart 1951).

Animals kept for long periods in artificial long days do not, however, show the usual pattern of annual oestrus, but, once their first oestrus is over, remain anoestrus indefinitely (Donovan 1967; Vincent 1970). Oestrus activity can be restored by transferring such animals for a time to short days and then returning them to long days (Donovan 1967). By contrast, animals kept in evening illumination do come into oestrus at about yearly intervals like the normal animal, but oestrus starts much earlier—in, for example, January (Herbert 1969). Ferrets kept continuously in short days also show synchronous recurrent periods of oestrus but not at yearly intervals (Vincent 1970), whereas those put into continuous light for long periods show intermittent oestrous activity at any time of the year without synchrony between different animals being evident (Thorpe 1967). Annual periodicity is also altered by exposing ferrets to alternating periods of long and short days. For example, animals put into each regime in turn for five months come into oestrus at ten-monthly intervals; if the two light periods last for two months each, ferrets will come into heat as often as three times a year (Vincent 1970).

Neural pathways involved in the response to light

The natural conclusion from the evidence summarized above is that oestrus is normally provoked, in the spring, by the increasing daylengths at this time of the year. However, although ferrets with both optic nerves divided in the autumn do not respond to artificial light, they do come into oestrus at about the same time as normal animals in the first spring after operation (Thomson 1951, 1954); in subsequent years, oestrus may occur at irregular intervals (Thorpe 1969). This indicates both that the retina contains the receptors for the response to light and that the timing of natural oestrus is not dependent upon the increasing daylength that immediately precedes it.

The effect of blinding is not reproduced by lesions of the optic tracts, superior colliculi, lateral geniculate bodies or the occipital cortex (Le Gros Clark, McKeown and Zuckerman 1939); the effect of dividing the accessory optic tracts, which recent work on rats (Moore *et al.* 1967) and monkeys (Moore 1969) suggests might be effective, has not yet been reported. There seems little evidence for direct nervous connexions between the retina and the hypothalamus either in the ferret or in several other species (Jefferson 1940; Kiernan 1967). Lesions of the hypothalamus, a presumed site of action of artificial light, do not prevent the effects of light on oestrus but themselves induce oestrus during winter (Donovan and

Van der Werff ten Bosch 1956*a*), although lesions placed elsewhere may have similar, though less pronounced, effects (Herbert and Zuckerman 1958).

The possibility that the pineal gland might be involved in the effect of light on oestrus in the ferret arose from the finding that bilateral superior cervical ganglionectomy, a procedure which removes the sympathetic innervation of the head and neck, has an effect similar to that of blinding (Abrams, Marshall and Thompson 1954; Donovan and Van der Werff ten Bosch 1956*b*). A search for the critical organ responsible for this finding excluded the effects of denervating the thyroid (Marshall 1963*b*) or the eyes (Marshall 1962). It has been shown that the pineal gland of the rat receives an extensive nerve supply from the ganglia (Rio del Hortega 1932; Owman 1964; Kappers 1965), and that this supply has to be intact if diurnal rhythms of various amines contained in the gland are to respond to experimental alterations in illumination (Wurtman, Axelrod and Fischer 1964; Wurtman *et al.* 1964; Fiske 1964). For many years speculation has existed that the pineal plays some part in reproduction, in particular in the onset of puberty (see Kitay and Altschule 1954), a process suggested as being comparable with the annual onset of oestrus in ferrets (Donovan and Van der Werff ten Bosch 1965).

Experiments have shown that the function of the pineal gland in the ferret appears to differ somewhat from that in the other mammalian species (mainly rodents) so far investigated. The studies described here are concerned with, firstly, the histology and histochemistry of the ferret's pineal and epithalamus with particular reference to features which seem to distinguish the ferret from other species and, secondly, with the effect of removing the gland or administering various methoxyindoles upon both light-induced and natural oestrus in ferrets.

METHODS

Histology and histochemistry

The histology of the normal pineal was studied in serial sections stained with either cresyl violet and luxol fast blue or Bodian's silver proteinate. Monoamines were demonstrated in pineals from anoestrous ferrets by the Falck and Owman (1965) technique (Trueman and Herbert 1970). Pineals were prepared for electron microscopy by perfusing ferrets through the ascending aorta with either 5 per cent buffered glutaraldehyde or a mixture of 1·25 per cent glutaraldehyde and 1 per cent paraformaldehyde (Palay *et al.* 1968), and postfixed in 2 per cent osmium. Acetylcholinesterase was demonstrated under the light microscope by the Koelle technique (Koelle and Freidenwald 1949) and under the electron microscope by the Lewis and Shute (1966) technique.

Studies on light-induced oestrus

Ferrets were kept in rooms fitted with light traps and temperature controlled at about 18 °C. They were illuminated either by daylight only, or by daylight supplemented by six hours of artificial light each evening (evening illumination: 16.00–22.00 hours B.S.T., 50–100 foot-candles) or wholly by artificial light for 14 hours/day (long days: 07.00–21.00 hours B.S.T., approx. 15 foot-candles); details are given below.

Animals were examined once weekly; onset of oestrus was defined as the first appearance of circum-vaginal oedema, and the end of oestrus as its first complete disappearance. They were weighed every four weeks.

Onset of oestrus was calculated (in weeks) from the day of first exposure to artificial light in experimental animals, and the same date was taken as the reference point for oestrus in animals kept in daylight.

Pinealectomy, superior cervical ganglionectomy and control operations were carried out as described previously (Herbert 1969).

Melatonin, 5-methoxytryptamine and 5-methoxytryptophol were prepared by dissolving 125 mg of each in a small quantity of propyl alcohol, and then diluting to 50 ml with arachis oil. Controls received a corresponding volume (0·2 ml) of diluent. Fresh solutions were prepared every four weeks. Doses used are given below.

Experiment 1: Animals were pinealectomized, ganglionectomized or control-operated between 8 October and 7 November (i.e. in early anoestrus) and put into evening illumination on 12 November. They remained in these conditions for up to three years.

Experiment 2: The same operations were made between 27 June and 9 August (i.e. during oestrus). The animals were put into evening illumination on 24 November (by which time they were anoestrous) and then transferred to long days on 26 January, in which they remained until after the end of the normal breeding season.

Experiment 3: Pinealectomies and control operations were made between 8 and 31 October, and the animals either put into long days on 20 November or left in daylight. Those in long days received either (*a*) melatonin, (*b*) 5-methoxytryptamine, (*c*) 5-methoxytryptophol or (*d*) control injections; 500 μg was given thrice weekly (body weight: approx. 800 g) subcutaneously, starting on the first day of exposure to artificial light and continuing for at least six months. Normal animals in daylight were also given (*a*), (*c*) or (*d*), starting on the same day as animals in artificial light.

During each experiment normal animals were kept in daylight as controls. The numbers of animals used are given in the section describing the results.

RESULTS

Histology and histochemistry

The ferret's pineal lies under the caudal aspect of the corpus callosum, in the position usual for carnivores (Fig. 1A).

Pinealocytes. The pinealocytes are distributed throughout the gland except for a caudal area, the pineal ganglion (see below), and do not form follicles. Fluorescent methods show that the pinealocytes contain high concentrations of a yellow fluorophore (probably 5-hydroxytryptamine, 5-HT) whose colour changes to greenish yellow after ganglionectomy. Substances expected to increase 5-HT (e.g. 5-hydroxytryptophan, 25 mg/kg) or decrease it (e.g. reserpine, 2·5 mg/kg) have no effect (Trueman and Herbert 1970). Electron microscopy shows that the cells give off a single process, whose destination has not been traced directly but is probably the perivascular space. The cytoplasm of the cells contains microtubules which are aligned into parallel bundles within the process. A variety of vesicles, some dense-cored, are found, particularly in the region of the Golgi apparatus.

Nerve fibres. A bundle of myelinated fibres attaches the cranial part of the gland to the habenular region, and the nervi conarii enter its caudal pole. After the Falck procedure intra-pineal fibres emit a bright green fluorescence (probably due to noradrenaline), particularly concentrated around blood vessels (Fig. 1B). The fibres of the n. conarii, but not those in the pineal stalk, fluoresce in the same way. No fluorescent fibres are visible after bilateral ganglionectomy or treatment with reserpine.

Pineal ganglion. A collection of neurons lies enmeshed in a matrix of nerve fibres and dendritic processes in the caudal part of the pineal gland. There are very few pinealocytes in this region (Fig. 1A). Neither the cell bodies nor the fibres of the pineal ganglion contain monoamines (Fig. 1B), and they cannot be made to fluoresce by treating animals either with L-dopa (100–150 mg/kg) or nialamide (300–500 mg/kg). They do, however, contain considerable amounts of acetylcholinesterase (Fig. 1C), which is not found elsewhere in the pineal. The electron microscopic appearance of the ganglion cells differs from that of pinealocytes: they are larger, and contain parallel arrays of rough endoplasmic reticulum and a deeply indented nucleus. Acetylcholinesterase activity occurs in the arrays of rough endoplasmic reticulum, as well as in shorter isolated lengths scattered throughout the cytoplasm and in strands running parallel to the

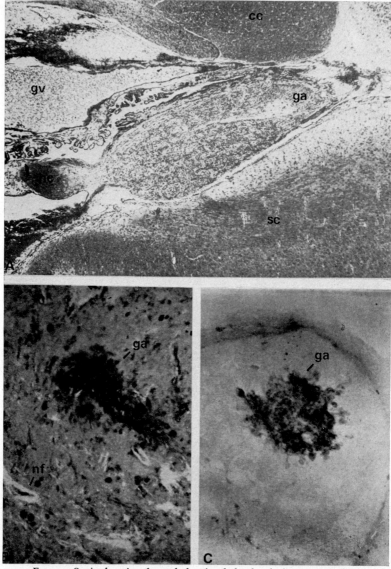

FIG. 1. A. Sagittal section through the pineal gland and adjacent area of the brain (× 32). The pineal ganglion (ga) appears as a pale area in the caudal part of the gland. cc: corpus callosum; gv: great cerebral vein; hc: habenular commissure; sc: superior colliculus.

B. The appearance of the caudal part of the gland after the Falck procedure for monoamines. The dark area is the pineal ganglion (ga). A bundle of nerve fibres (nf) is seen surrounding a blood vessel. Between the fibres and the ganglion the less intense fluorescence of the pinealocytes is visible. × 130 approx.

C. The appearance of the pineal ganglion (ga) in sections demonstrating acetylcholinesterase. A few other cholinesterase-positive cells are visible lying cranially (below, left) to the ganglion. × 130 approx.

nuclear membrane (G. D. S. Wright and J. Herbert, unpublished). Numerous synapses, some cholinergic, are observed in the pineal ganglion making contact with dendritic processes originating, presumably, from the ganglion cells. The synapses contain small (approx. 45 nm) electron-lucent vesicles and occasional larger (approx. 120 nm) ones with dense cores. The structure of these synapses seems to correspond to that described elsewhere in the central nervous system. Bilateral superior cervical gang-lionectomy has no detectable effect on them.

The habenula. The neurons in the medial habenular nucleus contain much acetylcholinesterase, and their ultrastructure resembles that of the pineal ganglion cells. The walls of blood vessels in the medial (but not the lateral) habenular nucleus are remarkable in containing a green fluorophore which has the characteristics of noradrenaline, and which disappears com-pletely after bilateral ganglionectomy or treatment with reserpine. Attempts to demonstrate that the synapses observed in the pineal ganglion are derived from the habenula have not so far been successful for technical reasons.

The pineal gland and the response to light

Effect of pinealectomy on light-induced oestrus. Removal of the pineal gland completely prevents the usual effect of artificial light in accelerating the onset of oestrus. There has been no exception in a total of 16 animals, studied in three separate experiments, and exposed either to evening illumination or to artificial long days. Pinealectomized animals under these conditions do, however, come into oestrus in the spring at about the same time as normal ferrets kept in daylight, and, in this, behave in a way similar to ganglionectomized or blinded animals exposed to artificial light (Figs. 2 and 4).

The exact relation between oestrus in normal ferrets in daylight and pinealectomized animals in artificial light has been variable. Six animals operated on during October–November and put into evening illumination, came into oestrus at the same time as controls (expt. 1); another six, operated on during October, and kept in long days, came in significantly earlier (expt. 3; $P < 0.001$), and a further four operated on during June–August and put first into evening illumination and then into long days came in significantly later (expt. 2; $P < 0.001$).

Parallel experiments show that the effect of bilateral ganglionectomy on the onset of oestrus is identical to that of pinealectomy (Fig. 2). Moreover, the interval between the onsets of the first and second oestrus in evening illumination after operation is much greater than one year (76·6 and 70·0 weeks respectively in pinealectomized and ganglionectomized ferrets),

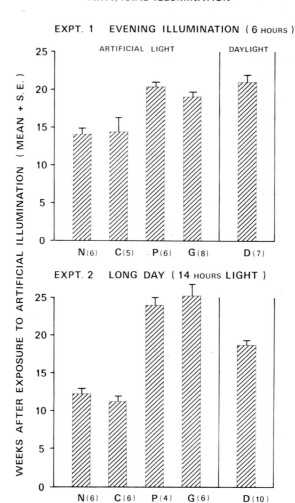

FIG. 2. The effect of either pinealectomy (P), ganglionectomy (G) or control operations (C) upon onset of oestrus in ferrets kept either in "evening illumination" (expt. 1, above) or "long day" (expt. 2, below), and compared with normal animals (N) kept either in artificial illumination or daylight (D). The numbers of animals are given in parentheses.

whereas intact animals kept in evening illumination continue to show annual periodicity (Fig. 3) (Herbert 1969).

These experiments show that the pineal is required if artificial light is to alter the timing of oestrus, but that oestrus still occurs in the pinealectomized ferret. Post-operative oestrus might either represent a delayed response to artificial light, or be a process independent of both environmental light and the pineal gland. The next experiment examines this point.

Effect of pinealectomy on oestrus in animals kept in daylight. Animals pinealectomized in the autumn and kept in daylight (expt. 3) come into oestrus at the normal time in the following spring, at a time not significantly different from control-operated or normal animals ($F = 0.24$;

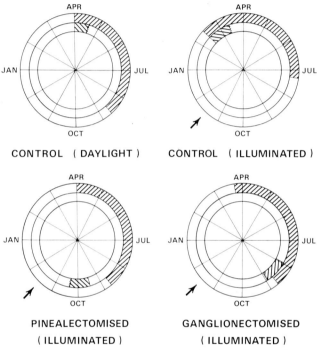

CONTROL (DAYLIGHT)   CONTROL (ILLUMINATED)

PINEALECTOMISED   GANGLIONECTOMISED
(ILLUMINATED)   (ILLUMINATED)

FIG. 3. The oestrous rhythm in normal, pinealectomized or ganglionectomized animals kept for two to three years in evening illumination; records for normal animals kept in daylight are also shown. The mean onset and duration of the oestrous period is indicated by the hatched area. The outer circle is the first year after operation, the inner the second. The arrow indicates the start of artificial illumination. The interval between the onsets of successive oestrous periods (mean weeks $\pm$ S.E.) was: normal, daylight: 51.3 ± 0.96; normal, illuminated: 52.5 ± 2.80; pinealectomized: 76.6 ± 3.96; ganglionectomized: 70.0 ± 0.58.

d.f. 27, 2; P = not significant) (Fig. 5). Whether oestrus in pinealectomized ferrets will continue to occur at annual intervals in succeeding years is not yet known.

This indicates that the pineal gland is not concerned in the onset of oestrus in the year following operation, but that it is necessary if the timing of oestrus is being altered by artificial light. It also suggests that

artificially illuminated, pinealectomized animals come into heat independently of environmental light in the same way as blinded ferrets.

*Effect of methoxyindoles on light-induced oestrus in pinealectomized or control-
operated ferrets.* A number of characteristic methoxyindoles, including
melatonin (Lerner, Case and Heinzelman 1959), 5-methoxytryptamine

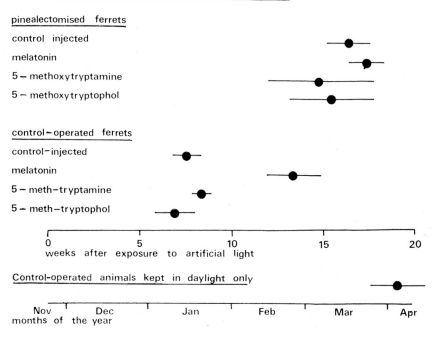

Onset of oestrus in pinealectomised and control ferrets in artificial light
during treatment with various methoxyindoles

Animals put into artificial light (long days : 14 L : 10 D)

pinealectomised ferrets

control injected

melatonin

5 — methoxytryptamine

5 — methoxytryptophol

control–operated ferrets

control–injected

melatonin

5 — meth–tryptamine

5 — meth–tryptophol

0   5   10   15   20
weeks after exposure to artificial light

Control-operated animals kept in daylight only

Nov   Dec   Jan   Feb   Mar   Apr
months of the year

6 experimental animals per group : 500 μg methoxyindole thrice weekly
means, standard deviations

FIG. 4. Onset of oestrus in ferrets kept in artificial light ("long days").
Pinealectomized animals (above) received either melatonin, 5-methoxy-
tryptamine, 5-methoxytryptophol or control injections. Shown
below are the effects of the same treatments given to control-operated
animals.

(i.e. the non-acetylated form of melatonin; Maickel and Miller 1968) and
5-methoxytryptophol (McIsaac, Taborsky and Farrell 1964) are found in
the rodent's pineal, and it seems likely that these are secreted into either
the blood or cerebrospinal fluid. Constant light diminishes the amount of
the enzyme (hydroxyindole-O-methyltransferase, HIOMT) forming

melatonin in rats (a nocturnal species) (Wurtman, Axelrod and Phillips 1963), but has the opposite effect on two diurnal species, the monkey (Moore 1969) and the hen (Axelrod, Wurtman and Winget 1964). There is, as yet, no information for the ferret or any other mammalian seasonal breeder.

Melatonin and other methoxyindoles decrease pituitary–ovarian function in rats (see Wurtman, Axelrod and Kelly 1968). But removal of the pineal in ferrets neither induces premature oestrus nor increases ovarian

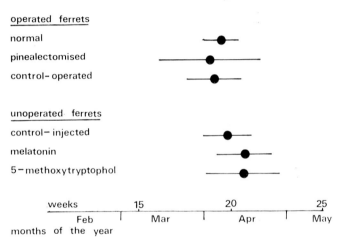

Onset of oestrus in pinealectomised & unoperated ferrets given methoxyindoles and kept in daylight

operated ferrets

normal

pinealectomised

control-operated

unoperated ferrets

control-injected

melatonin

5-methoxytryptophol

weeks   15   20   25

Feb   Mar   Apr   May

months of the year

6 animals per group (11 normals) 500μg methoxyindole thrice weekly means, standard deviations

FIG. 5. Onset of oestrus in pinealectomized animals kept in daylight (above) and in normal animals kept in daylight and given either melatonin or 5-methoxytryptophol (below).

weight (Herbert 1969), as it does in rats (Wurtman, Altschule and Holmgren 1959). Thus these substances might have stimulatory, rather than inhibitory effects on pituitary gonadotropins in ferrets.

However, none of the three compounds tested was able to restore the pinealectomized ferrets' response to artificial light, and all came into oestrus at the same time as control-injected pinealectomized ferrets ($F = 1 \cdot 56$; $d.f.$ 20, 3; $P =$ not significant) (Fig. 4). But both melatonin ($P < 0 \cdot 001$) and, to a lesser degree, 5-methoxytryptamine ($P < 0 \cdot 05$) delayed light-induced oestrus in control-operated animals. Melatonin-treated animals took almost twice as long as those receiving control injections to come into oestrus, but were still in oestrus earlier than control-operated animals kept in daylight ($P < 0.001$) or pinealectomized animals kept in long days ($P < 0.001$). 5-Methoxytryptophol had no effect (Fig. 4).

Thus it seems that none of the three substances is the one by which the pineal allows the pituitary to respond to light. But melatonin (and 5-methoxytryptamine) partially inhibit the oestrus-accelerating effect of light in animals with a pineal, whereas they have no effect on animals unable to respond to artificial illumination. To test whether the inhibitory effect was a specific one upon light-induced oestrus (as removal of the pineal seems to be), methoxyindoles were given to normal ferrets kept in daylight.

Effect of methoxyindoles on normal ferrets kept in daylight. Neither melatonin nor 5-methoxytryptophol, given thrice weekly from 24 November, had any effect upon the onset of oestrus in the following spring even though, by the time they had come into oestrus, these ferrets had received melatonin for longer than animals kept in long days. Both groups came into oestrus at the same time as normal and control-injected animals kept in daylight ($F = 1.70$; d.f. 25, 3; $P =$ not significant) (Fig. 5).

Pineal gland and the duration and termination of oestrus

Information on the role of the pineal and of methoxyindoles in regulating the duration of oestrus in ferrets is less complete. Neither ganglionectomy nor pinealectomy significantly alters the duration of oestrus in animals kept in either evening illumination or long day (Herbert 1969). Further data on animals treated with melatonin, or pinealectomized animals kept in daylight, are not yet available. However, there is evidence that removal of the pineal or the ganglia during oestrus may delay its termination in some animals kept in daylight (Herbert 1969).

GENERAL DISCUSSION

An intact pineal gland is a prerequisite for oestrus to be stimulated by artificial light in the ferret. Ganglionectomy has the same effect as pinealectomy, and also removes the noradrenergic nerve supply to the gland. It may thus be concluded that the effect of light is transmitted to the pineal by way of its autonomic nerve supply, though it is curious that, in the rat, noradrenaline itself stimulates the formation of melatonin-forming enzymes (Shein and Wurtman 1969), whereas electrical stimulation of the ganglia has the opposite effect (Brownstein and Heller 1968).

The role of the pineal in the onset of annual oestrus in the normal ferret exposed to daylight may be correlated with whatever part that the light plays, but what this is is still unclear. Since oestrus occurs in blinded, ganglionectomized or pinealectomized ferrets in the year after operation this means that the increasing daylength of that year is not responsible. If normal oestrus were entirely due to an "endogenous" rhythm, independent of light, then operated animals should come into oestrus, year after year, at the usual time. This they do not do. However, an endogenous rhythm with a period greater or lesser than a year may exist and be synchronized with the seasons by light, acting through the pineal, at some time during the previous year. On this argument, pinealectomized ferrets (and intact animals kept continuously in short days) come into oestrus in the years after experimental treatment because the endogenous rhythm is operating or, possibly, because the rhythm set up by exposure to annual changes in daylength before the experiment started takes some time to wane. But ferrets born and reared in short days can still come into oestrus (Thorpe 1967), which makes the latter explanation unlikely. Pinealectomy or ganglionectomy carried out during the previous summer may have a greater disrupting effect on spring oestrus than if performed later in the year because the animal's cycle has had more time to move out of phase with the environment.

Long days and continuous illumination (unlike short days) are not neutral stimuli (see Introduction), and therefore give no information about the existence of an underlying endogenous rhythm. Exposure to short days allows the ferret's pituitary to respond again to long days perhaps because some synthetic mechanism, itself independent of light, is able to restore the balance between synthesis and secretion in the absence of a stimulatory light regime. Since the pituitary appears, at least by cytological criteria, to contain little gonadotropin during the winter when secretion is minimal (Holmes 1960; Herbert, unpublished), this effect must occur at some other locus. If these conclusions are correct, then the oestrous periods of pinealectomized ferrets kept in daylight should, eventually, come to be out of phase with the seasons, and similar animals kept in long days should not be inhibited from showing recurrent periods of oestrus.

None of the three methoxyindoles investigated seems to be the critical substance linking the effect of light on the pineal with the pituitary. Melatonin has a depressive effect on the onset of oestrus (as in the rat) (Wurtman, Axelrod and Chu 1963) but only in intact animals exposed to artificial light. Its role in the normal ferret, if any, is obscure; it might be concerned with bringing oestrus to an end, though whether this can be induced by alterations in lighting is still undecided. It is interesting that melatonin has been found, in the rat, principally to decrease LH (luteinizing hormone), whereas 5-methoxytryptophol (which is ineffective in ferrets) has its main effect on FSH (follicle stimulating hormone) (Fraschini 1969). Yet the latter is the gonadotropin which, it has always been assumed, is the one principally concerned with the onset of oestrus. It is also noteworthy that removing the terminal acetyl group from melatonin (thus giving 5-methoxytryptamine) greatly reduces its potency in the ferret. The evidence suggests that, in the ferret, methoxyindoles inhibit not the secretion of gonadotropins *per se*, but the process by which this secretion is timed by light.

Had the dose of melatonin been larger, acceleration by light of oestrus might have been completely prevented. The dose used, an arbitrary one, was based on those (equally arbitrary) given to rats. If the pineal secretes substances directly into the cerebrospinal fluid, as has been suggested (Antón-Tay and Wurtman 1969; Sheridan, Reiter and Jacobs 1969), then the amounts acting directly on the central nervous system may be very much greater than would appear even from quite massive doses given systemically. Recently, a system of specialized cells in the ependyma lining the third ventricle in the region of the tuber cinereum has been observed in both ferrets and monkeys (Knowles, Kumar and Jones 1967; Knowles and Kumar 1969). These cells have a distinctive appearance under the electron microscope and send processes in the direction of the pituitary. They show marked cytological changes during the reproductive cycle, and may play a part in controlling the secretion of gonadotropin by detecting changes in the levels of oestrogen in the cerebrospinal fluid (Kumar and Thomas 1968); they, or cells like them, may equally detect other substances (e.g. monoamines and methoxyindoles) present in the cerebrospinal fluid.

A structure resembling the pineal ganglion of the ferret has not been described before, though nerve cells occur in the pineal gland of the monkey (Levin 1938; Le Gros Clark 1940). Whether or not it has any function is quite unknown. Their ultrastructure indicates that its neurons are unlikely to be vestiges of primitive photoreceptors but they may be derived from the medial habenular nucleus; alternatively, though less likely, they might be parasympathetic ganglion cells. They may make synaptic contact with the habenula (Trueman and Herbert 1970), where blood vessels contain high concentrations of noradrenaline which is derived either directly from the superior cervical ganglia, or from the pineal's autonomic supply. The role of the habenula in the function of the ferret's pineal gland merits further investigation.

Although many polycyclic rodents do not show well-defined breeding seasons, and thus differ from monoestrous seasonal breeders such as the ferret, the pineal may have analogous roles in both. Blinding hamsters (a nocturnal, polycyclic species), or putting them into continuous darkness, induces gonadal atrophy (Reiter and Hester 1966) which, however, only lasts about 20 weeks (Reiter 1969)—a period similar to that of oestrus in the ferret, and to that of testicular regression during the winter in normal hamsters kept in daylight (Mogler 1958; Czyba, Girod and Durand 1964). Whether blind hamsters show recurrent periods of "anoestrus" has not been reported. The duration both of anoestrus in hamsters and of oestrus in ferrets thus seems self-limiting under these conditions. The effect of darkness or blinding on hamsters is prevented by pinealectomy (Hoffman and Reiter 1965; Reiter and Hester 1966)—an effect comparable with the result of pinealectomy on light-induced oestrus in ferrets.

Putting rats into continuous light or darkness has greatly helped our understanding of the effect of illumination on the biochemistry and metabolism of the pineal, but has given little information on the biological function of the gland in this species, which is still obscure. But the action of light on rats is somewhat similar to that in ferrets in that it times the onset of oestrus (and ovulation) (Hemmingsen and Krarup 1937; Fiske 1941). Whether pinealectomized rats ovulate at the usual time (during the night) or whether they can still alter the time they ovulate in response to changed illumination, has not been reported. However, pinealectomy accelerates ovulation induced by pregnant mares' serum given eight hours after the start of the daily photoperiod, interpreted as indicating a facilitating effect of the operation on gonadotropin release (Dunaway 1969), but equally possibly due to small changes in the phase of the oestrous cycle in pinealectomized animals. The running activity of pinealectomized animals, unlike those blinded, is still able to adjust to changes in light, and the effect actually occurs rather more rapidly than in normal animals (Quay 1970).

The evidence suggests that the pineal is an essential component in the link between the environment and the pituitary in the ferret. There must be a physiological basis for the difference between species that breed seasonally and those that do so all the year round. It is tempting to look for this either in the pineal itself or in the way that the parts of the central nervous system which regulate the pituitary's function respond to substances secreted by the pineal.

SUMMARY

The female ferret normally comes into oestrus once a year in the spring, but putting anoestrous animals into artificial light advances the onset of oestrus to December or January. This effect of light is abolished by pinealectomy or superior cervical ganglionectomy, but operated animals kept in artificial light still come into oestrus in the spring. Subsequently, however, oestrus occurs at intervals greater than a year. Pinealectomy has no effect in the following year on the oestrus of animals kept in daylight.

Melatonin, 5-methoxytryptamine or 5-methoxytryptophol do not restore the response of pinealectomized ferrets to artificial light. But melatonin and, to a less degree, 5-methoxytryptamine, delay oestrus in normal animals exposed to artificial light, whereas they have no effect on animals kept in daylight.

The ferret's pineal contains large amounts of 5-hydroxytryptamine, and receives an extensive noradrenergic nerve supply from the superior cervical ganglia. The gland also contains a collection of neurons (the pineal ganglion) which contain, not amines, but acetylcholinesterase. The capillary walls of the medial habenular nucleus also contain noradrenaline, which is removed by ganglionectomy.

The evidence suggests that the pineal gland is an essential link in the connection between the environment and the pituitary gland in the ferret, though the way in which the pineal affects the timing of the secretion of gonadotropin remains obscure.

Acknowledgements

I am indebted to Sir Solly Zuckerman, F.R.S. for commenting on the manuscript, and to Mrs Sheila Rugman for her invaluable assistance.

REFERENCES

ABRAMS, M. E., MARSHALL, W. A. and THOMSON, A. P. D. (1954) *Nature, Lond.* **174**, 311.
ANTÓN-TAY, F. and WURTMAN, R. J. (1969) *Nature, Lond.* **221**, 474–475.
AXELROD, J., WURTMAN, R. J. and WINGET, C. M. (1964) *Nature, Lond.* **201**, 1134.
BEDFORD, DUKE OF and MARSHALL, F. H. A. (1942) *Proc. R. Soc. B* **130**, 396–399.
BISSONNETTE, T. H. (1932) *Proc. R. Soc. B* **110**, 322–336.
BROWNSTEIN, M. J. and HELLER, A. (1968) *Science* **162**, 367–369.
CZYBA, G., GIROD, C. and DURAND, N. (1964) *C.r. Séanc. Soc. Biol.* **158**, 724–745.
DONOVAN, B. T. (1967) *J. Endocr.* **92**, 105–115.
DONOVAN, B. T. and VAN DER WERFF TEN BOSCH (1956a) *J. Physiol., Lond.* **132**, 57P.
DONOVAN, B. T. and VAN DER WERFF TEN BOSCH (1956b) *J. Physiol., Lond.* **132**, 123–129.
DONOVAN, B. T. and VAN DER WERFF TEN BOSCH (1965) *Physiology of Puberty.* London: Arnold.
DUNAWAY, J. E. (1969) *Neuroendocrinology*, **5**, 281–289.
FALCK, B. and OWMAN, CH. (1965) *Acta Univ. lund. II* **7**, 1–23.
FISKE, V. M. (1941) *Endocrinology* **29**, 187–196.
FISKE, V. M. (1964) *Science* **146**, 253.
FRASCHINI, F. (1969) In *Progress in Endocrinology* (Proc. III Int Congr. Endocrinology), pp. 637–644, ed. GUAL, C. Excerpta Medica International Congress Series no. 184. Amsterdam: Excerpta Medica Foundation.
HAMMOND, J. (1951) *Nature, Lond.* **167**, 150–151.
HAMMOND, J. (1952) *J. agric. Sci. Camb.* **42**, 283–303.

HART, D. S. (1951) *J. exp. Biol.* **28**, 1–12.
HEMMINGSEN, A. M. and KRARUP, N. B. (1937) *Kgl. danske Videnstab. Selskab. Biol. Med.* **13**, no. 7.
HERBERT, J. (1969) *J. Endocr.* **43**, 625–636.
HERBERT, J. and ZUCKERMAN, S. (1958) *J. Endocr.* **17**, 433–444.
HOFFMAN, R. A. and REITER, R. J. (1965) *Science* **148**, 1609.
HOLMES, R. L. (1960) *J. Endocr.* **20**, 48–55.
JEFFERSON, J. M. (1940) *J. Anat.* **75**, 106–134.
KAPPERS, J. A. (1965) In *Structure and Function of the Epiphysis Cerebri (Progress in Brain Research* vol. 10), pp. 87–153, ed. Kappers, J. A. and Schadé, J. P. Amsterdam: Elsevier.
KIERNAN, J. (1967) *J. comp. Neurol.* **131**, 405–408.
KITAY, J. I. and ALTSCHULE, M. D. (1954) *The Pineal Gland—A Review of the Physiologic Literature.* Cambridge, Mass.: Harvard University Press.
KNOWLES, F. W. G. and KUMAR, T. C. A. (1969) *Phil. Trans. R. Soc. B* **256**, 357–375.
KNOWLES, F. W. G., KUMAR, T. C. A. and JONES, C. F. (1967) *Gen. comp. Endocr.* **9**, 526.
KOELLE, G. B. and FREIDENWALD, J. S. (1949) *Proc. Soc. exp. Biol. Med.* **70**, 617–622.
KUMAR, T. C. A. and THOMAS, G. H. (1968) *Nature, Lond.* **219**, 628.
LE GROS CLARK, W. E. (1940) *J. Anat.* **74**, 47–492.
LE GROS CLARK, W. E., McKEOWN, T. and ZUCKERMAN, S. (1939) *Proc. R. Soc. B* **126**, 449–468.
LERNER, A. B., CASE, J. D. and HEINZELMAN, R. V. (1959) *J. Am. chem. Soc.* **81**, 6084.
LEVIN, P. M. (1938) *J. comp. Neurol.* **68**, 405–409.
LEWIS, P. R. and SHUTE, C. C. D. (1966) *J. Cell Sci.* **1**, 381–390.
MAICKEL, R. P. and MILLER, F. P. (1968) *Adv. Pharmac.* **6A**, 71–77.
MARSHALL, W. A. (1962) *J. Physiol., Lond.* **165**, 27–28P.
MARSHALL, W. A. (1963a) *The role of light in the control of oestrus in ferrets.* Ph.D. thesis, University of Birmingham.
MARSHALL, W. A. (1963b) *J. Endocr.* **24**, 315–323.
McISAAC, W. M., TABORSKY, R. G. and FARRELL, G. (1964) *Science* **145**, 63.
MOGLER, R. K. H. (1958) Quoted by Reiter, R. J. and Fraschini, F. (1969) *Neuroendocrinology* **5**, 219–255.
MOORE, R. Y. (1969) *Nature, Lond.* **222**, 781–782.
MOORE, R. Y., HELLER, A., WURTMAN, R. J. and AXELROD, J. (1967) *Science* **155**, 220–223.
OWMAN, CH. (1964) *Int. J. Neuropharmac.* **2**, 105–112.
PALAY, S. L., SOTELO, C., PETERS, A. and ORKAND, P. M. (1968) *J. Cell Biol.* **38**, 143–201.
QUAY, W. B. (1970) *Physiol. Behav.* **5**, 353–360.
REITER, R. J. (1969) *Gen. comp. Endocr.* **12**, 460–468.
REITER, R. J. and HESTER, R. J. (1966) *Endocrinology* **79**, 1168–1170.
RIO DEL HORTEGA, P. (1932) In *Cytology and Cellular Pathology of the Nervous System*, vol. 2, pp. 635–703, ed. Penfield, W. New York: Hoeber.
SHEIN, H. M. and WURTMAN, R. J. (1969) *Science* **166**, 519–520.
SHERIDAN, M. N., REITER, R. J. and JACOBS, J. J. (1969) *J. Endocr.* **45**, 131–132.
THOMSON, A. P. D. (1951) *J. Physiol., Lond.* **113**, 425–433.
THOMSON, A. P. D. (1954) *Proc. R. Soc. B* **142**, 126–135.
THORPE, D. H. (1967) *Ciba Fdn Study Grp no. 26 The Effects of External Stimuli on Reproduction*, pp. 53–66. London: Churchill.
THORPE, D. H. (1969) *Gen. comp. Endocr.* **13**, 535.
TRUEMAN, T. and HERBERT, J. (1970) *Z. Zellforsch. mikrosk. Anat.* **109**, 83–100.
VINCENT, D. S. (1970) *Environment, pituitary and reproduction in the ferret.* Ph.D. thesis, University of Birmingham.
WURTMAN, R. J., ALTSCHULE, M. D. and HOLMGREN, U. (1959) *Am. J. Physiol.* **197**, 108–110.
WURTMAN, R. J., AXELROD, J. and CHU, E. W. (1963) *Science* **141**, 277.

WURTMAN, R. J., AXELROD, J., CHU, E. W. and FISCHER, J. E. (1964) *Endocrinology* **75,** 266–272.

WURTMAN, R. J., AXELROD, J. and FISCHER, J. E. (1964) *Science* **143,** 1328–1330.

WURTMAN, R. J., AXELROD, J. and KELLY, D. E. (1968) *The Pineal Gland*. New York and London: Academic Press.

WURTMAN, R. J., AXELROD, J. and PHILLIPS, L. S. (1963) *Science* **142,** 1071–1073.

DISCUSSION

Collin: I am very interested by your discovery of the pineal ganglion in the ferret. This proves that a pineal organ deprived of photoreceptor cells contains typical ganglion cells. In pineal organs of snakes (Vivien and Roels 1968) and birds (references in Collin 1969; Ueck 1970) where typical photoreceptors are not found, ganglion cells are present. The interpretation of the functional significance of these neurons is very difficult and I wonder whether during ontogeny some epithalamic structures are incorporated in the pineal, originating perhaps, in some cases, from the habenular ganglia? Dr Meiniel has studied the ganglion located just below the parapineal and connected to it in the parapineal complex of the lamprey (*Lampetra planeri*). He has termed it provisionally the "parapineal ganglion". In our electron microscopic studies we have shown that it contains the same components as those present in the left habenular ganglion. Furthermore the parapineal ganglion is connected to the left habenular ganglion by numerous nervous processes. So it seems that the parapineal ganglion does not belong to the parapineal organ but represents part of the left habenular ganglion. In the parapineal organ, the sensory ganglion cells are scarce and this fact is in agreement with the partial "rudimentation" of the direct sensory apparatus (Meiniel 1970). The results obtained by Dr Rüdeberg (1969) are different. In the parapineal of the trout (*Salmo gairdneri*) the photoreceptive apparatus is very poor. Dr Rüdeberg was able to find only three photoreceptor cells. Nevertheless, numerous ganglion cells are present in the parapineal. The parapineal tract also contains numerous axons which "run with the habenular commissure into the left habenular nucleus" (Rüdeberg 1969). The phylogeny and ontogeny of the parapineal in lower vertebrates are certainly interesting problems. These preliminary results from comparative anatomy suggest that during phylogeny some parts of the habenular components were incorporated in the parapineal, but this requires new studies. Such incorporation might be possible in the pineal. On this hypothesis, two situations could be present: either the nerve cells are moved as a group and constitute a ganglion in some animals; or they are progressively dispersed in the pineal during ontogeny, in other animals. What do you think, Dr Herbert, about the possibility that epithalamic structures are incorporated in the pineal?

Herbert: I think that that is the most likely interpretation. However, there are three possibilities: the first is that the pineal ganglion is a remnant of a more primitive photoreceptor mechanism. This doesn't seem very likely. The second possibility is that it is a collection of autonomic ganglion cells. The third possibility is that it is, as you say, related to or derived from the epithalamic region. Our evidence doesn't yet allow us to decide definitely between these three possibilities, but the ganglion cells may be connected with the habenula. There are nerve fibres apparently stretching between the two; the morphological characteristics of the cells in the ganglion are similar to those of the habenula; moreover, cells from both are cholinergic, and so are some of the synapses observed in the pineal ganglion under the electron microscope (G. D. S. Wright and J. Herbert, unpublished).

These facts favour the idea that the ganglion cells are epithalamic in connexion, if not in origin.

Collin: Would it be easy to obtain the different stages of the development in the ferret?

Herbert: This would be a very interesting thing to do.

Oksche: Is it possible to trace nervous pathways from the habenular ganglia to the pineal ganglion of the ferret in silver preparations? You described synaptic structures in your electron micrographs; perhaps some of the bundles originating in the habenular region could be traced in good silver preparations to this synaptic area of the pineal?

Herbert: We have tried to do this in three ways: first, by tracing fibres from the habenula. I myself am very diffident about drawing conclusions from trying to trace individual fibres in silver preparations, particularly when one is relying upon negative evidence, and silver impregnation of the fibres is not always consistent. But there does appear to be a tract running between the ganglion and the habenula.

In a second experiment, J. G. Malcomson and I (unpublished) destroyed the habenular nuclei on one side and tried to follow the subsequent degeneration. The question was whether fibres went from one side, entered the pineal and then doubled back to the other habenula, or whether they ended in the gland. If they did the former, and if you destroyed one side, you should get degeneration in the other habenula; in the second case, only in the pineal itself. This experiment was frustrated by the fact that the Nauta preparation shows degeneration very beautifully in the habenular commissure but as soon as the fibres enter the pineal impregnation stops immediately. Mitchell (1963) apparently found the same thing in the cat.

Now, we are trying to destroy one or both of the habenular nuclei and looking under the electron microscope to see whether the synapses in the pineal ganglion degenerate.

Kappers: Dr Herbert, did you observe degeneration of the intrapineal nerve cells after removal of both superior cervical ganglia?

Herbert: No, they looked normal (G. D. S. Wright and J. Herbert, unpublished).

Kappers: Would it perhaps be possible that these cells receive preganglionic fibres from the vagus?

Herbert: It is possible, but I think that Kenny's work (1961) requires confirmation.

Miline: Your results showing a connexion between the pineal gland and the habenular ganglion suggest that we should not reject the existence of an epithalamo-epiphysial complex or habenulo-pineal system (Roussy and Mosinger 1964; Kappers 1960). Have you any information about the relation between the pineal gland and the subcommissural organ? Do you find evaginations of the subcommissural organ in rosette forms in the parenchyma? Are there fibre connexions between the pineal ganglion and the subcommissural organ?

Herbert: Fibres entering the pineal seem to be derived both from the habenular commissure and from the region of the subcommissural organ. There are no follicles or rosettes in the pineal gland itself; the cells appear uniformly distributed, apart from in the pineal ganglion.

Oksche: Dr Herbert, would it be possible to remove only the distal part of the pineal containing the ganglion and then study fibre degeneration by the Nauta method in the more proximal stalk region? It is possible that the fibres you see in your neurohistological preparations originate in the nerve cells of the pineal ganglion; in the avian pineal there are numerous fibres in the pineal stalk, and a considerable number of them originate in the nerve cells in the dorsal wall of the pineal (Ueck 1970).

Herbert: I suppose anything is technically possible, although removing even the whole pineal from the ferret is not very easy because the gland lies beneath the corpus callosum (unlike in the rat). But what I said previously about the Nauta stain makes it an unsatisfactory method for studying the pineal gland. Neither would this sort of experiment resolve the origin of the synapses in the pineal ganglion. But it is certainly true that the axons from these ganglion cells must go somewhere.

Oksche: We have to exclude that the pineal pathway of the ferret doesn't run from the pineal ganglion to the nervous system. This seems to be a very important point.

Kelly: Dr Herbert, would you comment further on the morphology of the pinealocyte, particularly from two aspects? First, what is the situation of the pinealocyte processes and their organelles; are synaptic ribbons present anywhere within this organ? Secondly, what is the relationship of the pinealocyte and its processes to the perivascular spaces; is a continuous or partial astrocytic border present?

Herbert: We have never yet seen synaptic ribbons in the pinealocytes of the ferret. The second is a very interesting question. As I have pointed out, there are two areas in the ferret pineal, the ganglion and the parenchyma; the capillaries look different in the two areas. In the parenchyma they appear somewhat similar to those in the rat and other species except that the whole perivascular space is filled with endings. Some of these endings undoubtedly derive from the pinealocytes and others are autonomic, but we aren't yet sure which are which. One problem is that although there is a vast sympathetic nerve supply to the ferret's pineal, the number of dense-cored vesicles in the perivascular space is much fewer than that found in the rat. The space round the parenchymal capillaries contains little glial material; in the pineal ganglion there are few endings in the perivascular space but one can see fibrillary processes which seem to come from astrocytes, and which sometimes encircle the blood vessels. One question is, therefore, whether both ganglion and parenchyma are inside or outside the "blood-brain barrier", and we have some preliminary evidence on this. We gave ferrets trypan blue intraperitoneally for 10 or 14 days, then sectioned the brains, and studied them under dark-ground illumination. Our evidence so far suggests, surprisingly, that the whole of the pineal in this species is inside the blood–brain barrier, because trypan blue doesn't get in any part of it, although it can be seen in the external layer of the median eminence, the anterior pituitary, the area postrema and the choroid plexus (J. G. Malcolmson and J. Herbert, unpublished).

Kelly: Is the capillary endothelium fenestrated as in the rat pineal?

Herbert: No.

Kelly: This is a remarkable pineal organ and I hope that you will pursue it, particularly by looking at young stages, as Dr Collin suggested. You might be able to answer the question of compartmentation between the ganglion region and the parenchymal region in this way.

Wurtman: I would like to congratulate Dr Herbert on a beautiful piece of work and the development of a fascinating experimental model. Many of us working with the albino rat have had misgivings about the appropriateness of using that animal to study the effects of light on the pineal, and I think my misgivings have just increased several-fold.

I am trying to make some sense out of the fact that giving melatonin delays the onset of oestrus in ferrets exposed to light and pinealectomy also seems to have a delaying effect. Two experiments might be helpful. One would be to determine whether there is an annual rhythm in HIOMT activity in the ferret pineal, and to characterize the rhythm. We are doing this sort of study in three other annual breeders, namely the Waddell seal, the weasel and the sheep. All three species appear to have annual HIOMT rhythms. The precise characteristics of the rhythms vary somewhat, which is not surprising in view of the fact that the time of the annual oestrus is also somewhat different. Such studies in the ferret might give some indication of whether melatonin normally participates in the timing of annual oestrus. Secondly, in view of some of Dr Fiske's findings, the possibility should be considered that there is an annual rhythm in the sensitivity of the ferret brain to endogenous melatonin. Dr Fiske showed that the capacity of melatonin to increase pineal serotonin depended upon the time of day that it was administered (Fiske and Huppert 1968). If melatonin also affects serotonin levels in the ferret brain it might be interesting to see whether there is an annual rhythm in the dose–response relationship.

Herbert: Yes, or even a daily rhythm. We have no information on HIOMT; we have thought about doing this but, as you say, it seems difficult to assign a role for melatonin in the ferret and this has put us off. There is the possibility that melatonin might be concerned with ending oestrus in the autumn. I say this with no great conviction, for two reasons: first we have no evidence for it and, secondly, there's no satisfactory evidence that reduced light can bring oestrus to an end in the ferret.

As far as an annual rhythm in sensitivity to melatonin goes, the experiments I have described here are still in progress. The animals have been given melatonin for 6 months and we shall continue doing this for up to a year or so. We are particularly interested to see whether the timing of next year's oestrus is going to be affected by melatonin given this year.

Wurtman: One thing one might do is take animals that have been in oestrus for a month, two months, three months and then start them on melatonin.

Axelrod: It is obvious that the superior cervical ganglion is critical in the timing of the oestrous cycle, since it is very much involved with biogenic amines. Have you thought of measuring either serotonin or noradrenaline in the ferret pineal, around the clock and seasonally, also measuring acetylcholinesterase and also trying some pharmacological tests by giving atropine, carbachol, reserpine and things of that kind?

Herbert: We have not done any of the experiments you mention. Most of our attention is directed towards identifying the substance in the pineal which allows light to alter the secretory activity of the pituitary.

Axelrod: I would like to revert to the point I brought up earlier about the administration of melatonin. You have given a single injection three times a week. One doesn't know whether one has given an effective dose of melatonin all the time; this is the problem. You might have had melatonin present for just 2 or 3 hours in the entire week; thus you might have been giving an ineffective dose of melatonin.

Herbert: Two things make me think that our doses are effective. First, we got a positive effect in one kind of animal, namely intact ferrets exposed to artificial light, and therefore the negative effects in the others are likely to be due to the fact that melatonin doesn't do these things rather than to the dose being an ineffective one.

Secondly, we tried to minimize the rate of absorption by giving the melatonin in oil. We have no information about absorption of melatonin from oil but if we can extrapolate from the administration of steroid hormones, it's very likely that it was at least delayed.

Axelrod: Dr Owman has done a very nice study on the species differences in the distribution of catecholamines and tryptamine and 5-hydroxy-tryptamine in the pineal. Species differences in responsiveness to melatonin are of particular interest at the moment.

Owman: There is a considerable species difference with regard both to the identity of the amine stored in the parenchymal cells and to the concentration of serotonin in the cells, and also whether the gland has an adrenergic innervation and whether this innervation reaches the parenchyma or the pineal blood vessels (Owman 1965, 1968).

For example, in mice and rats we found a very rich adrenergic innervation to both vessels and parenchymal cells and a high concentration of serotonin in the parenchymal cells. In contrast to this the cat has no histochemically visible serotonin in the parenchymal cells although there is both a vascular and a parenchymal adrenergic innervation. The sheep and rabbit are similar to the cat, although the sheep and rabbit have almost no adrenergic innervation to the vessels; it innervates the parenchyma almost exclusively.

Guinea pigs have an almost exclusive adrenergic innervation to blood vessels and nothing to the parenchymal cells. In a species like the cow, there is no serotonin in the pineal and almost no adrenergic innervation at all in the gland, whereas the pig pineal, also with a very scarce adrenergic innervation, has huge amounts of serotonin.

The question is whether the conclusions drawn from experiments on one species, for example the rat, can be transferred to another species with completely different adrenergic innervation of the gland and amine concentrations in the parenchymal cells. In these respects the ferret pineal appears to resemble the rat pineal, with rather high amounts of serotonin,

or an indole, in the parenchymal cells and apparently an adrenergic innervation both to the vascular tree and to the parenchymal cells.

Herbert: I think not to the parenchymal cells; as far as we could see, it is
largely confined to the perivascular space, and preliminary electron
microscopic studies confirm this. Incidentally, it always seems to me that
the perivascular space is a peculiar place to have a nerve ending if you want
the latter to affect synthesis in the cell.

Owman: How do you explain the effect of ganglionectomy on the
pineal if you have no innervation of the parenchymal cells?

Herbert: The parenchymal cell processes and the autonomic nerve
endings are present together in the perivascular space.

Kordon: Coming back to Dr Wurtman's suggestion, F. Gogan from our
laboratory (1968) has shown that in a seasonal breeder like the duck,
hypothalamic thresholds to steroid feedback can undergo wide cyclic
variations; these variations seem to be light-dependent. By analogy, this
might support the idea that the sensitivity of neural structures towards
substances like melatonin can be affected by diurnal or seasonal variations.

We are very much interested by two of Dr Herbert's observations:
first, the opposite effects of pinealectomy in the ferret to those obtained in
most other species—an observation which has also been made, I think, in
the quail (Sayler and Wolfson 1968). Second, the fact that the effects of
pinealectomy are not completely reversible by giving melatonin. These
facts suggest the involvement of other pineal factors—the stimulatory
fraction described by Moszkowska, Ebels and Scemama (1965) in the first
case, and possibly non-indoleaminergic fractions in the latter—so that the
pineal of the ferret might be good material to make pineal fractionations.

Would you agree with the speculation that, among the different pineal
factors which have been described, some (for instance melatonin, or
stimulatory pineal principles) might have a predominant importance in
some species, whereas other factors might be more important in other
animals?

Herbert: Yes. The quail is somewhat similar to the ferret, but like many
other birds its reproductive cycle is much more dependent on light than
the ferret's. For example, quail kept on short days remain more or less
permanently anoestrous, or if males, in reproductive quiescence. This is
not so in many mammals, including the ferret (D. S. Vincent, unpublished).
Unfortunately, the evidence is that removing the pineal of the quail has
no effect on adults; they still come into oestrus or into reproductive condition if you put them into long days. This may be correlated with the
fact that, in birds, pineal enzymes (e.g. HIOMT) are found elsewhere than
in the pineal. But in young quail, the advancement of puberty which

occurs after putting them into long days seems to be at least partly inhibited by taking the pineal out (Sayler and Wolfson 1968).

REFERENCES

COLLIN, J. P. (1969) *Annls Stn Biol. Besse-en-Chandesse* suppl. 1, 1–359.

FISKE, V. M. and HUPPERT, L. C. (1968) *Science* **162,** 279.

GOGAN, F. (1968) *Gen. comp. Endocr.* **11,** 316.

KAPPERS, J. A. (1960) *Z. Zellforsch. mikrosk. Anat.* **52,** 163–215.

KENNY, G. C. T. (1961) *J. Neuropath. exp. Neurol.* **20,** 563–570.

MEINIEL, A. (1970) *J. Neuro-visc. Rel.* in press.

MITCHELL, R. (1963) *J. comp. Neurol.* **121,** 441–453.

MOSZKOWSKA, A., EBELS, I. and SCEMAMA, A. (1965) *C.r. Séanc. Soc. Biol.* **159,** 2298.

OWMAN, CH. (1965) In *Structure and Function of the Epiphysis Cerebri* (*Progress in Brain Research* vol. 10), pp. 423–453, ed. Kappers, J. A. and Schadé, J. P. Amsterdam: Elsevier.

OWMAN, CH. (1968) *Adv. Pharmac.* **6A,** 167–169.

ROUSSY, G. and MOSINGER, M. (1964) *Traité de neuroendocrinologie.* Paris: Masson.

RÜDEBERG, C. (1969) *Z. Zellforsch. mikrosk. Anat.* **96,** 548–581.

SAYLER, A. and WOLFSON, A. (1968) *Endocrinology* **83,** 1237–1246.

UECK, M. (1970) *Z. Zellforsch. mikrosk. Anat.* **105,** 276–302.

VIVIEN, J. H. and ROELS, B. (1968) *C.r. hebd. Séanc. Acad. Sci., Paris, Sér.* D **266,** 600–603.

FACTORS INFLUENTIAL IN DETERMINING THE GONAD-INHIBITING ACTIVITY OF THE PINEAL GLAND

Russel J. Reiter and Sandy Sorrentino, Jr.

Department of Anatomy, School of Medicine and Dentistry, University of Rochester, Rochester, New York

Animals vary considerably in the apparent sensitivity of their reproductive organs to the antagonistic action of the pineal gland when the latter is stimulated by light deprivation. In this regard, the neuroendocrine–gonadal axis of the golden hamster (*Mesocricetus auratus*) is considerably more labile than is this system in the albino rat (Reiter and Sorrentino 1970). An adequate explanation for the relative insensitivity of the hypothalamo-hypophysio-gonadal system in the albino rat to the activated pineal has not been provided, although a number of possible explanations have been advanced.

There are also differences in the reaction of the gonads of rats to the pineal according to their age. It is generally considered that the pituitary–gonadal axis of the maturing rat is more easily suppressed by the pineal or by pineal substances than is this system in adult animals. This difference is possibly due to the greater sensitivity of the hypothalamic feedback "centres" of immature animals to circulating hormones, both gonadal and extra-gonadal. At puberty, when the hypothalamic setpoint is adjusted to a higher level (that is, the nervous system becomes less sensitive) the ability of the pineal to interfere with gonadal functions becomes less pronounced. Thus, it is speculated that although the pineal in the adult rat maintains a high level of activity, the cells affected are more resistant to its hormonal products.

The purpose of the present report is to discuss experimental conditions under which the genital apparatus even of adult rats may be induced to atrophy under the influence of the pineal. Specifically, the mechanisms by which certain manipulations potentiate the gonad-inhibiting ability of the pineal are not understood. The list of potentiating agents is, however, becoming more extensive and undoubtedly others will be discovered. The ones considered here are those on which the most information is presently available.

ANOSMIA

Animals display a varying degree of dependency on olfactory stimuli for the maintenance of reproductive activity. It is usually considered that the olfactory sense merely serves to guide sexual behaviour. In some mice, however, olfaction plays a more central role in determining reproductive performance (Bronson 1968). In fact, Whitten (1956) observed involution of the ovaries and uteri of virgin female mice six weeks after surgical removal of the olfactory bulbs. Rats, on the other hand, experience fewer gonadal alterations after extirpation of the olfactory bulbs; Aron, Roas and Asch (1970) noted no disturbance in the frequency of spontaneous ovulation in anosmic rats although the ovaries of such animals may show slight morphological changes (Balboni 1967; Aron, Roas and Asch 1970). Reproductively, male rats seem to suffer little after removal of the olfactory bulbs (Reiter, Klein and Donofrio 1969).

There was virtually no evidence available which suggested a functional interplay between the olfactory system and the pineal gland until Miline, Devečerski and Krstić (1963) found that long-term olfactory stimulation led to rather striking changes in the pinealocytes; the changes observed were atrophic in nature and were exemplified by the reduction in the nuclear and nucleolar volumes. Prompted by these studies and the previously discussed work on olfactory–genital interactions, we investigated the gonad-inhibiting potential of the pineal in anosmic rats that were also deprived of light; the latter procedure was used as a stimulus for pineal activation (Wurtman, Axelrod and Kelly 1968). The combined operation of removal of the eyes and the olfactory bulbs resulted in a severe retardation in the growth of the reproductive organs and in the onset of puberty in both male (Reiter, Klein and Donofrio 1969) and female (Reiter and Ellison 1970) rats. When done singly, neither operation caused any pronounced delays in the sexual maturation of the animals. Removal of the pineal (also performed at 21 days of age) reversed nearly completely the atrophic response of the reproductive organs to combined blinding and anosmia.

The mechanisms whereby anosmia exaggerates the ability of eyelessness to induce gonadal regression are unknown, but several possible explanations exist. First, anosmia may further stimulate (in addition to the stimulation caused by blinding) the pineal to produce and secrete gonad-inhibiting factors. Secondly, the loss of olfaction may lower the threshold of sensitivity of the cells which are normally inhibited by the pineal substances. Thirdly, since both sight and smell are important for food intake, possibly the loss of both senses depressed food consumption to a level where malnourishment sensitized the pituitary–gonadal axis to the pineal antigonadotropic factor. Finally, dual sensory deprivation may have been such a severe stress that the gonads underwent a secondary atrophic response.

To check the validity of the first explanation, namely, stimulation of the pineal synthetic activity by anosmia, we measured the conversion of N-acetylserotonin to melatonin by determining concentrations of hydroxyindole-O-methyltransferase (HIOMT) in pineals of rats from which both olfactory bulbs had been removed. Compared to normal controls, the activity of this enzyme was not accentuated in anosmic rats with eyes. Furthermore, HIOMT levels in pineals of blinded, anosmic rats were not significantly higher than in animals that were blinded only (Reiter, Klein and Donofrio 1969; Reiter and Ellison 1970).

As an additional measure of pineal activity in anosmic rats, the amount of melatonin in pineals of such animals was quantitatively determined using a sensitive bioassay which was recently perfected by Ralph and Lynch (1970). In this method, melatonin is detected by measuring the dermal melanophore contraction in the skin of larval *Rana pipiens*. In both untreated and anosmic rats killed during the day, pineal melatonin was undetectable; when the animals were sacrificed during darkness, however, the quantities of melatonin in pineals of non-blinded and anosmic rats were readily measurable and the levels were similar in the two groups. Finally, the pineals of blinded and of blinded, anosmic rats contained equivalent amounts of melatonin.

Thus, judging from the levels of HIOMT activity and from the actual amounts of melatonin within the pineals of anosmic rats, it would appear that removal of the olfactory bulbs has little influence on the antigonado-tropic potential of the pineal. Inherent in this speculation, however, is the assumption that melatonin is *the* gonad-inhibiting factor derived from the pineal. Additional caution is warranted, since we know little about the factors which influence the secretory rate of pineal products.

The second possible explanation of how anosmia potentiates the gonad-inhibiting influence of the pineal in eyeless rats is less easily tested. Since axons of neurons located within the olfactory bulbs are widely distributed throughout the limbic system, including the hypothalamus (Scott and Pfaffmann 1967; Heimer 1968), and because the interruption of efferent olfactory pathways leads to chemical changes in various parts of the brain (Pohorecky, Larin and Wurtman 1969), it is difficult to predict the site at which anosmia may sensitize (lower the threshold of) the neuroendocrine axis to the pineal factors. The most frequently mentioned neural loci of action of the pineal inhibitory substances include the midbrain and medial basal hypothalamus (Antón-Tay *et al.* 1968; Fraschini, Mess and Martini 1968).

That a depression of food consumption in rats deprived of both their eyes and their olfactory bulbs may be operative in initiating gonadal changes seems unlikely in view of the following observations. In a recently

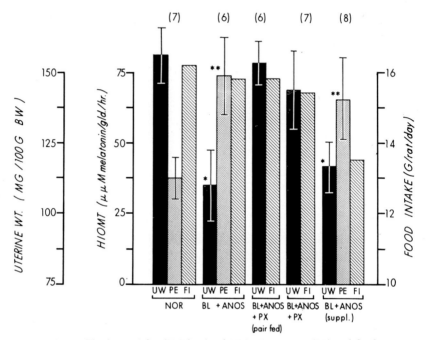

FIG. 1. Uterine weights (UW), pineal HIOMT content (PE) and food intake (FI) in five groups of adult female rats. Groups are numbered I to V from left to right. Animals of group III were pair-fed with those of group II. The rats of group V were given daily, in addition to the normal dry laboratory chow, the outer leaves of green lettuce (suppl.); supplementing the normal chow diet in this group accounts for the decrease in food intake which these animals showed; that is, the decrease in the amount of dry laboratory chow eaten. Vertical lines at the top of the bars signify the standard deviations. Number of animals per group is in parentheses at top. Animals were killed after 8 weeks of treatment. *, $P < 0.001$ compared with normal controls; **, $P < 0.05$ compared with normal controls. NOR, untreated rats; BL, blinded; ANOS, anosmic; PX, pinealectomized.

completed experiment, blinded, anosmic rats that were also pinealecto-mized were pair-fed with non-pinealectomized animals that also could neither see nor smell (Fig. 1). Throughout the duration of the study (8 weeks), the doubly sensorily deprived rats ate an amount of food (Purina laboratory chow) equivalent to that of unoperated controls, yet the uteri of these animals regressed markedly. The pair-fed animals which lacked a pineal maintained normal reproductive organ weights. Supplementing the diet of blinded, anosmic rats with fresh green lettuce did not ameliorate the uterine regression (Fig. 1). These data show that rats deprived of these two senses do not characteristically eat less than unoperated controls and thus reduced food intake does not account for the reproductive changes seen in animals treated in this manner. Food restriction may, in fact, act as a potentiating agent for the pineal; this subject is discussed later.

The final possibility is that blinded, anosmic animals were so severely stressed that the gonads degenerated secondarily. This proposition was not supported by observations of the pituitary–adrenal axis. The operations did not constitute a chronic stress to the animals since the adrenals were normal in size at the termination of the experiment (Reiter, Sorrentino and Ellison 1970). Furthermore, we have been unable to detect a significant change either in the basal levels of plasma corticosterone or in the diurnal variation in the levels of this constituent in the blood after blinding and removal of the olfactory bulbs (unpublished observations).

POSTNATAL HORMONE TREATMENT

The administration of either testosterone, oestrogen or stilboestrol to newborn rats interferes with the subsequent maturation of the hypothalamus and preoptic area (Gorski 1963; Barraclough 1967). In female rats, this treatment causes "masculinization" of the neural centres which regulate the cyclic release of gonadotropins; the effects in the male are much more subtle but, nevertheless, are detrimental to the growth of the reproductive organs. The most obvious untoward effects caused by the injection of these compounds usually are not apparent until after the animals reach puberty. Adult females, which had been exposed to exogenous hormones during the early postnatal period, exhibit persistent vaginal oestrus; concomitant with the vaginal cornification is the occurrence of stratified squamous metaplasia of the uterine epithelium (Reiter 1969a), a continual succession of large ovarian follicles, failure of ovulation and a lack of corpora lutea (Barraclough 1961; Gorski 1966). Males, under these conditions, have much smaller testes and accessory organs which also may exhibit meagre histological changes (Jacobsohn and Norgren 1965).

Several years ago, Kordon and co-workers (Kordon and Hoffmann 1967; Hoffmann, Kordon and Benoit 1968) observed that exposure of early androgen-treated male or female rats to nearly complete darkness drastically restricted the development of the reproductive organs and suppressed the changes that were characteristically associated with postnatal hormone treatment. These results seemed to be an obvious expression of an inhibition of the sexual organs by the activated pineal gland; when experimentally tested this proved to be the case. If female rats were sub-cutaneously injected with 1 mg of testosterone propionate (TP) when 5 days old and subjected to bilateral orbital enucleation 15 days later, the ovaries and uteri grew at a slower rate than normal and were generally infantile when the rats normally would have attained adulthood (Reiter 1970). Ovaries of animals treated in this manner contained reduced numbers of vesicular follicles, no corpora lutea and modest amounts of interstitial tissue; moreover, the frequency of cornified vaginal smears was

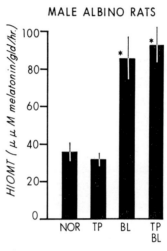

MALE ALBINO RATS

FIG. 2. Amounts of the melatonin-forming enzyme, hydroxyindole-O-methyltransferase (HIOMT), in pineals of male rats killed at 60 days of age. Vertical lines at top of bars indicate standard errors. Asterisks indicate values that differ significantly ($P < 0.001$) from those of un-treated control rats. Eight to 10 pineals per group. NOR, untreated animals; TP, animals subcutaneously injected with 1 mg testosterone propionate at 5 days of age; BL, rats that were blinded at 21 days of age.

reduced by 50 per cent (Reiter 1970), as was the incidence of uterine meta-plasia (Reiter 1969a). If such animals were either pinealectomized, or superior-cervical-ganglionectomized, all the signs of androgen-sterilization developed. Surgical removal of the superior cervical ganglia is usually equivalent to removal of the pineal itself (Reiter 1969b), since the essential innervation of the pineal is derived from these structures (Kappers 1969).

In male rats, as in females, the combination of early hormone treatment (either TP or oestradiol benzoate) and extirpation of the eyes markedly curtails the growth of the testes, the development of the germinal epi-thelium and the maturation of the interstitial cells (Reiter 1969b). These changes are overcome if the pineal gland is either ablated or denervated.

With regard to the degree of reproductive inhibition, early hormone treatment seems to be as effective as anosmia in potentiating the action of the pineal. As in the case of olfactory bulb removal, we have attempted to define whether TP exaggerates the pineal effect by acting directly on this organ or by an indirect action at another site. The results of a typical experiment are summarized in Fig. 2. The activity of the melatonin-forming enzyme was ascertained in pineals of four groups of male rats. As can be seen, TP treatment alone had no significant stimulatory influence on

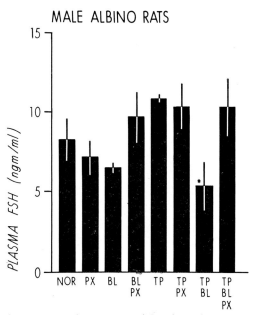

FIG. 3. Plasma FSH values, measured by the radioimmunoassay, in eight groups of male rats. Vertical lines at top of bars signify standard errors. All animals were killed at 60 days of age. Asterisk indicates mean which differed significantly ($P < 0.01$) from other groups that were treated with testosterone propionate. NOR, untreated animals; PX, pinealectomized; BL, blinded; TP, early postnatal treatment with 1 mg of testosterone propionate.

the ability of the pineal to produce melatonin. Likewise, the amount of enzyme in pineals of TP-treated, eyeless rats was not significantly different from that in animals that only lacked eyes, yet the reproductive organs of the former were infantile. These preliminary data led us to predict that treatment with TP, like the loss of smell, probably does not potentiate the pineal effect by acting directly on the organ itself (Reiter and Fraschini 1969). The same qualifications noted earlier in the discussion of anosmia apply to the speculations made here.

Considering the obvious decremental changes which the gonads undergo as a result of these treatments, one might anticipate equally apparent alterations in the pituitary and plasma levels of gonadotropins. Application of the radioimmunoassay technique to the measurement of plasma and pituitary concentrations of FSH and LH has yielded some worthwhile, but occasionally confusing, information. As an example, in a recently completed study it was found that the combination of TP administration and blinding insignificantly lowered plasma and pituitary levels of LH; this failure to induce a statistically significant change occurred in both sexes despite the fact that gonads were obviously hypotrophic. If we accept the idea that the pineal acts at the neural level to inhibit gonadotropins (Quay 1969; Reiter and Fraschini 1969), an alteration in the amount of LH would be expected. Findings such as these tend to complicate discussion of probable sites of action of the pineal substances. Under the same experimental conditions, plasma and pituitary levels of FSH were investigated. Again, neither sex showed any appreciable decline in the hypophysial content of FSH although, in males, the plasma concentration of this substance was significantly decreased after TP treatment and blinding (Fig. 3). Theoretically, studies on the amounts of the gonadotropins in the blood should distinguish between central and peripheral sites of action of the pineal substances, but, to date, results from our laboratory have been inconsistent.

NUTRITION

There are indications that nutrition may have a role in determining either the activity of the pineal gland or the sensitivity of the reproductive system to the gonad-inhibiting capacity of the pineal. Křeček and Palatý (1967) alluded to this in a recent paper. These workers reported that weaning male rats at 16 days of age (premature weaning) caused the weights of the seminal vesicles and the citric acid concentration of the same organs to be greatly depressed at the time the animals were killed (30–100 days of age). By comparison, prematurely weaned rats that had been pinealectomized (at 1 day of age) had seminal vesicles which were normal in both their size and citric acid content; this latter group was compared with normally weaned (21 days) males that had been sham-pinealectomized. Pinealectomy in normally weaned rats did not augment seminal vesicle weight or its citric acid content. The implication of these results is that the gonads of the prematurely weaned rats were more sensitive than normal to the pineal gland because they were undernourished for an indefinite time after being taken from their mothers.

In our laboratory as well, evidence has been accumulated which shows that undernourishment renders albino rats highly sensitive to the anti-gonadal factor from the pineal gland (Sorrentino, Reiter and Schalch 1970). Limiting the food intake (50 per cent of normal) of developing male rats, between the ages of 25 and 60 days, moderately depressed the maturation of the reproductive organs; when underfeeding was combined with light deprivation (blinding) the testes and accessory sex organs were approximately one-third and one-fifteenth their normal sizes, respectively. The marked lag in the development of the reproductive system in the latter group involved the pineal, since similarly treated rats that lacked a pineal had sexual glands that were consistently and significantly larger than those in underfed, eyeless animals. In this regard it may also be significant that the hypotrophic ovaries and uteri of underfed rats are stimulated to grow to their normal sizes by exposure of the animals to continuous illumination (Piacsek and Meites 1968), a known inhibitor of pineal function. To be more conservative, however, it should be remembered that not all of the sexual effects of constant light involve the pineal gland (Reiter and Fraschini 1969).

Experiments on the vole (*Microtus montanus*) have lent support to the idea that nutrition may have an influence on reproduction by way of the pineal. The studies referred to, however, indicate that the quality, in addition to the quantity, of the food may also be important (Pinter and Negus 1965; Negus and Pinter 1966). The reproductive organs of the meadow vole are sensitive both to the photoperiod and to dietary factors. Long daily periods of light (18 hours per day) stimulate growth of the reproductive system (Pinter and Negus 1965). Likewise, supplementing the diet with fresh green plants also stimulates the growth of the sexual organs of this species (Negus and Pinter 1966). It seems likely that the stimulatory effect of light is mediated through the pineal gland, but the question arose whether similar mechanisms were operative after dietary supplementation.

Dr Negus (personal communication) has recently informed us of the results of several experiments which were designed to test this possibility. Voles, which are strict herbivores, were fed Purina rabbit chow; experimental animals were fed the same diet but they received, additionally, the outer leaves of head lettuce. Equal numbers of control and experimental voles were placed in environments which provided either 8, 12 or 16 hours of illumination ("cool white" fluorescent lamps with an intensity of about 250 foot-candles) per 24-hour period. Regardless of the photoperiod conditions, supplementing the diet with lettuce resulted in significantly smaller pineal glands and larger reproductive organs. Furthermore, Negus noted that pineals of animals that received the supplement exhibited a 25 per cent reduction in HIOMT activity when compared to those of non-supplemented controls.

Undoubtedly, there are other potentiators of pineal function, for example possibly stress, reduced ambient temperature and hormonal feedback (Reiter and Fraschini 1969), but the evidence is too tenuous at this time to justify an extensive discussion. Of those we have considered here, namely anosmia, treatment with testosterone propionate and alterations in nutrition, not all can be considered to be normal modulators of pineal function but they may yield clues to the mechanisms and/or loci of action of pineal substances. It is certainly conceivable that under normal environmental conditions, more than the ambient photoperiod controls the gonad-inhibiting ability of the pineal.

Consider for example, animals in their natural habitat. In the fall of the year these animals are subjected to a variety of environmental changes, a number of which may assist in causing gonadal regression and several of which may accomplish this by acting, either directly or indirectly, through the pineal gland. Decreasing length of the photoperiod may in itself, at least in some species, be insufficient to induce total gonadal involution. Thus, reproductive regression may ensue only when the combination of circumstances is such that the pineal gland is active and the affected neural structures are sufficiently sensitive to become inhibited by the pineal substances. On this basis, it is not even necessary to assume that the activity of the pineal changes with the season of the year; it could be that the level of reproductive function is determined by the threshold of sensitivity of the neuroendocrine axis, merely being lower in winter than in summer.

This theory, as stated, is not applicable to all species, however. Some animals breed during seasons of the year when the length of daily illumination is the shortest while the midpoint of anoestrum coincides with the longest days of the year (Everett 1961). For the most part, the season of the year in which animals breed is dictated by the duration of gestation, since it is imperative that the young be born at a time that is conducive to optimal growth and maturation, namely in the spring. Because of this, some animals breed in the winter. Does this mean that the pineal is not involved in regulating the reproductive cycles in these species? Possibly in these animals short photoperiods are inhibitory rather than stimulatory to the pineal; this idea is not new since in some diurnal animals this is, in fact, the case (Wurtman, Axelrod and Kelly 1968). It is also not unlikely that in some animals the primary regulation of the pineal gland may be assumed by factors such as humidity, availability of food or water, and temperature.

Delayed implantation is another ploy by which animals may assure that their litters are born during the spring. In at least one species, the pineal may also be involved in this process. The western spotted skunk (*Spilogale putorius*), for example, breeds in September but nidation does not occur until the following April and the young are born about 1 month later (Mead 1969). The time of implantation can be advanced by exposing the animals to long daily photoperiods (14 hours of light per day) while nidation can be delayed even further by depriving the animals of photic stimuli. These data are strongly suggestive of an involvement of the pineal gland in the response.

Hence, it appears that light may operate in any of a number of ways to regulate reproduction. In this regard it should be realized that visible radiation has, with few exceptions (Wurtman and Weisel 1969), been considered only in its most general form. We must begin to look at lighting intensity and different wavelengths of light in relation to pineal function. The former may be particularly important in nocturnal animals that are also burrow dwellers. Also, the view that photic stimuli are the exclusive impellers of pineal function should be scrutinized. Finally, it must be borne in mind that a host of other factors may be important in determining, indirectly, the gonad-inhibiting capability of the pineal gland.

SUMMARY

The importance of qualitative and quantitative nutritional factors, anosmia and early postnatal hormone treatment in potentiating the anti-gonadotropic activity of the pineal gland has been considered. With one possible exception (quality of nutrition), it is surmised that these factors do not directly alter pineal biosynthetic or secretory activity but, presumably, act in an indirect manner to render the neuroendocrine axis highly susceptible to pineal substances. Under natural conditions, it is assumed that a host of external factors interact to regulate seasonal reproductive cycles, and gonadal regression (or, for that matter, regeneration) ensues only after all exteroceptive stimuli have been evaluated and summated. One important exteroceptive factor is environmental illumination (or lack of it) which, at least partially, influences reproduction by way of the pineal gland. It is not likely that this paper has exhausted the list of potentiating agents.

Acknowledgements

The authors are grateful to Dr C. L. Ralph and Dr H. J. Lynch for the assays of pineal melatonin and to Dr Robert Y. Moore for some of the HIOMT assays. The expert technical assistance of Mrs Anna Chornobil and Miss Ellen Jarrow is acknowledged. Work by the authors was supported by Grant HD-02937, U.S.P.H.S. and by a General Research Support

Grant from the University of Rochester. The first author is a U.S.P.H.S. Career Development Awardee (1 KO4 HD42398) and the second author is a U.S.P.H.S. Postdoctoral Fellow (1F024042856).

REFERENCES

Antón-Tay, F., Chou, C., Anton, S. and Wurtman, R. J. (1968) Science 162, 277.
Aron, C., Roas, J. and Asch, G. (1970) Neuroendocrinology 6, 109.
Balboni, G. C. (1967) Bull. Ass. Anat., Paris, 52, 160.
Barraclough, C. A. (1961) Endocrinology 68, 62.
Barraclough, C. A. (1967) Neuroendocrinology 2, 61–99.
Bronson, F. H. (1968) In Perspectives in Reproduction and Sexual Behavior, pp. 341–361, ed. Diamond, M. Bloomington: Indiana University Press.
Everett, J. W. (1961) In Sex and Internal Secretions vol. 1, pp. 497–555, ed. Young, W. C. and Corner, G. W. Baltimore: Williams and Wilkins.
Fraschini, F., Mess, B. and Martini, L. (1968) Endocrinology 82, 919.
Gorski, R. A. (1963) Am. J. Physiol. 205, 842.
Gorski, R. A. (1966) J. Reprod. Fert. suppl. 1, 67.
Heimer, L. (1968) J. Anat. 103, 413.
Hoffmann, J. C., Kordon, C. and Benoit, J. (1968) Gen. comp. Endocr. 10, 109.
Jacobsohn, D. and Norgren, A. (1965) Acta endocr., Copenh. 49, 453.
Kappers, J. A. (1969) J. Neuro-visc. Rel. suppl. IX, 140.
Kordon, C. and Hoffmann, J. C. (1967) C. r. Séanc. Soc. Biol. 161, 1262.
Křeček, J. and Palatý, V. (1967) Gen. comp. Endocr. 9, 466.
Mead, R. (1969) In Program of the Second Annual Meeting of the Society for the Study of Reproduction. p. 4.
Miline, R., Devečerski, V. and Krstić, R. (1963) Annls Endocr. 24, 377.
Negus, N. C. and Pinter, A. J. (1966) J. Mammal. 47, 596.
Piacsek, B. E. and Meites, J. (1968) Endocrinology 81, 493.
Pinter, A. J. and Negus, N. C. (1965) Am. J. Physiol. 208, 633.
Pohorecky, L. A., Larin, F. and Wurtman, R. J. (1969) Life Sci. 8, 1309.
Quay, W. B. (1969) Gen. comp. Endocr. suppl. 2, 101.
Ralph, C. L. and Lynch, H. J. (1970) Gen. comp. Endocr. 15, 334.
Reiter, R. J. (1969a) Anat. Rec. 164, 479.
Reiter, R. J. (1969b) In Progress in Endocrinology (Proc. III Int. Congr. Endocrinology), pp. 631–636, ed. Gual, C. Excerpta Medica International Congress Series no. 184. Amsterdam: Excerpta Medica Foundation.
Reiter, R. J. (1970) Acta endocr., Copenh. 63, 667.
Reiter, R. J. and Ellison, N. M. (1970) Biol. Reprod. 2, 216.
Reiter, R. J. and Fraschini, F. (1969) Neuroendocrinology 5, 219.
Reiter, R. J., Klein, D. C. and Donofrio, R. J. (1969) J. Reprod. Fert. 19, 563.
Reiter, R. J. and Sorrentino, S. Jr. (1970) Am. Zool. 10, 247.
Reiter, R. J., Sorrentino, S. Jr. and Ellison, N. M. (1970) Gen comp. Endocr. 15, 326.
Scott, J. W. and Pfaffmann, C. (1967) Science 158, 1592.
Sorrentino, S. Jr., Reiter, R. J. and Schalch, D. C. (1970) Neuroendocrinology in press.
Whitten, W. F. (1956) J. Endocr. 14, 160.
Wurtman, R. J., Axelrod, J. and Kelly, D. E. (1968) The Pineal. New York and London: Academic Press.
Wurtman, R. J. and Weisel, J. (1969) Endocrinology 85, 1218.

DISCUSSION

Mess: Dr Reiter, did you say that pinealectomy does not influence the depressive effect on the ovaries of giving oestrogens early in life?

Reiter: That is correct. Pinealectomy does not reverse the inhibitory effect of early hormone treatment on ovarian weight.

Mess: The decrease of ovarian weight after early androgen or oestrogen treatment might be due, as you have said, to the lack of corpora lutea, which itself is due to reduced LH production, as our experiments on animals with anterior hypothalamic lesions also showed. I don't find a parallelism between the two different types of anovulatory syndrome—that is, between your neonatally oestrogen- or androgen-treated rats and ours with superior hypothalamic lesions—as regards the response in weight and histology of the ovaries following pinealectomy.

Reiter: In your experiments the animals were pinealectomized as adults, and of course they ovulated within 12 days. Ours were pinealectomized at 21 days of age and killed after adulthood.

Wurtman: I wonder about the extent to which diurnal rhythms in plasma FSH or LH in animals that have not received testosterone or oestradiol might obscure whatever changes pinealectomy could produce? And not only diurnal rhythms but the recently discovered hourly rhythm in plasma LH levels in gonadectomized animals (Dierschke *et al.* 1970).

Reiter: Such rhythms could account for our results. We have variations within the groups which invalidate the statistical analyses, although levels always tended to be lower in the rats with small reproductive organs. The other conclusion would be that the site of action of the pineal substances is at the level of the gonads and thus plasma levels of hormones could be comparable in all groups. I personally find the peripheral site of action of pineal substances difficult to accept.

Martini: Dr Reiter, you are talking about a potentiating effect and you believe that this takes place somewhere in the brain? This pleases me very much, because my laboratory was the first to suggest that endocrine effects of the pineal hormones might all be mediated by the brain. I wonder whether this potentiating action might not be interpreted as due to some modification in the biochemistry of the hypothalamus or of the midbrain? Anosmia might modify brain stores of serotonin or of catecholamines.

Reiter: This has been done in Dr Wurtman's laboratory, of course! Anosmia and/or removal of the olfactory bulbs in rats causes widespread biochemical changes in the brain, including an increase in noradrenaline concentrations in the brainstem (Pohorecky *et al.* 1969).

Kordon: Dr Reiter, if I understood you properly, you interpret the effect of pinealectomy in your blinded animals as a removal of the high turnover of melatonin caused by blinding. I wonder whether another interpretation could not also be relevant. Neuroendocrine structures in the hypothalamus receive quite a variety of inputs, which they have to integrate in order to maintain the hormonostatic regulation of the animal. In species like the rat, the hormonostatic regulation is very rigid; that means that when you suppress one stimulus, or one input to the hypo-thalamus, the remaining inputs are able to compensate for the one you have removed; so that you have to disconnect most of the afferent stimuli to make the remaining ones really determinant for the hormonostatic regulation. For instance, in the rat, blinding alone is not enough to depress gonadotropic secretion significantly; you need additional treatments to obtain this effect, as for instance an interference with normal feedback mechanisms by postnatal testosterone treatment or possibly removal of the olfactory bulbs, as you reported, where no direct pineal involvement appears likely. In contrast to this, the hormonostatic regulation appears looser or less feedback-dependent in seasonal breeders, which exhibit much larger cyclic variations in gonadotropic secretion. In this situation, each particular stimulus or input has a greater relative importance. Could that not be the case in your blinded hamsters?

Reiter: Generally, I agree but I don't exactly see how it applies in the present case.

Herbert: Following Dr Kordon's point about species differences in stimuli, I would like to draw a parallel between findings on the pineal and those on sexual behaviour. In the two apparently very closely related species, the rat and the hamster, there is no doubt that olfaction plays a very large part in the sexual activity of both species. If you remove the olfactory bulb in the rat the effect on sexual activity is not particularly profound, but in the hamster sexual activity is completely abolished. This seems to bear out Dr Kordon's point about the number of different inputs and the relative importance of each in a given species when you remove one.

Miline: Two important reflexes influence the gonads, the opto-sexual reflex described by Benoit (1954) and the olfacto-sexual reflex (Aron and Aron 1950; Bruce 1967). The pineal gland and the rhinencephalon function in an integrated way. When the medial forebrain bundle is cut this integrity is disturbed, including the correlated circuits of the hippo-campus, amygdala and habenular nuclei. There are connexions between the rhinencephalon and the hypothalamus (Collin 1937). Have you seen any change in the hippocampus or in the habenular ganglion after these experiments? Secondly, do you think that the sensitivity of the pineal gland after removal of the olfactory lobes means that the connexions from the pineal to the hypothalamus are more sensitive than in normal rats?

Reiter: Yes; that, in essence, is what I meant. With regard to changes in the temporal lobes or the habenular nuclei after removing the olfactory bulbs, we did no biochemical studies on these regions, but we did look at some of the brains microscopically. We do not see any obvious structural alterations.

Kordon: You reported very nice experiments with the "Halasz type" hypothalamic cuts. Did you also study the effects of pinealectomy in animals with a complete hypothalamic deafferentation? This could tell us whether pineal factors are able to affect the hypothalamus directly without involvement of a neural relay.

Reiter: As you know, in the hamster all you have to do is blind the animal and the gonads atrophy; this is prevented by pinealectomy or superior cervical ganglionectomy (Reiter 1970). If we do a total hypothalamic de-afferentation in hamsters and blind them, the reproductive organs do not regress. There are several interpretations, one of which is that the site of action of the pineal substance is outside the hypothalamic cut and that we are cutting the axons of neurons that are normally inhibited by the pineal.

Kordon: What is the effect of the cut without blinding?

Reiter: Hypothalamic deafferentation has very little effect on the adult male hamster; in the male rat there is a slight depression of the weight of the accessory sex organs, but the animals are otherwise quite normal reproductively.

Wurtman: If you give melatonin to either the pinealectomized group or the pinealectomized and blinded group, does it have any inhibiting effect?

Reiter: In the hamster we have implanted melatonin in beeswax and, in other experiments, injected melatonin subcutaneously and we have never observed an inhibitory influence on reproduction. In immature rats we do get an effect with melatonin implanted in beeswax pellets; the onset of puberty is delayed. We get no effect with daily subcutaneous adminis-tration. Why specifically we don't get a response to melatonin in the hamster I don't know.

Wurtman: It would be interesting to see whether if you transect the fibres running from the raphe nucleus to the hypothalamus in the rat you would still observe effects of melatonin on puberty.

Martini: I am excited by these results. You find that a complete "hypo-thalamic deafferentation" has the same effect as pinealectomy. Your "hypothalamic deafferentation" interrupts all fibres coming from outside the hypothalamus; consequently the hypothalamus will no longer have nerve terminals rich in serotonin and catecholamines. It seems to me that your data are a further proof of the hypothesis put forward by Dr Motta at this meeting, namely that melatonin operates through an effect on aminergic mechanisms in the hypothalamus (see pp. 279–291).

Owman: We have recently published a study on the inputs into the pituitary system (Björklund *et al.* 1970). Five groups of monoamine-containing axons were seen to enter the median eminence and the neuro-intermediate lobe: a large group of dopamine axons, a large group of noradrenaline axons, two minor groups of catecholamine axons and a small group of scattered axons containing an unidentified fluorogenic substance. The fibres reached the basal hypothalamus by various pathways; some fibres entered the neural and intermediate lobe of the pituitary, some of them innervating cells in the intermediate lobe, some running to structures of unknown identity in the neural lobe.

Martini: In animals with a complete "hypothalamic deafferentation" there is no diurnal variation in plasma corticosterone levels; corticoids are rather high throughout the day (Halasz 1969). The suggestion again is that melatonin normally released by the pineal gland cannot cause the usual reduction of plasma corticosterone levels in the "deafferented" animals because their hypothalami are devoid of monoamine stores.

Wurtman: This is compatible with the studies of Steiner, Akert and Ruf (1969) and others on hypothalamic neurons whose physiological activity is inhibited by both dexamethasone and catecholamines.

Fraschini: What is known about effects of the pineal on growth hormone?

Reiter: We found that blinding depressed pituitary growth hormone in 60-day-old rats, and this effect was reversed by pinealectomy, as was the depression of growth hormone in blinded, anosmic rats. We detected no statistically significant changes in plasma growth hormone levels after any of the treatments (Sorrentino, Reiter and Schalch 1970).

REFERENCES

ARON, M. and ARON, C. (1950) *Eléments d'endocrinologie physiologique.* Paris: Masson.
BENOIT, J. (1954) *Bull. Acad. Natn. Méd.* **138,** 32–36.
BJÖRKLUND, A., FALCK, B., HROMEK, F., OWMAN, CH. and WEST, K. A. (1970) *Brain Res.* **17,** 1–23.
BRUCE, H. M. (1967) *Ciba Fdn Study Group No. 26 Effects of External Stimuli on Reproduction,* pp. 29–38. London: Churchill.
COLLIN, R. (1937) *L'innervation de la glande pituitaire.* Paris: Hermann.
DIERSCHKE, D. J., BHATTACHARYA, A. N., ATKINSON, L. E. and KNOBIL, E. (1970) *Endocrinology* **87,** 850–853.
HALASZ, B. (1969) In *Frontiers in Neuroendocrinology,* pp. 307–342, ed. Ganong, W. F. and Martini, L. London and New York: Oxford University Press.
POHORECKY, L. A., ZIGMOND, M. J., HEIMER, L. and WURTMAN, R. J. (1969) *Proc. natn. Acad. Sci. U.S.A.* **62,** 1052–1056.
REITER, R. J. (1970) *Am. Zool.* **10,** 247.
SORRENTINO, S., JR., REITER, R. J. and SCHALCH, D. S. (1970) *Neuroendocrinology* in press.
STEINER, F. A., AKERT, K. and RUF, K. (1969) *Brain Res.* **12,** 74–85.

THE EFFECT OF PINEALECTOMY ON PLASMA INSULIN IN RATS

Stefan M. Milcu, Lydia Nanu-Ionescu and Ioana Milcu

Institute of Endocrinology, Academia de Stiinte Medicale, Bucharest

In earlier studies of the part played by the pineal gland in carbohydrate metabolism we reported that a peptide extract of bovine pineal gland has an insulin-like effect on laboratory animals. This was characterized by hypoglycaemia, increased glucose tolerance (Milcou, Milcou and Nanu 1963; Milcu *et al.* 1961; Milcu and Milcu 1958; Milcu, Milcu and Damian 1951), an increase in hepatic and muscular glycogenesis after glucose loading (Milcu *et al.* 1966*b*, 1963), and an increase of the uptake of glucose *in vitro* and the respiratory exchange rate in diaphragm muscle of rodents previously injected with pineal extract (Milcu, Nanu and Marcean 1960*a, b*). The same extract prevented or greatly improved the impaired biochemical reactions in alloxan-diabetic rats (Milcou, Milcou and Nanu 1963; Milcu, Nanu and Marcean 1957).

Pinealectomy, by contrast, produced a biochemical syndrome characterized by diminished glucose tolerance (Milcu 1967; Milcu *et al.* 1964, 1965*b*), a decrease in hepatic and muscular glycogenesis (Milcu *et al.* 1965*a*, 1963), and increased blood pyruvate concentration (Nanu *et al.* 1969). The respiratory exchange rate *in vitro* and the glucose uptake in diaphragms of pinealectomized rats were depressed (Milcu *et al.* 1965*a*).

All these facts showed clearly that the pineal body played a part in carbohydrate metabolism and raised the problem of the response to endogenous insulin in experimental pineal syndromes.

The present paper is concerned with the changes observed in plasma insulin and insulin-like activity in pinealectomized rats, as well as in synergistic and anti-insulin systems in plasma.

MATERIALS, METHODS AND RESULTS

The investigations were carried out on pinealectomized, sham-operated and intact male Wistar rats. The surgical operations were performed according to Marcean's procedure, as described by Milcu and co-workers (1965*a*), on animals weighing 80–100 g. The experiments began three to four weeks after surgery. After a 48-hour fasting period (with water *ad libitum*) blood was collected in heparinized centrifuge tubes for determinations in the fasted state, and immediately afterwards glucose loading was begun. The animals received orally, over 5 hours, six equal hourly doses of glucose in 33 per cent aqueous solution, the total dose being 1 g per 100 g body weight. Blood was collected 30 minutes after the last dose of glucose. Blood sugar concentrations were measured both before and after glucose loading in 0·1 ml of whole blood by the Hagedorn-Jensen method (Loiseleur 1954). The following determinations were made on the blood plasma: (*a*) insulin-like activity (ILA), by both the rat epididymal fat-pad and diaphragm tests; (*b*) immunoreactive insulin (IRI); (*c*) suppressible insulin-like activity (SILA) and non-suppressible insulin-like activity (NSILA); (*d*) the effect on the exogenous insulin molecule; and (*e*) the effect on the biological activity of exogenous insulin.

Blood sugar level

The blood sugar levels before and after glucose loading in normal and pinealectomized rats are shown in Table I. In the control animals there was no significant modification of the fasting level after a glucose load. The pinealectomized animals showed a significant increase, indicating diminished glucose tolerance.

TABLE I

BLOOD SUGAR CONCENTRATIONS IN NORMAL AND PINEALECTOMIZED
48-HOUR FASTED AND GLUCOSE-LOADED RATS

Blood sugar (mg/100 ml)

Group	Fasting	Glucose loading	Modification after glucose loading Mean ± s.e.	P
Normal (9)	86±8	88±7	2±11	>0·80
Pinealectomized (9)	83±5	104±6	21± 7	<0·02

Values are the means ± s.e.
Number of animals in parentheses.

Plasma insulin-like activity by the rat epididymal fat-pad and diaphragm assays

Epididymal fat-pad test. The manometric bioassay method of Ball and Merill (1961) was used. The assay is based on the stimulating effect of insulin on the production of CO_2 from added glucose by the epididymal fat. Plasma dilutions (1:10) in Krebs Ringer bicarbonate–0·3 per cent glucose (KRBG) medium were assayed simultaneously with increasing quantities of beef insulin in KRBG medium containing 0·1 per cent gelatine; the corresponding insulin equivalents expressed in $\mu U/ml$ undiluted plasma were then calculated from the standard assay curve (percentage maximal responses against the logarithm of insulin concentration).

Diaphragm test. The rat hemidiaphragm procedure of Vallance-Owen and Hurlock (1954) was used, with preliminary shaking of the tissue in ice-cold buffer according to Brown and co-workers (1952). Plasma dilutions (1:6) in Krebs Ringer bicarbonate–0·1 per cent glucose medium were assayed simultaneously with increasing quantities of insulin in medium containing 0·1 per cent gelatine. The corresponding insulin equivalents in µU/ml of undiluted plasma were obtained from the standard curve plotted as the cube-root of the net glucose uptake against the logarithm of insulin concentration, according to Randle (1957).

The donors of both epididymal fat-pad and diaphragm tissues were Wistar, non-fasted, 100–120 g rats. Glucose in the incubation medium was estimated by the Somogy-Nelson method, as described by Loiseleur (1954). Each plasma sample was assayed in duplicate by every test. The assays were performed only on glucose-loaded rat plasma.

The results are presented in Table II. Plasma ILA determined by the two biological tests was significantly increased in the pinealectomized rats by comparison with the controls. No significant difference has been found between the average values observed in the two control groups—the normal and sham-operated rats. The ratios of the plasma ILA values obtained by the epididymal fat-pad test and the diaphragm test were 5·3 and 4·5 respectively in the control groups and only 1·4 in the pinealectomized group.

According to Antoniades (1966) and Antoniades and Gundersen (1961), we can consider the epididymal fat-pad ILA as "total" plasma insulin, the diaphragm ILA as "free" insulin and their difference as "bound" insulin.

TABLE II

PLASMA INSULIN-LIKE ACTIVITY (EXPRESSED IN EQUIVALENTS OF BEEF INSULIN, µU/ml) IN NORMAL, SHAM-OPERATED AND PINEALECTOMIZED GLUCOSE-LOADED RATS

Group	Fat-pad test	Diaphragm test	Difference
Normal (N) (7)	346±36	65·2±5	281±25
Sham-operated (S) (7)	307±25	65·6±4	242±15
Pinealectomized (P) (6)	513±55	360·0±20	153±40
Statistical significance of the differences between the means	P.N.<0·02 P.S.<0·05 S.N.>0·90	P.N.<0·01 P.S.<0·05 S.N.>0·90	

Values are the means ±s.e.
Number of animals in parentheses.

We can then say that the increases in the amount of total plasma insulin in pinealectomized rats were due to the "free" circulating form of the hormone.

Plasma immunoreactive insulin

The radioimmunochromatographic method of Yalow and Berson (1960) in an ascending system was used to assay plasma immunoreactive insulin. The method is based on the isotopic dilution principle and the property of free insulin (F) of being absorbed to the filter paper at the start of the chromatographic strip, while the antibody-bound insulin (B) migrates with the plasma proteins. Antiserum was obtained from guinea pigs immunized against beef insulin; ^{131}I-labelled beef insulin (Radiochemical Centre, Amersham) was used as a tracer. The final plasma dilution was

TABLE III

IMMUNOREACTIVE PLASMA INSULIN IN NORMAL AND PINEALECTOMIZED RATS
FASTED FOR 48 HOURS AND GIVEN A GLUCOSE LOAD

	Immunoreactive insulin ($\mu U/ml$ plasma)		
Group	*Fasting*	*Glucose loading*	*Increase after glucose loading*
Normal (9)	29 ± 8	105 ± 9	76
Pinealectomized (9)	12 ± 6	$155 \pm 13^{\star}$	143

Values are means $\pm$ S.E.
Number of animals in parentheses.
$\star$ The difference between the glucose loading mean values is statistically significant ($P < 0.001$).

$1:10$. The standard curve was made with crystallized beef insulin. The results are expressed in insulin equivalents as $\mu U/ml$ undiluted plasma.

The results are shown in Table III. It is evident that in the fasting state the pinealectomized rats had lower plasma IRI levels. After glucose loading an increase in the circulating IRI was observed in both the normal and pinealectomized animals; this increase reflects the stimulatory effect of the glucose on pancreatic insulin secretion, but in the pinealectomized group the plasma IRI reached a significantly higher level than in the control group.

Suppressible and non-suppressible plasma insulin-like activities

The insulin-like activity in plasma of normal and pinealectomized rats, in the presence of normal or anti-insulin guinea pig serum, was assayed by the diaphragm test. The test tissues were obtained from 18-hour fasted, 100–120 g male Wistar rats after decapitation. Quarter-diaphragms (60–70 mg) were used instead of hemidiaphragms; the four fragments of a diaphragm were placed in four incubation vessels containing Krebs Ringer

TABLE IV

SCHEME OF EXPERIMENTS TO DETERMINE PLASMA SILA AND NSILA IN NORMAL (N) AND PINEALECTOMIZED (P) RATS, BY THE DIAPHRAGM TEST

Incubation vessel no:	1	2	3	4
Contents (ml)				
KRBG medium	1·73	1·98	1·73	1·98
N or P rat serum	0·25	—	0·25	—
Normal guinea pig serum (GPS)	0·02	0·02	—	—
Anti-insulin GPS	—	—	0·02	0·02
Analysis				
Glucose before incubation	a	b	c	d
Glucose after incubation	a′	b′	c′	d′
Determinations				
Total glucose uptake (mg/g wet tissue/2 hours)	A(=a–a′)	B(=b–b′)	C(=c–c′)	D(=d–d′)
Plasma total (diaphragm) ILA	A–B			
Plasma NSILA				C–D
Plasma SILA		(A–B) — (C–D)		

bicarbonate–0·1 per cent glucose (KRBG) medium, plasma of normal or pinealectomized rats, and normal or anti-insulin guinea pig serum, according to the scheme shown in Table IV. The final dilution of the plasma was 1:8. Each plasma sample was assayed in duplicate. The results are expressed in mg glucose uptake from the medium per g of wet tissue for 2 hours.

The results are shown in Table V. It can be seen that after a 48-hour fasting period the pinealectomized animals showed some decrease of the total plasma insulin-like activity assayable by the diaphragm test; this decrease was due to a reduction of the suppressible fraction, which had an effect on glucose uptake by the diaphragm muscle which was 2·8 times less than that of normal rat plasma. The non-suppressible activity was moderately increased in the pinealectomized rats. After glucose loading the total

TABLE V

TOTAL, SILA AND NSILA PLASMA INSULIN-LIKE ACTIVITIES OF NORMAL AND PINEALECTOMIZED RATS FASTED FOR 48 HOURS AND GIVEN A GLUCOSE LOAD, ASSAYED BY THE DIAPHRAGM TEST

Insulin-like activity	Group	Glucose uptake (mg glucose/g wet tissue/2 hours)			
		Fasting (F)	Glucose load (G)	P (F.G.)	G/F ratio
Total	Normal	4·68±1·76	6·03±1·10	>0·50	1·28
	Pinealectomized	3·46±1·10	10·50±1·46	<0·01	3·03
SILA	Normal	2·73±1·50	6·02±1·90	>0·05	2·20
	Pinealectomized	0·96±1·00	7·81±1·50	<0·01	8·10
NSILA	Normal	1·95±1·00	0·01±0·56	>0·10	0·005
	Pinealectomized	2·50±0·58	2·69±1·58	>0·90	1·07

All values are means ± S.E. Nine normal and nine pinealectomized rats were used in this experiment for all determinations.

plasma ILA increased in both normal and pinealectomized rats, but the
increase was greater in the latter group. The glucose uptake of the diaphragm muscle after the glucose load was 1·28 times higher in the control
and 3·03 times higher in the pinealectomized rats than the corresponding
fasting values. The ILA increases were due in both cases to increases in the
suppressible fraction; the effect of this fraction was 2·2 times greater than
the fasting value in the control group and 8·1 times greater in the pinealectomized rats.

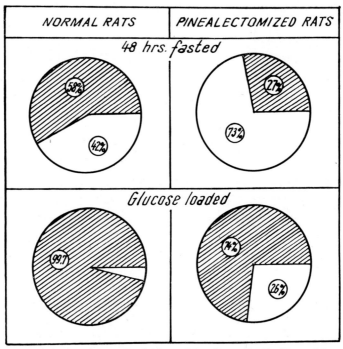

Fig. 1. The percentage distribution of the plasma insulin–like activity
between suppressible (hatched area) and non-suppressible (un-hatched
area) fractions in normal and pinealectomized rats fasted for 48 hours
and given a glucose load.

Figure 1 illustrates the percentage distribution of the plasma insulin-like
activity between the suppressible and non-suppressible fractions in normal
and pinealectomized rats in the two physiological states. It can be seen
that after a 48-hour fasting period in the normal animals 58 per cent of
plasma ILA was due to the suppressible fraction, while in the pinealectomized animals the non-suppressible fraction appeared to be responsible for
the major part of plasma ILA, namely 73 per cent of the effect. After
glucose loading the suppressible ILA fraction accounts for 99·7 per cent

of the total plasma ILA in the controls and for only 74 per cent in the pinealectomized animals, in which the remaining 26 per cent of plasma ILA was still due to the non-suppressible fraction.

Effect of plasma on the exogenous insulin molecule

We studied the effect on the labelled insulin molecule in various *in vitro* incubation conditions of plasma from normal, sham-operated and pinealec-tomized glucose-loaded rats. The plasma was analysed in the fresh state or after being kept one month at 4 °C or frozen; in the latter case the plasma was thawed just before use. 0·2 ml lots of 1 : 2 or 1 : 10 dilutions of plasma were incubated with 0·001 μg of beef or pig radioactively labelled insulin (50 μCi/μg specific activity) at 4 °C for 4 and 24-hour periods; after incubation the remaining free labelled insulin was separated from the degraded and plasma-protein-bound insulin by the Yalow-Berson chromatographic method (Yalow and Berson 1960). According to these authors the degraded and bound insulin molecules migrate with the serum proteins. The results are presented in Table VI as percentages of the total radioactivity on the chromatographic strip recovered in the protein zone. A correction for the degradation of labelled insulin in the absence of rat plasma was applied.

It can be seen from Table VI that when certain conditions in the experimental procedure were altered the proportion of labelled insulin which was degraded and/or bound varied, but no significant differences could be

TABLE VI

PERCENTAGES OF THE TOTAL RADIOACTIVITY RECOVERED IN THE ZONE OF PLASMA PROTEINS AFTER INCUBATION OF LABELLED INSULIN WITH PLASMA FROM NORMAL, SHAM-OPERATED AND PINEALECTOMIZED GLUCOSE-LOADED RATS

Experi-ment	Plasma state	Dilu-tion	Incu-bation time (hours)	Group		
				Normal	Sham-operated	Pinealectomized
1	Fresh	1:10	4	5·6±0·6	6·0±0·4	5·9±0·7
2	Fresh	1:10	24	10·6±0·3	10·6±0·7	10·5±1·0
3	Kept at 4 °C	1:10	4	5·6±0·3	5·7±0·8	5·5±0·9
4	Frozen–thawed	1:10	4	2·7±0·7	3·9±0·5	3·4±0·4
5	Frozen–thawed	1:2	24	21·0±1·7	20·7±1·0	20·7±1·3

Statistical significance between the means of the different experiments:

	Normal	Sham-operated	Pinealectomized
1–2	<0·001	<0·001	<0·001
1–4	<0·01	<0·01	<0·01

All results are expressed as means ± S.E.
Pig insulin labelled with [125]I (Radiochemical Centre, Amersham) was used in experiments 1–4 and beef insulin labelled with ^{131}I in our laboratory in experiment 5. Six animals per group were used in experiments 1–4 and 12 animals in experiment 5.

observed between the three experimental groups of normal, sham-operated and pinealectomized rats within the framework of the same experiment.

All these experiments indicate that pinealectomy does not modify the capacity of plasma to degrade and/or bind the exogenous insulin molecule in the rat.

Effect of plasma on the biological activity of exogenous insulin

The effect of incubating beef insulin with plasma of normal, sham-operated and pinealectomized glucose-loaded rats was assessed by the epididymal fat-pad assay as described by Doisy (1965); 0·1 ml lots of plasma, with and without 50 μU of crystallized beef insulin, were assayed simultaneously with 50 μU of pure insulin alone to determine recoveries with the same pad. In all cases the observed maximal percentage responses have been converted to insulin equivalents based on the response to 50 μU of crystallized insulin and the slope of standard assay curves. Recovery was determined by difference; thus, in μU, (plasma + 50 μU) − (plasma) = μU recovered. This value was subtracted from 50 (μU added insulin); thus, a positive or negative value was obtained, indicating respectively in μU of insulin either excess insulin-like activity due to a stimulatory effect of the rat plasma on insulin action, or the amount of added insulin which was neutralized in its action by inhibitory and/or antagonistic factors in the rat plasma.

The results are presented in Table VII. The standard error of the mean value in the group of normal rats was very high because of large variations in the effects of plasma from one individual to another; the average value was not significantly different from zero in this condition. Among the sham-operated animals some inhibitory effect was observed but without statistical significance. The activity of a significant quantity of added

TABLE VII

EFFECT OF PLASMA FROM NORMAL, SHAM-OPERATED AND PINEALECTOMIZED GLUCOSE-LOADED
RATS ON THE BIOLOGICAL ACTIVITY OF INSULIN (EPIDIDYMAL FAT-PAD ASSAY)

	Stimulatory (+) or inhibitory (−) effect, expressed as μU insulin	
Group	Mean + s.e. and significance of the mean	Significance of the difference between the means
Normal (N) (5)	$+1 \cdot 4 \pm 9 \cdot 18$ $P > 0 \cdot 80$	N.S. $> 0 \cdot 50$
Sham-operated (S) (5)	$-11 \cdot 1 \pm 3 \cdot 97$ $P > 0 \cdot 05$	P.S. $> 0 \cdot 05$
Pinealectomized (P) (5)	$-24 \cdot 0 \pm 3 \cdot 91$ $P < 0 \cdot 01$	P.N. $< 0 \cdot 05$

Number of animals in parentheses.

insulin was neutralized in the presence of plasma from pinealectomized rats.

This experiment led us to conclude that pinealectomy increases the plasma concentrations of insulin antagonistic and/or inhibitory factors in rats.

DISCUSSION

From the results presented here we can say that pinealectomized rats respond to oral glucose loading by a large increase in plasma insulin-like activity as well as in immunoreactive insulin. Besides this, our previous studies had proved that pinealectomized animals (rats, rabbits) had reduced glucose tolerance as well as a deficiency in liver and muscle glycogenesis (Milcu 1967).

Reduced glucose tolerance, associated with an increase in plasma insulin, is often seen in diabetic states in man. How can we explain this chemical diabetes-like syndrome in animals deprived of their pineals? The pineal produces, among other substances, an adrenal inhibitory factor, first described by Farrell in 1960 and later considered by Fabre and co-workers (1965) to be ubiquinone; however, its nature is still debated. In agreement with these facts are observations showing that pinealectomized animals develop (presumably by the elimination of the inhibitory factor) a hyper-functional adrenocortical syndrome. In the rat this was demonstrated most clearly by Kinson and Singer (1967) and Kinson, Wahid and Singer (1967) who found a significant increase in aldosterone in adrenal venous blood 17 days after pinealectomy and also an increase in corticosterone 30 days after surgery; the aldosterone increase was relatively larger, amounting to about three times the control values.

We believe that this adrenal hyperfunction, which because of its chronic character is not a negligible effect, could at least partially explain the diabetes-like symptoms seen in pinealectomized animals.

Of particular interest is the fact that the changes resulting from pinealect-omy in response to glucose loading are of the same type as those observed in glucocorticoid hypersecretion or after glucocorticoid or ACTH treatment. In man it has been reported that excess of these hormones produces im-paired glucose tolerance and also an abnormal increase in plasma insulin (Williams and Ensinck 1966; Berson and Yalow 1965; Perley and Kipnis 1966). The increased half-life of labelled insulin which was found by one of us in plasma from pinealectomized rats (L. Nanu-Ionescu, unpublished data) is consistent with one of the characteristic effects of ACTH, namely to inhibit degradation of the insulin molecule (Williams and Ensinck 1966).

Aldosterone as well as the glucocorticoids can produce diabetes-like phenomena in which there is an increase in plasma insulin and impaired glucose tolerance. Conn's observations in man prove that these phenomena appear in primary and secondary hyperaldosteronism (wrongly termed maturity diabetes) (Conn 1965). He considers the potassium loss in hyperaldosteronism to be the central phenomenon which could explain the diabetes-like syndrome. It is worth mentioning too that not only mineralocorticoids but glucocorticoids also eventually cause a potassium depletion, although a smaller one (Gaunt and Chart 1962).

However, can potassium depletion be shown to be a diabetogenic factor in rats, as in man? By prolonged feeding of rats with a potassium-deficient diet, Gardner and co-workers (1950) obtained signs of impaired carbo-hydrate metabolism which correspond to some of the changes that we observed in pinealectomized animals, namely impaired glucose tolerance and reduced glycogenesis in liver and muscle (Milcu 1967; Milcu et al. 1964, 1965a, b, 1963). The chronic hyperaldosteronism demonstrated by Kinson and Singer (1967) in pinealectomized rats suggests a potassium loss, which could explain the troubles mentioned above.

Several experimental observations are relevant here. Wurtman and co-workers (1960) measured urinary potassium in 36-day-old rats pinealec-tomized 10 days previously and obtained an increase of 31 per cent of the daily potassium output over the intact controls (5 in each group). Tanner and Hungerford (1962) similarly observed an increase of 27 per cent in the daily urinary potassium output of 5 pinealectomized rats between days 19 and 21 after operation, compared to 6 sham-operated controls. However, neither group of workers considered the differences significant. Our own studies (Milcu et al. 1966a, 1968) on larger groups of rats showed in two series of experiments that the loss of potassium is characteristic of pinealec-tomized rats. In our first experiment (1966), on 36 rats pinealectomized 30 days previously and 51 intact controls, we found a 42 per cent increase ($P < 0.001$) in daily potassium diuresis in the pinealectomized group. Two years later, using 10 pinealectomized and 24 control rats under apparently similar conditions, we found a potassium loss of 25 per cent, which was also significant ($P < 0.002$). We think that this potassium diuresis is an expression of chronic adrenal stimulation. It seems that changes of these orders of magnitude are not negligible and are the result of a chronic physiopathological process.

In connexion with the increase in plasma insulin, it is worth noting that Berson and Yalow (1965) found that the early maturity onset diabetes with moderately impaired glucose tolerance responded to glucose with the greatest increase in plasma insulin ever found by these authors, especially if glucose administration was repeated several times. These observations agree with our findings in rats, where a striking increase in plasma insulin is consistent with a moderately impaired glucose tolerance and is particularly evident after repeated glucose loading.

Concerning the increased insulin antagonists in the plasma of pinealectomized rats, it should be stressed that such factors seem to depend on the hypophysis and adrenals (Kipnis 1966; Williams and Ensinck 1966; Wright 1960), their increase again being consistent with the adrenal stimulation of pinealectomy.

The loss of potassium, the impaired glucose tolerance and the increase of plasma insulin in man in cases labelled as maturity onset diabetes (Conn 1965; Berson and Yalow 1965) could also be found in pinealectomized rats. In both cases, the phenomena are found together and seem to be determined by adrenal hyperfunction.

However, the question arises whether the diabetes-like symptoms of pinealectomy should be considered only as a reactive syndrome caused by the release of the adrenal gland from the pineal brake or whether we should also consider hormonal effects induced directly by the lack of a pineal hormone. We have not investigated this problem fully yet, but using our peptide extract of the beef pineal with its well-characterized hypoglycaemic effect, we obtained hypoglycaemia in adrenalectomized rats, which suggests a direct metabolic action of the pineal, which thus acts independently of adrenal inhibition (Milcou, Milcou and Nanu 1963). This observation raises the problem of the relationship (or perhaps identity) of the hypoglycaemic factor prepared by us (pinealine) and the pineal adrenal inhibitor. A first attempt to test the hypoglycaemic action of a pineal extract prepared according to the ubiquinone extraction procedure of Fabre and co-workers (1965) gave inconclusive results. The field of investigation of the specific metabolic effects of the pineal adrenal inhibitory factor remains open.

SUMMARY

The following changes in plasma insulin activity were found in pinealectomized rats:

(a) The plasma insulin-like activity determined by the epididymal fat-pad test and by the diaphragm test is significantly increased after glucose loading.

(b) The radioimmunochromatographic assay of immunoreactive insulin showed a decrease in plasma during starvation and a significant increase after glucose loading.

(c) The determination of the suppressible and non-suppressible insulin-like activity in plasma by the diaphragm test showed changes in the suppressible fraction similar to those observed in the radioimmunochromatographic assay. The non-suppressible activity was increased both in starvation and after glucose loading.

(d) When the effect of plasma from pinealectomized rats on labelled insulin was assessed by a radiochromatographic method, it was found that the pinealectomized rat had a normal plasma system of insulin degradation and/or binding.

(e) By contrast, using a biological assay, it was found that plasma of pinealectomized rats was able to neutralize *in vitro* the activity of an appreciable amount of insulin, owing to an increase in insulin antagonists.

The increase of the plasma insulin after pinealectomy in response to glucose loading may be attributed to the increased output of mineralo- and glucocorticoids following pinealectomy.

REFERENCES

ANTONIADES, H. N. (1966) In *Third Research Symposium of the American Diabetes Association*, ed. Lazarow, A. *Diabetes* **15**, 281–289.

ANTONIADES, H. N. and GUNDERSEN, K. (1961) *Endocrinology* **68**, 7–16.

BALL, E. G. and MERILL, M. A. (1961) *Endocrinology* **69**, 596–608.

BERSON, S. A. and YALOW, R. S. (1965) *Diabetes* **14**, 549–572.

BROWN, D. H., PARK, C. R., DAUGHADAY, W. H. and CORNBLATH, M. (1952) *J. biol. Chem.* **197**, 167–174.

CONN, J. W. (1965) *New Engl. J. Med.* **293**, 1135–1143.

DOISY, R. J. (1965) *Endocrinology* **77**, 49–53.

FARRELL, G. (1960) *Circulation* **21**, 1009–1015.

FABRE, L., BANKS, R. S., ISAAC, W. M. and FARRELL, G. (1965) *Am. J. Physiol.* **208**, 1275–1280.

GARDNER, L. I., TALBOT, N. B., COOK, C. D., BERMAN, H. and URIBE, C. (1950) *J. Lab. clin. Med.* **35**, 592–602.

GAUNT, R. and CHART, J. J. (1962) In *Handbuch der experimentellen Pharmakologie*, pp. 514–569, ed. Eichler, O. and Farah, A. Berlin: Springer.

KINSON, G. and SINGER, B. (1967) *Neuroendocrinology* **2**, 283–291.

KINSON, G., WAHID, A. K. and SINGER, B. (1967) *Gen. comp. Endocr.* **8**, 445–454.

KIPNIS, D. (1966) In *Third Research Symposium of the American Diabetes Association*, ed. Lazarow, A. *Diabetes* **15**, 281–289.

LOISELEUR, J. (1954) *Techniques de Laboratoire*, I, p. 795. Paris: Masson.

MILCOU, S. M., MILCOU, I. and NANU, L. (1963) *Annls. Endocr.* **24**, 233–254.

MILCU, I. (1967) *Proc. Congresul de Endocrinologie, Bucureşti*, pp. 37–46.

MILCU, I., DAMIAN, E., IONESCU, M. and POPESCU, I. (1966a) *Studii. Cerc. Endocr.* **17**, 547–550.

MILCU, I., DAMIAN, E., POPESCU, I. and IANAS, O. (1968) *Studii Cerc. Endocr.* **19**, 283–287.

MILCU, S. M. and MILCU, I. (1958) *Medizinische* **17**, 711–715.

MILCU, S. M., MILCU, I. and DAMIAN, E. (1951) *Comunle Acad. Rep. pop. rom.* **1**, 683–687.

MILCU, I., NANU, L. and MARCEAN, R. (1957) *Endocrinologia* **2**, 138–147.

MILCU, I., NANU, L. and MARCEAN, R. (1960a) *Studii Cerc. Endocr.* **11**, 461–466.

MILCU, I., NANU, L. and MARCEAN, R. (1960*b*) *Studii Cerc. Endocr.* **11**, 467–475.

MILCU, I., NANU, L., MARCEAN, R. and IONESCU, V. (1964) *Rev. Roum. Endocr.* **1**, 203–208.

MILCU, I., NANU, L., MARCEAN, R. and IONESCU, V. (1965*a*) *Studii Cerc. Endocr.* **16**, 17–24.

MILCU, I., NANU, L., MARCEAN, R. and IONESCU, V. (1966*b*) *Omagiu C. I. Parhon*, pp. 299–302. Bucureşti.

MILCU, I., NANU, L., MARCEAN, R. and SITARU, S. (1961) *Studii Cerc. Endocr.* **2**, 719–729.

MILCU, I., NANU, L., MARCEAN, R. and SITARU, S. (1963) *Studii Cerc. Endocr.* **14**, 651–655.

MILCU, I., NANU, L., MARCEAN, R. and SITARU, S. (1965*b*) *Revue Roum. Endocr.* **2**, 27–33.

NANU, L., MARCEAN, R., IONESCU, V. and MILCOU, I. (1969) *Revue Roum. Endocr.* **6**, 141–147.

PERLEY, M. and KIPNIS, D. M. (1966) *New Engl. J. Med.* **274**, 1237–1241.

RANDLE, P. J. (1957) *Ciba Fdn Coll. Endocrinol. 11 Hormones in Blood*, pp. 115–132. London: Churchill.

TANNER, W. D. and HUNGERFORD, G. F. (1962) *Proc. Soc. exp. Biol. Med.* **109**, 388–390.

VALLANCE-OWEN, J. and HURLOCK, B. (1954) *Lancet* **1**, 68.

WILLIAMS, R. H. and ENSINCK, J. W. (1966) *Diabetes* **15**, 623–654.

WRIGHT, P. H. (1960) *Lancet* **1**, 951–954.

WURTMAN, R. J., ALTSCHULE, D., GREEP, R. O., FALK, J. L. and GRAVE, G. (1960) *Am. J. Physiol.* **199**, 1109–1111.

YALOW, R. S. and BERSON, S. A. (1960) *J. clin. Invest.* **39**, 1157–1175.

DISCUSSION

Singer: Both aldosterone and corticosterone probably cause a potassium loss; insulin of course causes an increase in the rate of entry of potassium into cells. Have you demonstrated a fall in plasma potassium in these animals? I presume the total body potassium has fallen.

Milcu: In both experimental series reported in our paper we found not only a significantly increased potassium diuresis but a diminution in extra-cellular potassium too (which illustrates the plasma loss). This diminution was 10 per cent in one experiment ($P < 0.02$, in 37 animals) and 9.1 per cent (not significant, in 13 animals) in the other.

Singer: This loss of potassium need not mean that insulin is not having its normal effect, because as far as I know, the effect of insulin on potassium transfer into muscle and other tissues is independent of its action on carbo-hydrate metabolism. It is possible that with the corticoids having an antagonistic effect on carbohydrate metabolism, insulin levels may be affected. However, I am very doubtful that potassium loss associated with raised aldosterone and corticosterone levels is causing the diabetic-like state in your animals. It may be just a concomitant.

Milcu: We are led to believe that there is a causal relationship between the potassium loss and the diabetic-like state by investigations which were especially concerned with this correlation. I mentioned Gardner's investi-gation in the rat, in which chronic potassium depletion led to impaired glucose tolerance as well as liver glycogen loss (Gardner *et al.* 1950). Conn's very consistent investigations in man have shown that in cases labelled as maturity-onset diabetes accompanied by hyperaldosteronism and potassium loss, loading with potassium salts has corrected the impaired glucose tolerance as well as the insulin secretion defect to the same degree as the extirpation of an aldosterone-producing adrenal adenoma (Conn 1965).

Sagild (quoted by Conn), using an orally administered ion-exchange resin, has obtained potassium depletion accompanied by a considerable decrease in carbohydrate tolerance in normal man. That is why we stressed the correlation between the potassium loss and the diabetic-like state in our paper.

Wurtman: Dr Milcu, you have evidence of an antagonist in the plasma of pinealectomized animals that reduces the activity of added insulin by 27 per cent. You also showed that in pinealectomized animals not all the insulin-like activity was really insulin, so pinealectomy seems to have two opposing effects: it causes the presence of both an insulin antagonist and a molecule with insulin-like activity. Can you speculate about what kinds of compounds might act at skeletal muscle or at other insulin target organs to potentiate the effect of insulin? Are there compounds that are known to do this?

Milcu: The antagonists and synergists of insulin are found in the circulation and they can be shown in different ways. As Grodsky and Forsham (1966) state, most insulin antagonists, with the exception of antibody, do not act on the insulin molecule but are hyperglycaemic agents such as hormones or poorly identified plasma substances.

We identified plasma insulin synergists only biologically, as insulin-like activity that is not suppressed by insulin antiserum. The chemical nature of the so-called "non-suppressible insulin-like activity" is still unknown.

Wurtman: Dr Cegrell has shown the presence within the pancreas of cells that contain serotonin and dopamine (see Falck and Owman 1968) and Porte and Williams (1966) have shown that catecholamines act directly upon the pancreas to decrease their sensitivity to glucose and decrease the insulin secretion. I don't know if anyone has studied the effect of serotonin on insulin secretion. Is there any possibility that pineal compounds that act on brain serotonin might also act directly on pancreatic serotonin or dopamine and in so doing, modify the secretion of insulin from the pancreas?

Owman: A general influence directly on the pancreatic cells is possible.

Wurtman: Is it known whether serotonin has an inhibitory effect like noradrenaline or adrenaline on the secretion of insulin from the pancreas?

Owman: Serotonin has been shown to inhibit the secretion of insulin from the hamster pancreas *in vitro* (Feldman and Lebovitz 1970).

Singer: Have you investigated the possibility that other substances which are antagonistic to insulin, such as growth hormone or glucagon, are present in excess?

Milcu: No, not yet. We hope to do this.

Nir: An explanation in terms of an adrenocortical effect doesn't appeal to me, because we know that the effects of pinealectomy on corticosterone are transitional and very small, and in order to get a diabetogenic effect by giving ACTH or corticosterone we need to give enormous amounts. A more likely possibility is some direct effect on the secretion of the pancreatic cells.

Milcu: In our paper we were interested not only in the increase in corticosterone but especially in the aldosterone increase, which produced the diabetic symptoms by potassium loss, as I mentioned.

Nir: We found no effect of pinealectomy on the blood corticosterone concentration after 30 days, but even if you accept Dr Singer's finding that after 30 days you get increased blood corticosterone, this would still not explain the diabetogenic effect.

Singer: The maximum secretory capacity of corticosterone which we observed 30 days after pinealectomy was approximately doubled, as compared with sham-operated animals. Did you follow this effect with time; was this something that wore off with time? It might be interesting to see if it has a similar time course to the changes in adrenocortical function which we have observed.

Milcu: No, we haven't studied this.

Wurtman: Has anyone examined the corticosterone secretion rate around the clock in pinealectomized animals? We know that in some patients with Cushing's disease the plasma cortisol levels may be "normal" at the time of day when cortisol levels are normally high. Their problem is that cortisol levels stay up throughout the 24-hour period. It is tempting to speculate that pinealectomy might not only raise the maximum level but also block the diurnal decline.

Fiske: As I indicated earlier, we have measured corticosterone levels after denervation of the pineal by removal of the superior cervical ganglia. Young adult female Sprague Dawley rats purchased from the Charles River Laboratories were used in this work. The plasma corticosterone concentration was measured at only two times in the photoperiod, that is, when the corticosterone level is customarily high, 4 p.m., or low, 9 a.m., in animals housed in light from 6 a.m. to 6 p.m. Not only was the diurnal rhythm maintained in both groups, but the maximal and minimal values of corticosterone in ganglionectomized rats also did not differ significantly from those found in sham-operated animals.

Miline: Dr Milcu, were your results the same in male as female rats?

Milcu: We have only studied male rats.

Miline: We sacrificed adult male rats six months after epiphysectomy. Interscapular brown tissue and periglandular brown tissue around the adrenal glands is greatly increased. The adrenal glands are very hyperplasic, both medulla and cortex (zona fasciculata and zona reticularis). Šćepović and his co-workers (Šćepović 1963; Šćepović *et al.* 1965) have studied the behaviour of the supraoptic nucleus and of the nephron in epiphysectomized adult male rats. The neuroglandular cells of the supraoptic nucleus are very hypertrophic; the juxtaglomerular apparatus shows hyperplasic changes; the nephrocytes are also increased in the pars proximalis.

Can you explain this correlation between an accumulation of adipose tissue and the insulin-like reactivity?

Milcu: We know that insulin stimulates lipid synthesis, so this is a possible explanation. There might be other factors too. But it is also possible that both hyperinsulinism and hypercorticism in the pinealecto-mized animals might augment lipogenesis.

Singer: Was the total body nitrogen lower in pinealectomized rats?

Milcu: We did only the opposite experiment, with negative results, by injecting pineal extract in young rats (unpublished data). In a test (devised for the anabolic function of growth hormone) which consists in measuring the accumulation of urea in blood after intravenous administration of an amino acid mixture to nephrectomized rats, we found a diminution of urea formation in rats injected with pineal extract and an increase in urea in pinealectomized ones (Milcu *et al.* 1969).

Singer: This would fit in with a catabolic effect of hyperglucocorti-coidism.

REFERENCES

CONN, J. W. (1965) *New Engl. J. Med.* **293**, 1135–1143.
FALCK, B. and OWMAN, CH. (1968) *Adv. Pharmac.* **6A**, 211–231.
FELDMAN, J. M. and LEBOVITZ, H. E. (1970) *Endocrinology* **86**, 66–70.
GARDNER, L. I., TALBOT, N. B., COOK, C. D., BERMAN, H. and URIBE, C. (1950) *J. Lab. clin. Med.* **35**, 592–602.
GRODSKY, G. M. and FORSHAM, P. H. (1966) *A. Rev. Physiol.* **28**, 347–380.
MILCU, I., NANU, L., MARCEAN, R. and IONESCO, V. (1969) *J. Endocr.* **45**, 175.
PORTE, D., JR. and WILLIAMS, R. H. (1966) *Science* **152**, 1248–1249.
ŠĆEPOVIĆ, M. (1963) *Korelativna histofiziologija epitalamo-epifiznog kompleksa i nadbubrega.* Habilitacioni rad, Medicinski fakultet, Sarajevo.
ŠĆEPOVIĆ, M., MILOŠEVIĆ, Z., KNEŽEVIĆ, N. and HRNJIČEVIĆ, M. (1965) *Acta anat.* **61**, 475.

GENERAL DISCUSSION

ROLE OF SEROTONIN IN THE PINEAL

Owman: I would like to offer a suggestion about the significance of pineal serotonin which might be worth considering until the next pineal meeting. We all agree that melatonin in the pineal gland is an active substance which fulfils several criteria for a hormone, and we know that serotonin is a precursor of melatonin. However, there is much evidence that only a relatively small portion of pineal serotonin is directly engaged in the synthesis of melatonin, and a considerable proportion of the serotonin may thus have some other role in the gland. During the last few years it has been found that several other endocrine cell systems are capable of producing and storing high amounts of various amines (Falck and Owman 1968; Pearse 1968a, b; Aures, Håkanson and Owman 1969; Håkanson 1970): (a) the various types of enterochromaffin and enterochromaffin-like cells in the gastric mucosa contain serotonin, dopamine, histamine, tryptamine and perhaps also 5-methoxytryptamine and acetylcholine; (b) the A cells and B cells in the islets of Langerhans store serotonin and dopamine; (c) the thyroid C cells contain serotonin, tryptamine and probably also acetylcholine; (d) a substance, probably identical with tryptamine, has been demonstrated in some of the pituitary endocrine cells; (e) finally, there are preliminary indications that some kind of amine mechanism may be operating in the parathyroid cells.

It is well established that all these various systems of cells store different kinds of polypeptide hormones: the gastro-intestinal hormones, insulin, glucagon, calcitonin, pituitary polypeptides, parathyroid hormone. In view of these findings I would think it very reasonable to assume that the high concentration of serotonin in the pineal gland reflects the presence in this endocrine structure also of some yet unidentified protein or polypeptide hormone which would perhaps help to explain several of those pineal effects that cannot be immediately ascribed to melatonin. We have direct experimental evidence on the calcitonin-producing cells that the amine is somehow involved in hormone release mechanisms within the cell (Melander, Owman and Sundler 1970). It is possible that the amine changes the permeability of membranes within the cell and, for example, facilitates the release of lysosomal enzymes or opens the cell membrane for the release of the polypeptide.

Martini: Dr Owman's idea will make many people here happy, including Madame Moszkowska and Professor Milcu!

Axelrod: It is known that in the adrenal gland catecholamines are involved in the release of two proteins, dopamine-β-hydroxylase and chromogranin (Viveros, Arqueros and Kirshner 1969), and also we have found that there are large amounts of circulating dopamine-β-hydroxylase, which is part of the storage granule (Weinshilboum and Axelrod 1970). Most of this comes not from the adrenal gland but from the sympathetic nerve terminal, so there is an intimate association of, if not serotonin, at least a catecholamine, with the release of a specific protein.

Kordon: Dr Owman's suggestion is a very appealing one, but I am somewhat disturbed, if we are to allow this hypothesis, by the fact that in *in vitro* systems, addition of serotonin does not interfere with the release of pituitary hormones (Moszkowska 1965; Scemama 1970), whereas substances that affect membrane permeability or changes in the ionic concentration of the medium have a very marked effect on this release (Samli and Geschwind 1968; Jutisz and De La Llosa 1970).

Owman: I don't think this is so disturbing, because in some cells we know that there is a concomitant presence of a polypeptide and an amine, and we have indications that there is a functional interrelation between the amine and the polypeptide. It may make a considerable difference whether the amine operates within the cell itself or has an exogenous action on the surface of the endocrine cells.

Kordon: Even if it is taken up, as is labelled 5-HT into the pituitary?

Owman: Certain of the pituitary cells contain a fluorogenic amine; others do not, although after administration of various precursor amino acids they can be seen to synthesize and store the corresponding amine, which is then visible in the fluorescence microscope. We think that such a model imitates the presence of some endogenous amine which we cannot yet demonstrate with available histochemical methods. The 5-HT which is taken up follows the mechanisms used by the endogenous substance and it's not necessary that the 5-HT has the same function within the cell as the unknown amine which is normally stored there.

Milcu: It seems difficult to explain all the physiological effects of the pineal only by melatonin and indole derivatives in general. All our results—hypoglycaemia and many other metabolic effects as well as the reduction of 17-ketosteroids in rabbit urine—were obtained using pineal peptides, which are not believed to contain melatonin (Milcu 1967).

Martini: Has anybody considered the possibilities (1) that there might be a "carrier" for melatonin; and (2) that the pineal gland might contain both melatonin and the protein (or the peptide) that acts as a "carrier"?

Milcu: The pineal peptides prepared by us do not contain melatonin.

Kappers: Has anyone here new information on the role of lipids, especially of phospholipids, in the mammalian pineal? Pineal lipid chemistry is important because the quantity of pineal lipids is a parameter of pineal activity. In the 1963 meeting, J. Zweens (1965) showed that the pineal lipid content fluctuates with the phases of the oestrous cycle in the rat and is influenced by the amount of circulating gonadotropins. I have the feeling that the relation between pineal lipids and pineal secretory activity has been somewhat neglected by pinealologists.

Milcu: We have carried out some experiments in rats on the action of pineal peptides on the uptake of ^{32}P by phospholipids from different areas of the central nervous system. We found an increased uptake in the cerebellum, cortex and bulb (Milcu *et al.* 1957).

Kappers: I am really wondering whether more is now known about the biochemical role that pineal lipids, and especially phospholipids, play in the secretory function of the pinealocyte or in the process of extrusion of its secretory products. Evidently more studies are needed here.

EFFECT OF MELATONIN ON SEROTONINERGIC SYSTEMS

Shein: The work reported by Dr Antón-Tay in collaboration with Dr Wurtman (see pp. 213–220) has an especially promising potential for making the pineal more interesting to people who are not primarily endocrinologists. Are Dr Wurtman or Dr Antón-Tay willing to speculate on the possible functional or behavioural significance of their finding that melatonin can stimulate the content of serotonin in serotonin-containing neurons in the midbrain and elsewhere? Specifically, in view of studies by Jouvet (1969) and others which implicate serotoninergic neurons in sleep mechanisms, I wonder about the effects of administering melatonin on the cycles of REM sleep and on the ratio of REM sleep to non-REM sleep. Also, in view of the pharmacological studies which correlate drug-induced reversals of depressed mood with elevation in serotonin concentrations in the brain, I wonder about the effects of administering melatonin chronically upon mood and affective behaviour.

Antón-Tay: In collaboration with Dr A. Fernández-Guardiola and José Luis Díaz (in preparation) we have started a systematic study of the effects of melatonin on brain activity in man. So far we have given an intravenous injection of 1·25 mg per kg to normal volunteers and to a few epileptic patients. We have also given 1·25 g of melatonin daily by mouth for 4 weeks to two patients with Parkinson's disease. In volunteers receiving melatonin we have seen an increase of EEG alpha activity and increased

EEG synchronization. The subjects fell asleep very easily and reported vivid dreams during this time. REM cycles seemed to be more frequent. They also reported a feeling of well-being and moderate elation, and that they experienced unusual visual imagery. In epileptic patients we found the same EEG and mental changes, and in the two Parkinsonians besides these same mental changes and changed EEG patterns we saw a striking amelioration of all the signs and symptoms of the syndrome.

Wurtman: At the present time melatonin may be the only hormone that has been shown to exert a major effect on an enzyme in the brain. Cortisol induces many enzymes in the liver but has only been shown to induce two enzymes in the brain; one of these is tryptophan hydroxylase in the brainstem and the effect is minor, and this enzyme is probably not rate-limiting (Azmitia and McEwen 1969). The other is phenylethanolamine-*N*-methyltransferase in the olfactory bulb (Pohorecky *et al.* 1969) and the effect here too is minor. Thyroxin has major effects on brain development but I know of no evidence that thyroxin *per se* has any effect in inducing specific enzymes in the adult brain. Unlike other hormones studied, melatonin apparently does just this. Moreover, it induces an enzyme, pyridoxal kinase, that causes the formation of a compound (pyridoxal phosphate) that is a critical co-factor not only in serotonin biosynthesis but also in the formation of GABA and, very likely, the catecholamines as well. We have emphasized the effect of melatonin on serotoninergic neurons simply because this is the first neurotransmitter that melatonin was shown to affect. In the same manner, we have emphasized the effect of the pineal on neuroendocrine functions simply because this was the first group of functions to be examined in relation to the pineal, but I would anticipate that the next symposium on the pineal may be concerned with other neurotransmitter substances in the brain and with other neurophysiological functions quite unrelated to neuroendocrinology.

Axelrod: Dr Fiske has made a very interesting finding on the relationship between melatonin and serotonin in the pineal.

Fiske: It is important to know when melatonin is being administered in respect to the photoperiod. We (Fiske and Huppert 1968) have found that pineal serotonin levels continue to vary characteristically with the photoperiod if rats are given daily injections of melatonin, in microgramme amounts, at the onset of darkness. This is the time when endogenously produced melatonin is normally released. If, however, melatonin is administered in the eighth hour of the light period, when little if any melatonin is being secreted, the serotonin rhythm of the pineal is blocked. Since Dr Antón-Tay and his colleagues (Antón-Tay *et al.* 1968) have shown that melatonin affects serotoninergic neurons in the brain, our results may be interpreted as an indication that melatonin affects signals in the brain necessary for the maintenance of such rhythmic functions of the pineal as its production of serotonin.

Shein: Another area that we have not discussed is the possible role of the pineal in immature animals. I am reminded of the situation with the thymus, where for years people were not interested because removal of the thymus in adult animals seemed to have little obvious effect. Finally the thymus was removed in immunologically immature animals and very obvious persistent immunological deficiencies were found. If one removed the pineal from foetal animals it would be interesting to see whether the pinealectomy altered the normal development of, for example, serotoninergic neurons in the brain, or the normal development of some portion of an endocrine organ.

Owman: Some years ago I did foetal pinealectomies *in utero* on rats and, indeed, very "spectacular effects" appeared (in the epithelial cells of the ileum: Owman 1963, 1964), but the results are difficult to interpret because they do not yet fit into any accepted functional model. I say "not yet" since I certainly hope that the gap between our knowledge about the adult and the developing or foetal pineal will be bridged.

Martini: Another critical thing to do is to find a sensitive method for measuring melatonin. I am thinking of a competition binding assay or a radioimmunoassay.

Wurtman: There are considerable problems in trying to estimate melatonin secretion in humans. Firstly, if melatonin is normally secreted into the cerebrospinal fluid, data on the fate of radioactive melatonin given intravenously or intraperitoneally tell us nothing about the fate of the endogenously secreted indole. Secondly, we don't yet know what compound to measure in the urine as the best index of melatonin secretion. The situation is a little analogous to the examination of brain noradrenaline 10 or 15 years ago. At that prehistoric date, many people interested in the biochemistry of schizophrenia tried to relate the course of the disease to urinary noradrenaline levels. One reason why they discovered so little about schizophrenia or brain noradrenaline is that very little of the catecholamine is excreted into the urine unchanged; it must all be metabolized first. Without knowing how much melatonin is metabolized prior to excretion, and the nature of the chief metabolites, we are unable to develop a method to estimate melatonin secretion.

Axelrod: In the rat melatonin is metabolized by 6-hydroxylation.

Wurtman: But this is systemically administered melatonin, not melatonin in the cerebrospinal fluid.

Axelrod: Yes, but melatonin won't be metabolized in the brain.

Antón-Tay: It has been shown (Jones, McGeer and Greiner 1969) that tracer doses of [^{14}C]melatonin administered to schizophrenic patients have practically the same fate as in rats. I have tried to see whether melatonin injected into the cerebrospinal fluid or in direct contact with brain homogenates has a different fate. It seems that new compounds are formed by the brain. Thus, if melatonin goes to the cerebrospinal fluid it could have a different fate.

Axelrod: You would have picked this up even after systemic administration. If it went into the brain and was metabolized there, some minor metabolite would have been detected in the urine, unless the amount is very small. I don't think there is evidence for a metabolite.

Martini: Another possibility is to discover which enzymes metabolize melatonin and to provide us with a good inhibitor of these enzymes.

Axelrod: We have described the enzyme that metabolizes melatonin, and W. M. McIsaac has found very potent inhibitors not of the metabolism of melatonin but of the *in vitro* formation of melatonin; it would be interesting to see the physiological consequences of preventing the formation of melatonin.

Wurtman: The metabolism of melatonin *in vivo* can be inhibited by chlorpromazine (Wurtman, Axelrod and Antón-Tay 1968).

Axelrod: Anything that inhibits the microsomal enzymes should also inhibit the metabolism of melatonin.

Arstila: There are good indications from the work of Bentley (1963) and others that for instance oxytocin can diffuse from the serosal surface of the frog bladder through the layer of basement membrane, collagen fibrils and fibrocytes and affect the sodium transport of the epithelium. Therefore I do not think that on a morphological basis we can rule out the possibility that melatonin could reach the ventricles.

Mess: It is a crucial question whether pineal hormones are secreted into the bloodstream or are secreted directly into the cerebrospinal fluid. It would not be very difficult in a larger species such as the sheep or dog or even the rabbit to cannulate the big veins coming from the pineal gland, to see the content of melatonin or serotonin in the blood leaving the pineal body, for example in the night when the pineal gland is activated. This could answer this question—provided that an assay method has been developed.

Secondly, are there any pharmacological or biochemical data giving direct evidence that melatonin and the other members of the indoleamine series are able to cross the blood–brain barrier? Both these points seem to me to be crucial. As an anatomist and histologist I have to agree with Dr Kappers, because the electron microscopic and histological evidence is almost all in favour of secretion via the capillary system, but the physiological results of Professor Martini's group indicating pineal secretion directly into the cerebrospinal fluid are very convincing too. We have to find the biological cause of this contradiction.

Wurtman: There is no blood–brain barrier for melatonin but it concentrates in the brain a hundred times better if it is placed in the cerebrospinal fluid.

Kappers: This pharmacological finding is, in itself, no reason for accepting that, under physiological circumstances, the pineal secretory products are extruded into the cerebrospinal fluid! Once more I should like to stress that all light and electron microscopical data point to the extrusion of the pineal products into the general blood circulation.

Wurtman: The essential experiment requires a large animal whose pineal makes a lot of melatonin. One then should stimulate the sympathetic nerves to the pineal and measure the melatonin in the venous blood coming from the pineal and cerebrospinal fluid from the cisterna magna.

Kappers: Perhaps a bioassay method could be used to demonstrate characteristic pineal compounds such as melatonin in the blood of the confluens sinuum.

Wurtman: I agree that a chromatography method followed by bioassay is the most hopeful. The problem with isotope methods is that you cannot give a radioactive precursor for melatonin and get the pineal to label itself, because such a tiny fraction of all the tryptophan in the body goes to the pineal. When melatonin emerges from the pineal both the amine and the oxygen are blocked because it is N-acetylated and O-methylated.

The pineal does us the favour of being out of the brain; it is not within the brain in the way that the hypothalamic releasing factor cells are. In this sense it's much more like the adrenal medulla. It is possible to isolate the adrenal medulla, stimulate the cholinergic nerve leading into it and measure the adrenaline released into the venous blood. This gives one some idea of its normal physiology. This same study of input–output relations must now be done for the pineal.

Fraschini: With Dr Z. Kniewald we have recently tried to establish a gas chromatographic procedure for the estimation of melatonin in the plasma and in the pineal gland. The preliminary results obtained so far look very promising. It was possible to measure melatonin in the peripheral blood during the night (when its synthesis is activated) but not at 6 p.m. following a prolonged period of exposure to light.

Kordon: Since a specific serotoninergic mechanism seems to be inhibitory to the hypothalamic control of sexual behaviour (Meyerson 1964), it would be worthwhile investigating whether melatonin or pinealectomy are also able to affect behavioural responses. On the other hand—and also in view of a possible mediation of melatonin effects by serotonin—one of Dr Fraschini's results raises a problem. In most of his experiments, melatonin was supplied directly to the median eminence—a structure which contains serotoninergic terminals, but apparently no cell bodies. Is it likely that melatonin could affect serotonin metabolism at that level, without being in contact with the cell bodies at all?

Wurtman: Is serotonin synthesized in the terminals, just as noradrenaline is?

Owman: Yes, it is. I would think it possible to have effects of melatonin mediated on the terminals as well as on the cell bodies.

Antón-Tay: Dr Kordon has shown that median eminence tissue can synthesize [^{14}C]serotonin from [^{14}C]tryptophan *in vitro*. Moreover, melatonin may be promoting some other biochemical or neurophysiological change in the neural population that is sensitive to melatonin.

Milcu: The doses of melatonin often used in experiments (of the order of a hundred microgrammes) seem to me to be very large. According to Prop and Kappers (1961) a rat pineal contains only about 5×10^{-4} µg of melatonin.

Martini: The pineal might not be a gland which stores the compound it has made.

Axelrod: If you inject melatonin, after 30 minutes it has all gone from the circulation. After giving one injection, no matter how much you give, it will disappear very fast.

Nir: The possibility remains that it could be stored.

Axelrod: Not that I know of, except in the pineal gland itself, but not much there; the ovary has a little.

Milcu: It is important to distinguish between a pharmacological effect and a physiological effect of melatonin.

BEHAVIOURAL EFFECTS OF PINEAL PRINCIPLES

Martini: In collaboration with Dr M. C. Fioretti, we have recently studied some non-endocrinological effects of pineal principles. First of all, we have evaluated whether melatonin, 5-hydroxytryptophol, 5-methoxytryptophol and 5-hydroxytryptamine might modify the duration of barbiturate-induced sleep in rats. Pineal indoles and methoxyindoles have been injected intraventricularly; pentobarbitone (3 mg/100 g body weight) has been injected intraperitoneally.

Figure 1 clearly indicates that intraventricular injections of melatonin

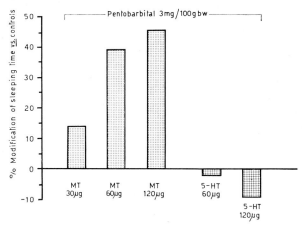

FIG. 1 (Martini). Effect of intraventricular injections of melatonin (MT) and of serotonin (5-hydroxytryptamine, 5-HT) on pentobarbitone-induced sleep in male rats.

are able to prolong the effect of pentobarbitone. It is also apparent that this effect of melatonin is dose-related.

Figure 2 shows that 5-methoxytryptophol is also able to potentiate the activity of barbiturates. However, the potentiating effect of this methoxy-indole is somewhat lower than that of melatonin. The effect of 5-methoxy-tryptophol, like that of melatonin, is dose-related. 5-Hydroxytryptophol is much less effective than either melatonin or 5-methoxytryptophol in increasing the duration of sleep in barbiturate-treated animals. Serotonin is completely ineffective.

These data suggest that pineal principles (and particularly melatonin and 5-methoxytryptophol) may exert a sedative effect on the central nervous

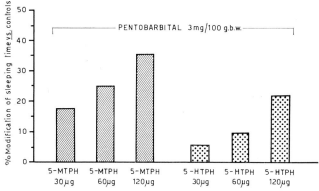

FIG. 2 (Martini). Effect of intraventricular injections of 5-methoxy-tryptophol (5-MTPH) and of 5-hydroxytryptophol (5-HTPH) on pentobarbitone-induced sleep in male rats.

system. Additional evidence indicating that pineal hormones may interfere with brain activity has already been reported at this meeting.

In another set of experiments performed with Dr M. C. Fioretti, we have studied whether melatonin might influence the acquisition or the extinction of a conditioned avoidance response. In these experiments melatonin was injected subcutaneously in a daily dose of 250 µg/rat.

Figure 3 shows that the acquisition of the conditioned response is quite similar in the controls and in the melatonin-treated animals. By contrast,

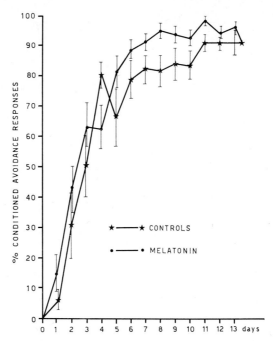

FIG. 3 (Martini). Effect of subcutaneous injections of melatonin (250 µg/rat per day) on the rate of acquisition of an avoidance response in normal male rats.

the extinction of the learned avoidance response is significantly facilitated in animals chronically treated with melatonin (Fig. 4).

These data might be taken to prove once more an effect of melatonin on the central nervous system. However, another interpretation is also possible. Dr Motta has shown (see pp. 279–291) that melatonin suppresses the secretion of ACTH. De Wied (1969) has repeatedly reported that ACTH is able to retard the extinction of avoidance responses. Consequently, one might also suggest that the effect of melatonin reported here is not direct in nature, but mediated by the suppression of the secretion of ACTH.

Axelrod: We (Quinn, Axelrod and Brodie 1959; Axelrod, Reichenthal and Brodie 1954) found that we could prolong the sleeping time after barbiturates with compounds such as SKF 525 and oestradiol. The reason was that these drugs block the metabolism of phenobarbitones by liver microsomal enzymes. Melatonin is also metabolized by the same group of enzymes in the liver which metabolize barbiturates (Kopin *et al.* 1961). Dr Wurtman has shown that if you give pentobarbitone you can induce the metabolism of melatonin (Wurtman, Axelrod and Antón-Tay 1968).

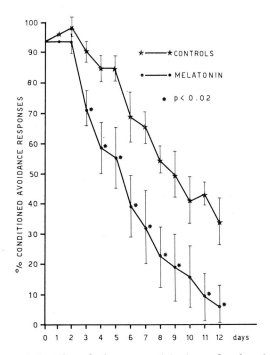

Fig. 4 (Martini). Effect of subcutaneous injections of melatonin (250 μg/rat per day) on the rate of extinction of an avoidance response in normal male rats.

All the compounds that are active in prolonging the sleeping time are metabolized by this microsomal enzyme, methoxytryptophol for example, while serotonin is not. The prolongation of the sleeping time might be due to melatonin blocking the metabolism of the barbiturate, therefore.

Wurtman: The fact that placing serotonin in the cerebrospinal fluid did not have the same effect as melatonin need not mean that serotonin is not involved, for the following reason. W. Feldberg and others who have put serotonin in the cerebrospinal fluid and studied its effects on sleep or body

temperature have postulated that serotonin is not acting as a neurotransmitter; that is, it is not entering the brain and doing what serotonin normally
does; rather it is acting on receptors near the ventricular surface (like the
area postrema) that are washed with cerebrospinal fluid. It's quite possible
that melatonin is affecting serotonin synthesis and turnover in brain loci
which are involved in sleeping, whereas serotonin placed in the cerebrospinal fluid either lacks this effect or antagonizes its own effect by direct
effects on receptors in the area postrema.

Herbert: Professor Martini, you might consider substituting MSH for
ACTH as the critical substance in the learning experiments. Bertolini and
co-workers (1969) injected a number of peptides into the cerebral ventricles
of male rabbits and found that MSH was as effective as ACTH in inducing
"sexual excitement". We know of course that melatonin has a pronounced
effect on MSH.

Martini: Actually what is important for the behavioural effects is the
chain of seven amino acids from 4 to 10, which are common to both ACTH
and MSH; so you might be quite right.

Shein: In order to investigate whether serotonin is the mediator of the
sleep induced by melatonin in Professor Martini's experiments, it might be
worthwhile trying an inhibitor of serotonin synthesis, *p*-chlorophenylala-
nine for example, to see whether melatonin would still have similar
sleep-inducing effects in the presence of both depressed serotonin levels and
inhibited serotonin synthesis.

ROLE OF THE PINEAL IN COLD ADAPTATION

Miline: We have studied the part played by the pineal in the regulatory
system controlling adaptation to cold (Miline 1969; Miline *et al.* 1969,
1970). One group of normal adult male rats and one group of epiphysectomized adult male rats were exposed to an external temperature of
3°–10 °C for two weeks. The pineal gland is very sensitive to cold.
After one week there was an increase of the activities of succinic dehydrogenase, monoamine oxidase, alkaline and acid phosphatases and adenosine
triphosphatases in the pineal gland. In electron micrographs two characteristics were seen: dilatation of the Golgi zone and the appearance of secretion
granules; and the presence of a large number of synaptic ribbons. The
supraoptic nucleus of normal rats after exposure to cold showed various
depressive changes, including blockade of neurosecretory granules. The
nuclei of the neuroglandular cells were reduced in volume. In epiphysectomized rats exposed to cold there was hypertrophy of the neuroglandular
cells, hypertrophy of the nuclei and nucleoli, migration of nucleoli into

the cytoplasm and the appearance of vacuoles in the cytoplasm. In the pars nervosa of the hypophysis after exposure to cold of normal rats there is blockade and stasis of neurosecretory material, but after epiphysectomy large numbers of neurosecretory granules are mobilized. The epiphysectomized rats are more sensitive to cold than normal rats.

The question arises of the part played by the changes in the pineal gland in the regulation of adaptation to cold. Are they the result of stress due to cold or a manifestation of a specific active intervention of the pineal in the interplay of the nervous and endocrine systems under the influence of cold? Among the responses of the organism to a changed environmental temperature, the behaviour of the hypothalamus, which is a fundamental relay in thermoregulatory reflexes (Laborit 1966), is particularly important under stress conditions because of the hypothalamo-epiphysial connexions. In rats with intact pineal glands exposed to low temperatures, the neuroglandular cells of the supraoptic nucleus show signs of reduced activity. In epiphysectomized rats, the supraoptic nucleus shows signs of increased activity under the influence of cold. These results indicate correlated functioning of the pineal gland and hypothalamus during stress by cold. Since the pineal gland is responsible for the behaviour of the supraoptic nucleus at low temperatures, it follows that the pineal gland is active in the response to these environmental factors.

These results show that the mechanism of the effects of low temperatures on the diencephalon is complex and that the pineal gland is to be considered as integrated in the regulatory system for adaptation to cold.

CONTROL OF CIRCADIAN RHYTHMS

Nir: We have heard about the different circadian rhythms found in the pineal. In the rat pineal the "phasing" of some rhythms like that of serotonin, through the synchronizing influence of external lighting, resembles the regulation by lighting of other circadian rhythms. These similarities would suggest that the nervous route which transmits lighting information regulating pineal function might also transmit lighting information that influences other circadian rhythms. To see whether this is so we decided to explore a possible link between the pineal and a peripheral circadian rhythm. The secretion of urinary 17-ketosteroids was chosen for investigation.

We examined the 17-ketosteroids excreted in urine of adult female rats in two periods of time: a 12-hour light period and a 12-hour dark period. A definite rhythm could be seen in the quantities excreted, both of urine and 17-ketosteroids, during the dark and light periods. The dark period values were approximately twice those of the light period. We then pinealectomized the animals in the hope that the rhythm would be abolished, but were disappointed because nothing changed, neither the diuresis nor the output of 17-ketosteroids.

Consequently we decided to study whether these rhythms could be affected before they were established. Immature 21-day-old female rats were pinealectomized and their diurnal diuresis and 17-ketosteroid excretion followed for 8 weeks. We found that in the pinealectomized animals the rhythm was evident much earlier (between 3 and 5 weeks) than in the sham-operated and intact controls (between 5 and 7 weeks). This may imply that the pineal normally acts as a kind of gear for the circadian rhythm of 17-ketosteroids. By removing the gland the rhythm is generated much earlier. This may be the first example of the pineal controlling a circadian rhythm other than its own.

Wurtman: There seems to be some debate in the literature about the age at which the adrenal cortical rhythm normally develops in the rat. Dr Fiske has done a lot of work with this.

Fiske: We (Fiske and Leeman 1964) found that the 24-hour rhythm in circulating corticosterone was not evident in 16 to 18-day-old Sprague Dawley rats (Charles River Laboratories) of either sex but was detectable in animals 20 to 22 days of age. The sex differences in corticosterone secretion occur later.

Wurtman: So it starts much earlier in Wellesley, Massachusetts than in Jerusalem!

Nir: This is different from our experiments. We have been determining not the blood corticosterone levels around the clock, but the total urinary 17-ketosteroids excreted during a 12-hour period of light and a 12-hour period of darkness. In our experiments a significant difference was evident at a certain age which was earlier in the pinealectomized animals than in the controls, but this does not mean that the blood corticosterone rhythm could not have been established before that. Our finding may be associated with the accelerated sexual maturation known to occur in pinealectomized rats.

Fiske: Allen and Kendall (1967) have reported similar results to ours; they found diurnal differences in plasma levels of corticosterone in rats 25 to 30 days of age.

LIGHT INPUT TO THE PINEAL

Wurtman: There is increasing interest in identifying the photoreceptors that mediate the effect of light on the mammalian and avian pineal. There has been some physiological evidence that early in life light can affect the pineal in the blinded mammal (Zweig, Snyder and Axelrod 1966), with a suggestion that there might be an extraretinal photoreceptor. What are the minimal criteria for accepting the existence of an extraretinal photoreceptor? Secondly, suppose one did a spectral sensitivity curve and found that the ability of light to inhibit HIOMT in the intact animal was, for example, greater for blue light than for yellow-green (that is, the most sensitive part of the spectrum for vision). How should one interpret this differential sensitivity of HIOMT?

Dodt: We have no idea about extraretinal photoreception in mammals. Nobody has shown any light sensitivity other than that mediated by the lateral eyes. This, however, does not exclude that light, especially ultraviolet radiation, produces some change in chemical compounds; on the other hand, ultraviolet light is heavily absorbed by blood and skin and other tissue, so I don't see any possibility for ultraviolet radiation to reach the pineal body. In blinded ducks Benoit and Assenmacher (1959) have shown that red light is more effective for neurovegetative reactions, which means that blood transmits mainly long-wavelength light either to unidentified photoreceptor structures within the brain or to unidentified chemical compounds located at some unknown site.

In answer to your second question, the photoreceptive capacity of light receptors within the lateral eye of higher vertebrates is well known. In nocturnal animals, wavelengths between violet and yellow are mainly effective; in day animals, wavelengths between blue-green and red are effective.

Wurtman: But if we were to find the opposite, that blue is more effective than yellow light in acting indirectly on the pineal, in terms of what is known about the photopigments in the photoreceptor cells, is there a rod or a cone that contains a photopigment that you would expect to be maximally responsive in the blue portion of the spectrum?

Dodt: In the light-adapted retina there are some photoreceptors especially sensitive to blue light, in the frog and the rabbit for example. Besides this, all photopigments in mammals are more sensitive to wavelengths between ultraviolet and blue than to red, where light absorption slows down linearly with the increase of wavelength. The high sensitivity of all photopigments to short wavelengths is due to the absorption within the β-band. However, you will get lower absorption there than by exposing the animals to lights between blue-green and yellow, because of absorption within the α-band.

Wurtman: So if somebody does observe that blue light is more effective than yellow in inhibiting the pineal, it would be very unusual.

Kordon: Similar results have been obtained by Professor Benoit and co-workers (1966). They showed that the retinal receptors involved in photostimulation of the gonads in the duck are only affected by red radiation, and practically unresponsive to other wavelengths, in contrast to the visual receptors, which are maximally sensitive to yellow light.

Wurtman: Of course this was a bird, not a mammal, and once one gets into that portion of the red one has to worry about heat effects.

Kordon: There were no heat effects in this experiment, since infrared wavelengths were eliminated by the use of interference filters with a very small bandwidth.

Oksche: There is a gap between our understanding of the functions of the pineals of vertebrates and those of mammals. We know the outer segment structure; we know the chromatic and achromatic reactions of the lower vertebrate pineal, as shown by Professor Dodt; we know from Dr Owman that there is serotonin in the epiphysis of fishes and frogs (Owman and Rüdeberg 1970; Owman, Rüdeberg and Ueck 1970) but what is the biological significance of these responses and substances and how do we have to understand Dr Menaker's experiments that locomotor rhythms are controlled by the pineal (Gaston and Menaker 1968)? If we compare for example the hypophysis of the lamprey with that of the rat, they are structurally very different but there is a clear-cut outline of hypophysial functions, and I do not yet see this clear-cut outline for the pineal systems *in toto*, perhaps because we do not know the *biological* significance of all the light-dependent reactions of lower vertebrate pineals. Are they transformed into some kind of neuroendocrine mechanism—that is, pigmentary responses, colour changes? Are they conducted to some extrapyramidal locomotor or phototactic system? This is still unknown.

REFERENCES

ALLEN, C. and KENDALL, J. W. (1967) *Endocrinology* **80**, 926–930.

ANTÓN-TAY, F., CHOU, C., ANTON, S. and WURTMAN, R. J. (1968) *Science* **162**, 277–278.

AURES, D., HÅKANSON, R. and OWMAN, CH. (1969) *J. Neuro-visc. Rel.* **31**, 337–349.

AXELROD, J., REICHENTHAL, J. and BRODIE, B. B. (1954) *J. Pharmac. exp. Ther.* **112**, 49–54.

AZMITIA, E. C., JR. and MCEWEN, B. S. (1969) *Science* **166**, 1274–1276.

BENOIT, J. and ASSENMACHER, I. (1959) *Recent Prog. Horm. Res.* **15**, 143–164.

BENOIT, J., LAGE, C. DA, MUEL, B. *et al.* (1966) *C.r. hebd. Séanc. Acad. Sci., Paris, Sér. D* **263**, 62.

BENTLEY, P. J. (1963) *Gen. comp. Endocr.* **3**, 281–285.

BERTOLINI, A., VERGONI, W., GESSA, G. L. and FERRARI, W. (1969) *Nature, Lond.* **221**, 667–669.

DE WIED, D. (1969) In *Frontiers in Neuroendocrinology*, pp. 97–140, ed. Ganong, W. F. and Martini, L. New York and London: Oxford University Press.

FALCK, B. and OWMAN, CH. (1968) *Adv. Pharmac.* **6A**, 211–231.

FISKE, V. M. and HUPPERT, L. C. (1968) *Science* **162**, 279.

FISKE, V. M. and LEEMAN, S. E. (1964) *Ann. N.Y. Acad. Sci.* **117**, 231–243.

GASTON, S. and MENAKER, M. (1968) *Science* **160**, 1125–1127.

HÅKANSON, R. (1970) *Acta physiol. scand.* suppl. 340, 1–134.

JONES, R. L., McGEER, P. L. and GREINER, A. C. (1969) *Clin. chim. Acta* **26**, 281–285.

JOUVET, M. (1969) *Science* **163**, 32–41.

JUTISZ, M. and DE LA LLOSA, M. P. (1970) *Endocrinology* **86**, 761–768.

KOPIN, I. J., PARE, C. M. B., AXELROD, J. and WEISSBACH, H. (1961) *J. biol. Chem.* **236**, 3072–3075.

LABORIT, H. (1966) *Thermorégulation et la système nerveux végétatif.* Basel: Karger.

MELANDER, A., OWMAN, CH. and SUNDLER, F. (1970) *Histochemie* in press.

MEYERSON, B. (1964) *Acta physiol. scand.* **63**, suppl. 241, 5.

MILCU, I. (1967) *Proc. Congresul de Endocrinologie, Bucureşti*, p. 221.

MILCU, S. M. *et al.* (1957) *Comunle Acad. Rep. pop. rom.* **7**, 491.

MILINE, R. (1969) *Int. J. Biometeorology* **13**, suppl. 1, 6.

MILINE, R., DEVEČERSKI, V., ŠIJAČKI, N. and KRSTIĆ, R. (1970) *Hormones* in press.

MILINE, R., WERNER, R., ŠĆEPOVIĆ, M., DEVEČERSKI, V. and MILINE, J. (1969) *Bull. Ass. Anat., Paris* **145**, 289–293.

MOSZKOWSKA, A. (1965) In *Structure and Function of the Epiphysis Cerebri* (*Progress in Brain Research* vol. 10), pp. 564–575, ed. Kappers, J. A. and Schadé, J. P. Amsterdam: Elsevier.

OWMAN, CH. (1963) *Q. Jl exp. Physiol.* **48**, 402–407.

OWMAN, CH. (1964) *Acta endocr.* **47**, 500–516.

OWMAN, CH. and RÜDEBERG, C. (1970) *Z. Zellforsch. mikrosk. Anat.* **107**, 522–550.

OWMAN, CH., RÜDEBERG, C. and UECK, M. (1970) *Z. Zellforsch. mikrosk. Anat.* **111**, 550–558.

PEARSE, A. G. E. (1968a) *Proc. R. Soc. B* **170**, 71–80.

PEARSE, A. G. E. (1968b) *J. Histochem. Cytochem.* **17**, 303–313.

POHORECKY, L. A., ZIGMOND, M., KARTEN, H. and WURTMAN, R. J. (1969) *J. Pharmac. exp. Ther.* **165**, 190–196.

PROP, N. and KAPPERS, J. A. (1961) *Acta anat.* **45**, 90.

QUINN, G. P., AXELROD, J. and BRODIE, B. B. (1959) *Biochem. Pharmac.* **1**, 152–159.

SAMLI, M. H. and GESCHWIND, I. I. (1968) *Endocrinology* **82**, 225.

SCEMAMA, A. (1970) In *Neuroendocrinologie*, ed. Benoit, J. and Kordon, C. Paris: Centre National de la Recherche Scientifique.

VIVEROS, O. H., ARQUEROS, L. and KIRSHNER, N. (1969) *Science* **165**, 911–913.

WEINSHILBOUM, R. and AXELROD, J. (1970) *Pharmacologist* **12**, 214.

WURTMAN, R. J., AXELROD, J. and ANTÓN-TAY, F. (1968) *J. Pharmac. exp. Ther.* **161**, 367–372.

ZWEENS, J. (1965) In *Structure and Function of the Epiphysis Cerebri* (*Progress in Brain Research* vol. 10), pp. 540–551, ed. Kappers, J. A. and Schadé, J. P. Amsterdam: Elsevier.

ZWEIG, M., SNYDER, S. H. and AXELROD, J. (1966) *Proc. natn. Acad. Sci. U.S.A.* **56**, 515–520.

SUMMARY OF SYMPOSIUM

R. J. WURTMAN

It is very difficult to summarize the content of a meeting in which information bombs keep bursting to the last minute before the summary, but it might be useful to attempt to consider where the pineal was at the time of the last big meeting (Kappers and Schadé 1965), what the major discoveries have been since, and what we can agree on as a consensus statement of pineal function in 1970. Then perhaps we can try to identify the major gaps in our knowledge and the critical experiments which remain to be done.

The 1963 meeting in Amsterdam was an exciting time because many of us discovered that people working in a variety of different disciplines had almost simultaneously turned their attention to the pineal during the previous four or five years and had come up with hard facts. Indeed, the "hard facts" enunciated at Amsterdam were to form the basis of what has taken place during the ensuing seven years.

Some of these "hard facts" included the following. First, it was clear by 1963 that the pineal was not one, but at least two organs (Kelly 1962). Within the vertebrate kingdom the pineal could be a photoreceptive structure or a quite different secretory structure: there had been an extraordinary evolution from photoreceptive to secretory pineals and although it is not yet known whether the photoreceptive cell specifically evolved into the secretory cell or whether there are two cell types throughout phylogeny, it was certain that pineal organs could not automatically be labelled as glands. Secondly, thanks largely to studies by Dr Ariëns Kappers, it was recognized that even though the mammalian pineal originates embryologically as part of the brain and even though it lies within the cranium and is connected to the brain by a stalk, the pineal is not really part of the brain in the adult mammal but instead receives its sole neuronal input from the peripheral autonomic nervous system (Kappers 1960). This strange relationship between the pineal and the nervous system turned out to be very important in subsequent studies of pineal physiology.

In 1963 it had been known for three or four years that the pineal contained at least one unique chemical, melatonin, which was discovered by Dr Lerner in his attempt to identify the pigment-cell-lightening factor in bovine pineal extracts (Lerner, Case and Heinzelman 1959). Repeated attempts to relate melatonin to pigmentation in people and other mammals have since yielded disappointing results (Wurtman, Axelrod and Kelly 1968). However, this discovery of melatonin was of great importance, inasmuch as it provided the first hard, biochemical fact about the pineal. Soon after, it was shown that the pineal not only contained melatonin but also could synthesize melatonin. Moreover, as Axelrod and Weissbach demonstrated, *only* the pineal could make melatonin in mammals, because *only* the pineal had the methylating enzyme, hydroxyindole-O-methyl-transferase (HIOMT), that catalysed the terminal step in melatonin bio-synthesis (Axelrod *et al.* 1961).

In 1963 it was known on the basis of several decades of studies (sum-marized by Kitay and Altschule in 1954) that the mammalian pineal had an inhibitory effect on gonad growth and gonad weight: Fiske and others had also shown that environmental lighting stimulated the growth of the rat (Fiske 1941) but depressed pineal weight (Fiske, Bryant and Putnam 1960). Hence it had been possible for us to hypothesize several years earlier that light stimulated the gonads, whatever that meant, by inhibiting the synthesis or release of some gonad-inhibiting substance made in the pineal (Wurtman *et al.* 1961). The suggestion had not yet been made that melatonin was that gonad-inhibiting substance, but one could see it on the horizon. By 1963 it had been shown that melatonin had some effects upon the weight and function of the rat gonads (Wurtman, Axelrod and Chu 1963). However, these effects were hardly dramatic, and it was not clear what to make of them.

In 1963 it was already recognized that the pineal contained very large amounts of biogenic amines, but especially serotonin (Giarman and Day 1959). Moreover, pineal serotonin was unusual in that it was present not only within parenchymal cells but also within the terminals of pineal sympathetic nerves (Bertler, Falck and Owman 1964). (This was and remains terribly unusual; I don't know of any other locus in the body where serotonin is present in peripheral nerve endings.) It had been shown that pineal sympathetic nerves take up radioactive noradrenaline (Wolfe *et al.* 1962) and it was therefore suggested that noradrenaline was the neurotransmitter released by them as well as by other sympathetic nerve endings. It had not yet been shown that the pineal sympathetic nerves actually contained the endogenous catecholamine. Soon it was to be shown that they did (Zieher and Pellegrino de Iraldi 1966; Wurtman and Axelrod 1966) and then the question could be considered of which biogenic mono-amine, serotonin or noradrenaline, was the pineal sympathetic neuro-transmitter.

It is apparent to all who have attended the present meeting that since

1963 many major advances have been made in our knowledge of the pineal. Almost all of those advances were built on the facts enunciated at Amsterdam.

It has since been shown that environmental lighting, acting indirectly by the eyes, controls pineal biosynthetic activity. It was initially demonstrated that light controlled the synthesis of melatonin in the rat pineal by depressing the activity of the enzyme hydroxyindole-O-methyltransferase (HIOMT) (Wurtman, Axelrod and Phillips 1963). Subsequently, it was shown that environmental lighting affects other enzymes in the pineal, first aromatic L-amino acid decarboxylase (Snyder *et al.* 1965), more recently the N-acetylating enzyme (Klein, Berg and Weller 1970; Klein *et al.* 1970). It was shown that the pathway by which light reached the pineal ultimately depended on its exotic sympathetic innervation, such that if one deprived the pineal of sympathetic nervous signals (either by cutting these nerves or decentralizing the superior cervical ganglia) the pineal was functionally cut off from environmental lighting (Wurtman, Axelrod and Fischer 1964). So it became apparent that the pineal of mammals continues to be related to light even though it is no longer directly photoreceptive: it is now dependent on the lateral eyes and, ultimately, on its sympathetic nerves, for information about the state of environmental lighting.

Soon it was shown that the effects of constant light and constant darkness upon pineal function were simply an exaggeration of daily rhythms in pineal function, the normal 12 hour light/dark, on/off cycle that reflected itself in changes in pineal biosynthetic activity, in HIOMT activity (Axelrod, Wurtman and Snyder 1965) and in the serotonin content (Quay 1963) of the pineal. The serotonin rhythm in the pineal was found to be fundamentally different from the rhythm of the melatonin-forming enzyme, HIOMT, in that the latter rhythm was completely dependent upon environmental lighting for its existence whereas the serotonin rhythm persisted in animals that were deprived of a cyclic photic input. Soon thereafter, it was demonstrated that the central nervous pathways that mediated the effect of light and dark on the pineal were fundamentally different from the pathway that mediated the effect of light on vision, and that the pathway leading ultimately to the pineal involved the inferior accessory optic tracts (Moore *et al.* 1968). It was also shown that not only did denervating the pineal (by bilateral superior cervical ganglionectomy) block *its* response to light but it also suppressed some of the effects of light on the gonads (Wurtman *et al.* 1967). This provided further evidence that changes in pineal secretory patterns in response to light and darkness mediated at least some of the gonadal responses to light and darkness.

13*

Around 1964 or 1965 it was shown that another experimental animal, the hamster, showed much greater changes in gonad weight in response to environmental lighting and to removal of the pineal than the albino rat (Hoffman and Reiter 1965). This was gratifying for several reasons: first it is clearly much better to work with a 10-fold change than a 20 per cent change. Secondly, there are some fundamental and unresolved, almost philosophical problems engendered by using albino animals as models for studying effects of light and dark on neuroendocrine physiology. A variety of subsequent studies on the pineals of many species of vertebrates suggest that most, if not all, show some biochemical response to light; I am not aware of a single bird or mammal that has been studied which has not shown some change in HIOMT activity in response to environmental light. On the other hand, we were unable to detect any effect of light and dark on melatonin synthesis in the frog. A large body of indirect evidence has by now accumulated showing that the pineal does participate in effects of light and dark on gonad function, probably by changing its rate of methoxyindole biosynthesis.

Several years ago Owman (1964) showed that the presence of serotonin within pineal nerves was very likely an artifact caused by the very high concentration in nearby pinealocytes: if one removed the pineal from its normal position and put it somewhere else among sympathetic nerves, so long as the pineal continued to make large amounts of serotonin the sympathetic nerves near it would take on the fluorescence characteristics of serotonin. This suggested that pineal neuronal serotonin might not necessarily be important in pineal function. Subsequent studies using organ culture methods have demonstrated that the neurotransmitter that appears to mediate the sympathetic control of melatonin synthesis is not serotonin at all, but noradrenaline (Axelrod, Shein and Wurtman 1969; Wurtman et al. 1969). This is a source of some relief to neuropharmacologists, inasmuch as it allows us to return to a simpler representation of the postganglionic sympathetic nervous system; Bishop Occam would be pleased that all sympathetic nerves once again can be thought to use the same transmitter.

Several years ago it was shown that if one implanted melatonin within the brain, or, more recently, one placed melatonin within the lateral ventricles, one thereby produced significantly greater physiological effects than if one gave the indole systemically (see Fraschini, Collu and Martini 1971). This has also produced a gratifying amplification of the physiological responses associated with the pineal. It has, however, raised a nagging question that I hope someone will answer soon, of whether melatonin is physiologically secreted into the cerebrospinal fluid or into the bloodstream.

To my knowledge, there is only one other hormone yet demonstrated to be released into the cerebrospinal fluid, the anti-diuretic hormone. I still think that a study that I suggested earlier should be done, namely to determine whether stimulating the pineal sympathetic nerve causes an increase in melatonin elaboration into the venous blood draining the brain, or into the cerebrospinal fluid, or into both. In any event, it was shown that the amount of melatonin that entered and remained within the brain was at least a hundred times greater if melatonin was placed in the cerebrospinal fluid than if it was placed in the blood (Antón-Tay and Wurtman 1969), and these direct and indirect studies conspired to generate a hypothesis that seems to have won fairly wide acceptance here, namely that the most likely locus of melatonin action is on the brain itself. This is in contrast to the assumption some of us made in 1963 that melatonin might act on the periphery, on the basis of evidence that radioactive melatonin was concentrated in the ovaries (Wurtman, Axelrod and Potter 1964). We should have known better than to assume that the site in which a hormone is concentrated is necessarily the site at which it acts.

Around this time, it was shown that not only was melatonin taken up in the brain, but also that it was concentrated within certain areas of great neuroendocrine interest, namely the midbrain and the hypothalamus (Antón-Tay and Wurtman 1969). Moreover, melatonin was shown to exert marked chemical effects upon these brain areas. Melatonin was first shown to affect the amounts of serotonin present within the midbrain, the hypothalamus and the telencephalon (Antón-Tay et al. 1968). More recently it has been shown to affect the levels of another putative neurotransmitter, GABA, and, perhaps more important, of an enzyme, pyridoxal kinase, which is involved in the synthesis of serotonin, GABA and probably other neurotransmitters as well (Antón-Tay 1971). This interest in the possibility that melatonin produces its endocrine effects by acting on the brain coincided with the realization that the administration of the indole also led to other physiological effects that must involve the brain. About five years ago the first paper was published showing that melatonin affected the electroencephalogram (Marczynski et al. 1964). Melatonin has since been shown by several laboratories to affect sleep and behaviour.

Over the past few years we have been fortunate to witness some nice "coupling" experiments in which one laboratory shows that taking out the pineal does one thing and another shows that giving melatonin does the opposite. This begins to look like legitimate endocrinology. For example, Antón-Tay and I show that melatonin causes an increase in brain serotonin in certain regions; Kordon and Glowinski show that pinealectomy causes a decrease. Martini and his collaborators show that melatonin causes an increase in the sensitivity of the brain to barbiturates; Nir and his colleagues show that pinealectomy seems to decrease the lethality of barbiturates. Mess shows that pinealectomy can *cause* ovulation in animals with supra-chiasmatic lesions, while melatonin can block this effect. Melatonin also appears to block ovulation in normal animals provided it is given before the critical period, and as Kordon has shown, this critical period has been shown to bear some special relationship to brain serotonin levels. It has been shown by several laboratories using a variety of rodent species that pinealectomy accelerates spontaneous vaginal opening; here too, melatonin appears to block the effect.

The past few years have seen the development of better physiological assay systems for studying the effects of pinealectomy or of pineal com-pounds on the gonads. There is first the recognition, initially attributable to Reiter and Hoffman, that some species of animals show bigger responses to light/dark effects or to melatonin than others. Secondly, it has been recognized that many of the functions that the pineal influences are also influenced by other inputs—cold, olfaction, light/dark, neural inputs, and circulating testosterone levels, for example. The more the investigator can standardize or simplify or remove these inputs, the more sensitive his preparation is likely to be to the effects of melatonin or pinealectomy. We have seen some strange types of experimental animals presented here, animals that differ very much from the animals that God put on the earth, but animals which are in consequence far more sensitive than their natural counterparts to the effects of melatonin and pinealectomy.

During all this time, the growth of the pineal has involved not only true pinealologists but many other scientists who were not primarily concerned with the pineal but liked to use it because it's there, it's convenient and it has some particular attributes that make it especially useful for their purposes. For example, there have probably been as many papers written on synaptic vesicles in the pineal as on any other organ, even though there are very few synapses in the pineal, and I suspect that many pharmacolo-gists think of the pineal simply as a bag of serotonin or a bag of synaptic vesicles. The pineal has been very convenient for studying indole metabo-lism and its responses to drugs; the pineal is a lot easier to remove in one uncontaminated piece than a particular brain region that contains serotonin. I also suspect that as much is known about the comparative evolution of pineal cells in their transformation from a photosensitive to a secretory function as about any other type of cell. The pineal became an interesting object for study in this regard not only because it's the pineal but also because one sees these dramatic changes. So I suspect that the popularity of the pineal has grown apace not only because the accumulation of hard data has made more of us more willing to invest time in studying it, but also because many people who have had no particular commitment to it have elected to use it for their own disciplinary interests.

I would like to propose a formulation of mammalian pineal function, *circa* 1970, that we might all be able to accept. Light, acting through the eyes and the brain and the sympathetic nervous system, affects the pineal. One thing that light does to the mammalian pineal is to decrease the activity of the melatonin-forming enzyme; it also affects other enzymes. In the process light inhibits the synthesis of melatonin. Melatonin acts on the brain by influencing the synthesis or release of one or more neurotransmitters; in so doing it also modifies neuroendocrine function.

This formulation begs several very important questions. I said "light": is it only light that affects the pineal? I think most of us would doubt this; evidence has been presented here that cold, stress, hormones and other inputs can also affect the pineal function. Moreover, one should not talk about "light" as though it were a homogeneous entity that existed in two states: on and off. There are different spectra of light in nature and very different spectra in laboratories illuminated by commercial fluorescent and incandescent sources (Wurtman and Weisel 1969).

Secondly, we beg the question of other pineal hormones. This has turned out far more than any of us anticipated to be a melatonin meeting. It certainly was not that by design; it reflects the fact that more good work has been done on melatonin and other methoxyindoles than on most other compounds in the pineal. As enthusiastic as most of us are for melatonin, it would be a great mistake to forget the possibility that peptides and phospholipids and other compounds with potential biological activity might also be made and secreted by the pineal. Here one thinks of the thyroid. What gland has been better studied than the thyroid, and yet three or four years ago it was still possible to discover an additional thyroid hormone, thyrocalcitonin, that turns out to have great physiological significance. So we should keep an ear open for new information on other compounds made by the pineal; some of these might also have biological activity. I doubt we will be so lucky as to be presented with another low molecular weight compound whose synthesis is regulated by an enzyme found exclusively in the pineal.

Other questions that this formulation begs include other physiological actions of melatonin or other methoxyindoles on the brain which might be as important as, or more important than, their neuroendocrine effects. Many of us entered pineal research from careers in endocrinology; hence we quite naturally looked first for endocrine effects of pineal compounds. Also, much of the interest in the pineal was generated 97 years ago by the observation of its involvement in an endocrine syndrome (precocious puberty in a child with a pinealoma; Kitay and Altschule 1954). It may turn out that the effects of melatonin or its possible therapeutic uses may be far more important in non-endocrine than in endocrine areas. We should keep this possibility in mind when we design experiments on the pineal. Another question that we beg is the possibility that melatonin or methoxyindoles might act at other sites besides the brain. I privately suspect that the brain is the major site of action; however, there are investigators who report effects of melatonin on testicular metabolism, thyroid metabolism and elsewhere.

One of the major gaps in our knowledge concerns phylogenetic changes in pineal cytology. Is there a "basic" pineal photoreceptor cell which, in the course of evolution, has transformed itself into a secretory cell? Have there instead always been two "clones" of pineal cells, or even two distinct pineal organs, such that in different species one cell or organ predominates? I suspect this question is amenable to analysis and Dr Kelly has suggested some experimental ways of approaching it.

A similar question has to do with the function of ganglion cells within avian pineals, and now within ferret pineals. If these pineals lack photoreceptors, then what are the ganglion cells for? They are not doing what ganglion cells in pineals normally do, that is, they are not transmitting information about light to the brain, because they are not receiving any such information to start with. Do they receive efferent inputs? Do they send out afferent inputs? Also, in the mammal, what is the retinal photoreceptor that mediates the effect of light on the pineal? What is its action spectrum? After Professor Dodt's comments I would be especially interested in examining the possibility that blue light has an effect on HIOMT synthesis in the pineal. The action spectrum for the biochemical responses of the mammalian pineal awaits examination. Do non-retinal photoreceptors really exist in immature mammals, or are the reported effects of light on serotonin rhythms in blind newborn animals related to direct photochemical effects on the brain?

The pineal receives its nervous input from the superior cervical ganglion, which is one of many ganglia of the sympathetic nervous system. In general, people tend to think of the tone of the sympathetic nervous system as being controlled as a unit. Should we then expect to discover that light affects the tone of the sympathetic nerves to the blood vessels in the leg, or the tone of the preganglionic sympathetics to the adrenal medulla? I don't think anybody has examined these questions in experimental animals; it has, however, been shown that light and vision affect noradrenaline excretion in humans. The fact that light exposure has an effect on the flow of impulses through the superior cervical ganglion should now allow us to get further information about its relation to sympathetic nervous function in general. It should be possible to determine whether discrete control exists within the sympathetic nervous system; that is, are various regions of the sympathetic nervous system each influenced primarily by one kind of input, photic input for the superior cervical ganglion, an orthostatic input for the sympathetic nerves to the legs, and so on?

Are there really true cholinergic nerve endings in the pineal, or do the agranular vesicles described here simply reflect technical difficulties in displaying the granules? If cholinergic terminals exist, where do their axons come from? Is it possible, as has been suggested here, that noradrenaline from sympathetic nerve terminals might influence the N-acetylating enzyme, whereas the cholinergic input might affect HIOMT? We have a new degree of freedom if cholinergic nerves to the pineal really do exist. We also have the possibility of explaining why there can be two types of diurnal rhythms within the pineal: those that disappear when the day/night cycle is replaced by continuous darkness and those that persist. This paradox has not been explicable until now. Physiologically, the very important question of pineal input/output relations remains to be explained. Perhaps this is the central question of pineal physiology. How much of what does the pineal secrete, where and in response to what? Does the pineal secrete melatonin? Does it secrete serotonin? Does it secrete either of these indoles into the bloodstream or the cerebrospinal fluid? Does it secrete them in response to nerve impulses? Does the hormonal milieu—the plasma oestrogen levels and other hormonal factors—influence the input/output relations in the pineal? Is it possible that adult animals secrete less—or more—melatonin in response to a given neuronal input than do immature animals? Which brain neurons are the targets for pineal secretions? We have seen evidence that melatonin affects the serotonin levels and GABA levels in brain and affects the activity of an enzyme involved in synthesizing these, but I think none of us would any longer accept the notion that a change in the levels of a neurotransmitter within a neuron necessarily implies a change in the functional activity of that neuron. It suggests it but it doesn't prove it. Does melatonin affect the physiological activity of "serotoninergic" neurons?

The problem of studying the effects of melatonin on the brain is not dissimilar from the "classical" neuroendocrine problem of studying the effects of cortisol. How do we identify specific central neurons that respond to cortisol? We can give radioactive cortisol and see where it localizes. However, this approach has led us down blind alleys far more often than it has helped us—one thinks, for example, of melatonin concentrating in the ovary or phenobarbitone concentrating in the liver. Another possibility is to apply cortisone or dexamethasone directly to brain neurons and study the effects of such local applications on their electrophysiological activity. Perhaps someone will examine the effects of applying melatonin to midbrain raphe neurons. We can study the effects of cortisol or of melatonin on neurotransmitter synthesis and turnover. This sort of study has been done with gonadectomy and noradrenaline; it has been shown that gonadectomy accelerates the synthesis and turnover of brain noradrenaline. The important point is that we must now ask the same questions that any neuroendocrinologist asks in attempting to explain the effects of hormones on the brain. Here too we have the good fortune that melatonin has already been shown to do something that no other hormone has been shown to do, that is, to affect a brain enzyme in a major way.

In conclusion, I leave this meeting with very great optimism. I expected this to be a good meeting because seven years is a long time and there was a lot to say, but I am amazed at the quantity and the quality of the new information that has emerged. The meeting has been held at a good time; the pineal and melatonin are more and more topical. I am only concerned that the advance of knowledge in this field is so rapid and the number of people that could be invited to a subsequent meeting is so great, that it may never again be possible to hold a small multidisciplinary meeting on the pineal. This will be a great tragedy. The necessity of learning enough to understand practitioners of widely divergent disciplines has, I submit, been of critical importance to many of us working in this field. This was most striking during the discussion of Dr Herbert's paper on the ganglion cells in the ferret pineal: how the consideration of what these cells were and what their neurotransmitter was and what their physiological function might be touched the special interests of almost every one of us. The opportunity to meet and communicate with each other has, I submit, been a great source of strength in the development of pinealology. I hope that subsequent pineal meetings will also include this multidisciplinary grouping.

REFERENCES

ANTÓN-TAY, F. (1971) This volume, pp. 213–220.
ANTÓN-TAY, F., CHOU, C., ANTON, S. and WURTMAN, R. J. (1968) *Science* **162**, 277–278.
ANTÓN-TAY, F. and WURTMAN, R. J. (1969) *Nature, Lond.* **221**, 474–475.
AXELROD, J., MACLEAN, P. D., ALBERS, R. W. and WEISSBACH, H. (1961) In *Regional Neurochemistry*, pp. 307–311, ed. Kety, S. S. and Elkes, J. Oxford: Pergamon Press.
AXELROD, J., SHEIN, H. M. and WURTMAN, R. J. (1969) *Proc. natn. Acad. Sci. U.S.A.* **62**, 544.

AXELROD, J., WURTMAN, R. J. and SNYDER, S. H. (1965) *J. biol. Chem.* **240**, 949–954.
BERTLER, A., FALCK, B. and OWMAN, CH. (1964) *Acta physiol. scand.* suppl. 234, 1–18.
FISKE, V. M. (1941) *Endocrinology* **29**, 187–196.
FISKE, V. M., BRYANT, G. K. and PUTNAM, J. (1960) *Endocrinology* **66**, 489–491.
FRASCHINI, F., COLLU, R. and MARTINI, L. (1971) This volume, pp. 250–273.
GIARMAN, N. J. and DAY, N. (1959) *Biochem. Pharmac.* **1**, 235.
HOFFMAN, R. A. and REITER, R. J. (1965) *Science* **148**, 1609.
KAPPERS, J. A. (1960) *Z. Zellforsch. mikrosk. Anat.* **52**, 163–215.
KAPPERS, J. A. and SCHADÉ, J. P. (ed.) (1965) *Structure and Function of the Epiphysis Cerebri* (*Progress in Brain Research* vol. 10). Amsterdam: Elsevier.
KELLY, D. E. (1962) *Am. Scient.* **50**, 597–625.
KITAY, J. and ALTSCHULE, M. D. (1954) *The Pineal Gland—A Review of the Physiologic Literature.* Cambridge, Mass.: Harvard University Press.
KLEIN, D. C., BERG, G. R. and WELLER, J. (1970) *Science* **168**, 979–980.
KLEIN, D. C., BERG, G. R., WELLER, J. and GLINSMANN, W. (1970) *Science* **167**, 1738–1740.
LERNER, A. B., CASE, J. D. and HEINZELMAN, R. V. (1959) *J. Am. chem. Soc.* **81**, 6084.
MARCZYNSKI, T. J., YAMAGUCHI, N., LING, G. M. and GRODZINSKA, L. (1964) *Experientia* **20**, 435–437.
MOORE, R. Y., HELLER, A., BHATNAGAR, R. K., WURTMAN, R. J. and AXELROD, J. (1968) *Archs Neurol., Chicago* **18**, 208–218.
OWMAN, CH. (1964) *Int. J. Neuropharmac.* **2**, 105–112.
QUAY, W. B. (1963) *Gen. comp. Endocr.* **3**, 473–479.
SNYDER, S. H., AXELROD, J., WURTMAN, R. J. and FISCHER, J. E. (1965) *J. Pharmac. exp. Ther.* **147**, 371–375.
WOLFE, D. E., POTTER, L. T., RICHARDSON, K. C. and AXELROD, J. (1962) *Science* **138**, 440–442.
WURTMAN, R. J. and AXELROD, J. (1966) *Life Sci.* **5**, 665–669.
WURTMAN, R. J., AXELROD, J. and CHU, E. W. (1963) *Science* **142**, 1071–1073.
WURTMAN, R. J., AXELROD, J., CHU, E. W., HELLER, A. and MOORE, R. Y. (1967) *Endocrinology* **76**, 798–800.
WURTMAN, R. J., AXELROD, J. and FISCHER, J. E. (1964) *Science* **143**, 1328–1330.
WURTMAN, R. J., AXELROD, J. and KELLY, D. E. (1968) *The Pineal.* New York and London: Academic Press.
WURTMAN, R. J., AXELROD, J. and PHILLIPS, L. S. (1963) *Science* **142**, 1071–1073.
WURTMAN, R. J., AXELROD, J. and POTTER, L. T. (1964) *J. Pharmac. exp. Ther.* **143**, 314–318.
WURTMAN, R. J., ROTH, N., ALTSCHULE, M. D. and WURTMAN, J. J. (1961) *Acta endocr., Copenh.* **36**, 617–624.
WURTMAN, R. J., SHEIN, H. M., AXELROD, J. and LARIN, F. (1969) *Proc. natn. Acad. Sci. U.S.A.* **62**, 749–755.
WURTMAN, R. J. and WEISEL, J. (1969) *Endocrinology* **85**, 1218–1221.
ZIEHER, L. M. and PELLEGRINO DE IRALDI, A. (1966) *Life Sci.* **5**, 155–161.

INDEX OF AUTHORS*

Numbers in bold type indicate papers; other entries are contributions to discussions.

*Author and subject indexes prepared by William Hill.

INDEX OF SUBJECTS

Printed by William Clowes & Sons Limited, London, Colchester and Beccles